Depression as a Systemic Illness

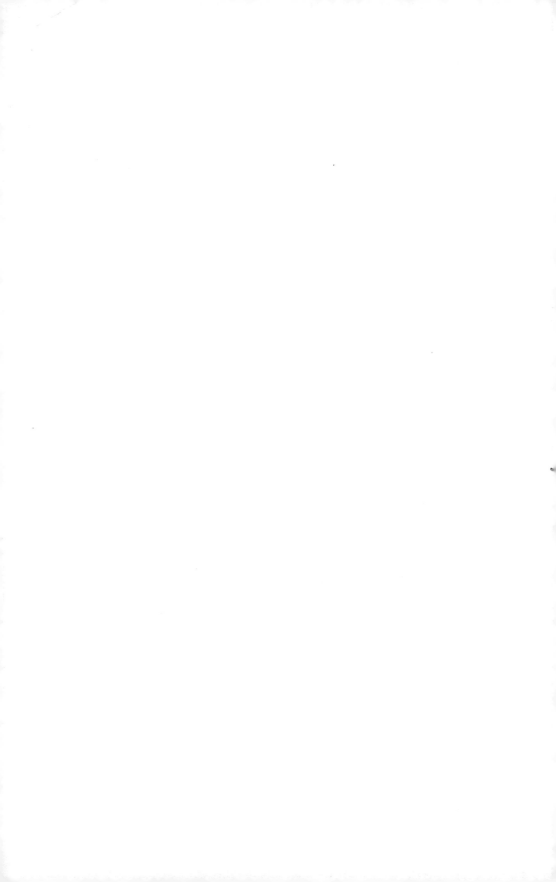

Depression as a Systemic Illness

Edited by

James J. Strain, MD
Professor of Psychiatry
Professor of Medical Education
Master Teacher
Icahn School of Medicine at Mount Sinai
New York, New York

Michael Blumenfield, MD
Sidney E. Frank Distinguished Professor Emeritus of
Psychiatry and Behavioral Sciences
New York Medical College
Valhalla, New York

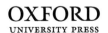

OXFORD
UNIVERSITY PRESS

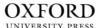

OXFORD
UNIVERSITY PRESS

Oxford University Press is a department of the University of Oxford. It furthers
the University's objective of excellence in research, scholarship, and education
by publishing worldwide. Oxford is a registered trade mark of Oxford University
Press in the UK and certain other countries.

Published in the United States of America by Oxford University Press
198 Madison Avenue, New York, NY 10016, United States of America.

CIP data is on file at the Library of Congress
ISBN 978–0–19–060334–2

3 5 7 9 8 6 4 2

This material is not intended to be, and should not be considered, a substitute for medical or other
professional advice. Treatment for the conditions described in this material is highly dependent
on the individual circumstances. And, while this material is designed to offer accurate information
with respect to the subject matter covered and to be current as of the time it was written, research
and knowledge about medical and health issues is constantly evolving and dose schedules for
medications are being revised continually, with new side effects recognized and accounted for
regularly. Readers must therefore always check the product information and clinical procedures with
the most up-to-date published product information and data sheets provided by the manufacturers
and the most recent codes of conduct and safety regulation. The publisher and the authors make no
representations or warranties to readers, express or implied, as to the accuracy or completeness of
this material. Without limiting the foregoing, the publisher and the authors make no representations
or warranties as to the accuracy or efficacy of the drug dosages mentioned in the material. The
authors and the publisher do not accept, and expressly disclaim, any responsibility for any liability,
loss or risk that may be claimed or incurred as a consequence of the use and/or application of any of
the contents of this material.

Printed by Sheridan Books, Inc., United States of America

I would like to dedicate this book to my wife, Dr. Gladys Witt Strain, for her continuing support and loving interest in my efforts for more than half a century, and to my three sons: Drs. Jay, Jeffrey, and Jamie Strain, who have contributed to my academic efforts over the years. Finally, I would like to dedicate this volume to Mrs. Cynthia Green Colin, who has witnessed and fostered my academic growth and accomplishments over the past 35 years, not only through her funds—the Green Fund, the Malcolm Gibbs Fund—but even more importantly, through her intellectual and steadfast support of the concepts and ideas that I have tried to promote.

—JJS

I would like to dedicate this book to my wife, Dr. Susan Blumenfield, and our three children, Jay, Bob, and Sharon, for their support and encouragement in all my various professional endeavors over the years. I would also include my four grandchildren, Lucy, Leo, Nia, and Obi, with the thought that someday one or more of them might be making contributions to this important and fascinating area of study.

—MB

This book is dedicated to our beloved colleague and friend: Dr. Jimmie Holland who passed away December 24, 2017. Jimmie was a person of all seasons: Mother, grandmother, teacher, practitioner, researcher and devoted to the care of patients and staff. She was a remarkable leader at Memorial Sloan Kettering Cancer Center and revolutioned the psychological care of cancer patients not only in the United States but through out the world. Through her continuing effort she influenced cancer hospitals to have psychiatrists on their staff. She came up with a sixth vital sign: "distress" to be asked every patient the staff would encounter. Jimmie began psycho-oncology journals, wrote the first text book in the field, and initiated at least two international societies to address the psychological needs of patients with cancer. And, still she had the capacity to be compassionate, loving, caring, a friend, and thoughtful to all of those she encountered. We will miss you Jimmie and are grateful to have known you, worked with you, and to have seen you excel in bringing psychological care to the cancer community. Your chapter in this volume is another testimony to the gifts you gave the world.

Table of Contents

Foreword

Depression occupies the minds and work of people of diverse disciplines. Prior to the introduction of anti-depressive treatments, depression was widely treated with interventions like electric-convulsive therapy (ECT). In the mid-1900s, the first monoamine oxidase inhibitors (MAOIs) and tricyclic antidepressants (TCAs) were introduced. For decades subsequently, much research focused on such treatments. Depression was considered a mental disorder. The focus on these antidepressants was followed over the next five or six decades with few new developments.

This book stresses the breadth of the topic, describing depression as a systemic illness, not just a mental illness. The best thinking today is that there are new tools and concepts in research, awareness of multiple causes, multiple kinds of depression, and increasing recognition of the mechanics and physiology that produce them. The book creates an optimistic and innovative approach to understanding and treating depression.

Brain plasticity is remarkable. Much current focus has been on brain action. However, this text uniquely conceives of depression as systemic, resembling other non-psychiatric chronic illnesses such as diabetes, hypertension, asthma, congestive heart failure, etc.

New research techniques have generated a conviction that integrating diverse lines of research enhances the promise for advances in understanding the disorder of depression. Another conviction among depression experts is that clinicians and scientists should focus on earlier stages of the disorder. Early intervention appears to produce better outcomes. Also, there is a greater focus on the continuing effects of depression.

Brain plasticity and recognition of depression's pervasive impact throughout the body—McEwen's "allostatic load"—has induced scientists to examine enduring and long-term effects of depression. More depressive episodes and longer periods of depression appear to be correlated with more serious states of depression.

Contributory causes are multiple—genetics, family history, adverse childhood development, environmental stress, etc. Depression is highly heterogeneous. For example, when youth have persistent anxiety and/or depression as well as mental lability, subclinical mania, accompanied by parents with early-onset bipolar disease, 50% of such children also develop bipolar disease.

The systemic nature of depression with the many interconnections also results in omnipresent comorbidity. This new text explores, e.g., cancer, heart disease, and neurological disorders in this regard.

New treatment approaches being developed make use of neuroimaging, brain stimulation, and substances like ketamine. The latter produces rapid improvement in mood rating in patients resistant to typical antidepressants, but it may have a minimal lasting effect if not serially repeated; it is not as yet FDA-approved for depressive disorders.

There are five different types of transcranial medical stimulation (TMS). In some, TMS generates brain tissue regrowth over four- to six-week periods. Treatments like cognitive behavioral therapy work on circuits. Interpersonal therapy, too, is being used in creative ways in underdeveloped countries. One emphasis is looking for interventions that may foster synaptic plasticity and connections.

The enthusiasm of many scientists is palpable. Some assert "a scientific revolution in mood disorder research is anticipated." Encouraged by advances in cancer treatment through precision medicine, some foresee possible application of precision medicine to depression. The rich knowledge being developed from neuroimaging has led to "neuro-imaging phenotypes," which means an imaging picture shared widely by many depressed patients.

These developments are significant for education. The impact on training, the impor-tant role of primary health care professionals, the potential of psychoeducation are per-tinent educational issues. Should primary care physicians not be able to diagnose and care for "garden variety" depressive disorders, and then, if necessary, refer refractory patients on to more experienced clinicians? Medical school curricula and residency training will need to be altered for non-psychiatric physicians to have sufficient skills to accomplish this.

Depression deserves recognition as an illness of major proportions. It affects vastly different body systems. The World Health Organization ranks it as exacting the great-est burden of illness on the world population. Innovative treatments and ideas provide optimism.

Considering it a systemic illness represents a change from the former perspective that brought patients with depression brief interludes of relief with ECT, psychotherapy, and/ or drugs while ignoring the long-term course and its biological accompaniments. We deal with a longstanding illness that needs enduring attention. If treated early, and if one can modify the number, intensity, and length of episodes, we will be likely to produce improved outcomes.

This formulation of depression as a systemic illness, not just a mental illness, may also be welcomed, recognizing the many decades in which psychiatric illness and treatment suffered from stigma. Outstanding innovative leaders from many fields grasping the breadth of depression's impact are working together, accumulating vast data and mani-festing enthusiasm about possible major strides going forward.

This rich book brings experts together and covers extensively the biological, psycho-logical, endocrinological, genetic, and imaging aspects of depression. This collabora-tion by outstanding scientists and clinicians represents probably our greatest hope for real improvement in the management of depression. It is well described here. While not minimizing how much has to be done, this is an uplifting book, given the excellence of its contributors and their laboratories, and the proliferation of new and imaginative tools and concepts to advance the effort to bring depression under control.

Herbert Pardes, MD
Executive Vice Chairman of the Board of Trustees of New York–Presbyterian
New York University Hospital of Columbia and Cornell.
Former Director of the National Institutes of Mental Health
Former President of the American Psychiatric Association
Former Dean and Chair of Psychiatry Columbia-Presbyterian School of Medicine
Former Chair of Psychiatry at Downstate School of Medicine, New York;
University of Colorado School of Medicine.

Acknowledgments

First, I would like to acknowledge the colleagues who have contributed to this volume and the exploration of a unique concept: *depression is a systemic illness, and not just a mental disorder*. Their focus to bring this concept to the front and center is the hallmark of this book, and our hope is that we may influence the global community to examine unique ways to not only understand the phenomenon of depression, but explore models to enhance its detection and treatment. With the knowledge from the World Health Organization that depression is the illness with the greatest burdens of health in the world—it is incumbent that we move from the halls of academia to the real world where people suffer and sometimes end their lives because of this ubiquitous illness. New ways must be found to determine its presence, new models for physicians to execute evidence-based care, and the incorporation of the patient as a key resource in actualizing advanced methods to identify, screen, be present for care, and follow through with recommendations. As said earlier, my wife and sons have been steadfast supporters of these efforts, and Jay, my eldest son, has worked with me on these projects since he was 14 years old and even now that he is a trained trauma surgeon. And I hasten to mention again Cynthia Green Colin, Emeritus Trustee of the Mount Sinai Medical School and Hospital, without whose unwavering support this book, the countless studies, the hundreds of lectures given at home and abroad, and the development of an electronic medical record—when such documentation was virtually unknown—would not have been possible to accomplish.

Finally, I want to acknowledge the natural laboratory that the Icahn School of Medicine at Mount Sinai has afforded to me; the opportunity to develop and test methods to enhance the knowledge base of countless physicians of all specialties, nurses, residents, and students with regard to promoting the psychological care of the medically ill. The patients, the students, doctors in training, nurses, social workers, and ethicists have all supported the creation of a *center of excellence* for encouraging better care. My hope is this book will continue to promote that effort.

—*James J. Strain*

I would like to acknowledge my colleague and friend Dr. Jim Strain, who originated the concept of this book and not only gave birth to it while we were co-editing an earlier book on psychosomatic medicine, but nurtured and brought it to fruition with his unique creativity and energy. It has been an honor and privilege to work with him. I also want to acknowledge all my many teachers, colleagues, and students over the years, who, along with our patients, have taught me about the mind, emotions, physical functioning, and illness. We have learned so much over the past 50 years, and yet there is so much more on the horizon.

—*Michael Blumenfield*

Prologue

James J. Strain, MD

DEPRESSION AS A SYSTEMIC DISEASE

This book is intended to make two major points. One of them is the increasing accumulation of evidence that depression should be thought of as a systemic disease and not simply as an "emotional" or "mental" disorder. The second point is that, because of this evidence, medical education needs to change so that wider arrays of physicians are trained to recognize and treat this systemic illness, especially the non refractory depressions, which increasingly presents in their practices.

Chapters in this book, presenting data supporting the hypothesis that depression is a systemic disease, describe the biological parameters of depression and its effects on cortisol, the hypothalamic-pituitary-adrenal axis, cytokines, glucose metabolism, platelet activity, etc., and how they affect physiological systems, promoting an allostatic load that can exacerbate somatic morbidity. Inflammation has been recently implicated as a possible mechanism or accompaniment of major depressive disorders and is an important focus of contemporary research.

"Neuropsychiatric research has pivoted from investigation of monoaminergic mechanisms to novel mediators, including the role of inflammatory processes. Subsets of mood disorder patients exhibit immune-related abnormalities, including elevated levels of proinflammatory cytokines, monocytes, and neutrophils in the peripheral circulation; dysregulation of neuroglia and blood-brain barrier function; and disruption of gut microbiota. The field of psychoneuroimmunology is one of great therapeutic opportunity . . . such as peripheral cytokine targeting antibodies, microglia and astrocyte targeting therapies . . . producing findings that identify therapeutic targets for future development"[1] (p. 1–14). Furthermore, disruptions may occur in a neuroimmune axis that interfaces the immune system and the central nervous system that controls behavior. Evidence has been found in patients and animal models of depression that demonstrates how the peripheral immune system acts on the brain to alter responses to stress and vulnerability to mood disorders.[2] It follows that this ubiquitous disorder could and should be initially screened for, diagnosed, and treated by the primary care physician (PCP). Another important reason for the necessary and essential move to PCPs for care of depression is that in most countries, even developed ones, there are not enough psychiatrists to participate in collaborative care—and now there is a strong *headwind* in the United States to address effective mental health care via the medical doctors available—most often the PCP.

It is interesting to note that family practice residencies include training for the screening, diagnosis, treatment, and assessment of outcome for depression, while standard internal medicine residencies—the source of most of our PCPs—do not have similar pedagogical expectations.[3] It is stunning that of the 8 million annual ambulatory care visits for depression, PCPs see more than one half.[4] And, equally stunning, PCPs prescribed more than 70% of the antidepressants in the United States[5]—even though they may not have had the training of the family practitioner, let alone the more intensive focus of residencies in psychiatry.

Possibly reflecting that fact, although PCP practices have established care-management processes for such common diseases as asthma, diabetes, hypertension, and congestive heart failure, they have not done so for depression. This is despite the fact that today, screening, diagnostic, and treatment phases for depressive illness, and also assessment of meaningful outcomes, can be assisted by teams, such as social workers and nurse physician assistants; and new technologies, e.g., screening devices, algorithms, electronic health records (EHR), telemedicine and SKYPE interviews for consultative review (second opinions).

The World Health Organization (WHO) in March 2017 stated that depression is the illness causing the greatest burden of health in the world. Heart disease is the greatest burden for mortality.[6,7] There is an increased recognition of the important relationship between depression and heart disease: it is now widely understood that depression is a risk factor for worsening heart disease greater than smoking. The unsurprising adverse effects that depression can have on many illnesses will be described in detail in this volume.

Because patients are reluctant to go to psychiatrists as a result of the stigma of mental health disorders, and because there are too few psychiatrists in the world anyway, many patients will not be diagnosed, and many, even if identified, are under-treated if treated at all. This is a crisis in health care worldwide that should—indeed, must—lead to important changes in how medicine is practiced, how doctors are trained, and how systems of care need to be transformed. In order to provide assistance for this hugely burdensome illness in developed as well as developing countries, major changes are required in the education of physicians, in particular the primary care physician (PCP). They are the *gateway* for the patient's access to diagnosis and treatment. The training of PCPs to recognize and treat these illnesses should be a major academic focus. We need to move from a *collaborative care model* (the current framework for mental health care in the medical setting)—to the *medical model* where the PCP is an autonomous physician working with his/her team for the care of depression, although, as for other illnesses, occasionally referring to a specialist.

There are three helpful ways to understand depressive disorders in the medically ill:

1. The first is outside the focus of this book: namely, as psychologically depressive reactions to the stressors of medical illness (possibly leading to non-compliance, giving up, feelings of guilt and shame, and even to self-harm);
2. The second way is to understand how depressive disorders can biologically adversely affect physical disease and processes—that they may have a significant and negative

effect on the body and on bodily function because of their effects on allostatic load and consequent biological stresses on body functions. Most of the arguments in in the early chapters emphasize this aspect of understanding.

3. The third way of understanding shows how some somatic-dysfunctions and medical treatments, including pharmacological agents, can lead biologically to the occurrence of depression and somatic physiological changes (e.g., interferon, medications utilized for HIV) (see Chapter 10 on drug–drug interactions). These reactions are not "psychological" in that they are not the patient's psychological response to a medical illness or physical limitation, e.g., demoralization or stresses from having cancer or having coronary artery disease; reactive depressive disorders; adjustment disorders, major depressive disorders from the stressors of physical illness. They are direct effects of body dysfunction and medications on the structure of the brain.

Though less stressed in the supportive chapters, the third way demonstrates the *bidirectionality* of depressive disorders, and it deserves emphasis, since it supports the two major points of this volume: that major depressive disorders are *systemic diseases* and that the PCP needs to be trained to understand why this common systemic disorder could and should be within their domain of competence. Several examples of this bidirectionality of depression will be presented in the chapters that follow. However, these chapters will not be an *all*-inclusive inventory of the innumerable somatically or pharmacologically induced affective disorders that may occur.

Finally, a new model to approach the identification and management of depression is sorely needed, as has been uniquely developed with comprehensive guidelines for such illnesses as stroke, sepsis, delirium, and decubitus ulcers—illustrated in the concluding chapter. A possible approach with an innovative electronic health record and currently available technology, such as the smartphone, the health kiosk, newly developed apps, telemedicine, SKYPE, etc., illustrate how the PCPs and their staff can be assisted to access essential information and guidelines, which, at the same time, will lessen the demands on the physicians' time.

It is my hope that this book may save lives, or at the least make some lives better.

REFERENCES

1. Pfau ML, Menard C, Russo SJ. The inflammatory mediators in mood disorders: therapeutic opportunities. *Annu Rev Pharmacol Toxicol.* 2018;58(14):1–14.
2. Hodes GE, Kana V, Menard C, Merad M, Russo SJ. Neuroimmune mechanisms of depression. *Nat Neurosci.* 2015;18:1386–1393.
3. American Academy of Family Physicians (AAFP). Reprint No. 270. www.aafa.org/dam/aafp/documents/medical_education_residency/program_directors/reprint270_mental.pdf.
4. Bishop TF, Ramsay PP, Casalino LP, Bao Y, Pincus HA, Shortell SM. Care management processes used less often for depression than for other chronic conditions in US primary care practices. *Health Aff (Millwood).* 2016;35(3):394–400.

5. Faghri NMA, Boisvert CM, Faghri S. Understanding the expanding role of primary care physicians (PCPs) to primary psychiatric care physicians (PPCPs): enhancing the assessment and treatment of psychiatric conditions. *Ment Health Fam Med.* 2010;7(1):17–25.

6. Mathers CD, Loncaar D. Projections of global mortality and burden of disease from 2002 to 2030. *PloS Med.* 2006;3(11):2011–2029.

7. Global Burden of Disease. *Lancet* 2016;388:1459–1544.

Contributor List

Michael Blumenfield, MD
Sidney E. Frank Distinguished Professor
Emeritus of Psychiatry and Behavioral
Sciences, New York Medical College,
Valhalla, New York, N.Y.

Patricia Casey, MD
Professor of Psychiatry, University of
Dublin, Dublin, Ireland

Eduardo A. Colón Navarro, MD
Chief of Psychiatry, Hennepin County
Medical Center Rochester, Minn.;
Professor of Psychiatry, University of
Minnesota; Chairman Department of
Psychiatry, Hennepin County Medical
Center, Minneapolis, Minn.

Kelly L. Cozza, MD
Psychiatry Clinical Clerkship Director,
Department of Psychiatry Scientist,
Center for the Study of Traumatic Stress,
Uniformed Services University of the
Health Sciences, Bethesda, Md.

Bradleigh Hayhow, MD
Fellow of the Royal Australian and
New Zealand College of Psychiatrists
(FRANZCP), Hon. Academic Fellow,
Melbourne Neuropsychiatry Centre, The
University of Melbourne Clinical Senior
Lecturer, Department of Psychiatry, The
University of Western Australia, Perth,
Western Australia

Jimmie Holland, MD
Department of Psychiatry and Behavioral
Sciences, Memorial Sloan Kettering
Cancer Center, New York, N.Y.

Andres M. Kanner, MD
Professor of Clinical Neurology,
Director, Comprehensive Epilepsy
Center; Head, Epilepsy Division,
Department of Neurology, University
of Miami, Miller School of Medicine,
Miami, Fla.

Nicole Mavrides, MD
Department of Psychiatry and Behavioral
Sciences, Center on Aging, University
of Miami Miller School of Medicine,
Miami, Fla.

Bruce S. McEwen, PhD
Alfred E. Mirsky Professor, Laboratory
of Neuroendocrinology, The Rockefeller
University, New York, N.Y.

Daniel C. McFarland, DO
Division of Network Medicine Services,
Department of Medicine, Memorial
Sloan Kettering Cancer Center, West
Harrison, N.Y.

Eric G. Meyer, MD
Department of Psychiatry, Uniformed
Services University of the Health Sciences,
Bethesda, Md.

Charles Nemeroff, MD, PhD
Department of Psychiatry and Behavioral
Sciences, Center on Aging, University
of Miami Miller School of Medicine,
Miami, Fla.

Eric J. Nestler, PhD, MD
Head of Brain Institute, Icahn School
of Medicine at Mount Sinai; Fishberg
Department of Neuroscience and
Friedman Brain Institute, Icahn School of
Medicine at Mount Sinai, New York, N.Y.

Robert M. Post, MD
Bipolar Collaborative Network,
Bethesda, Md.

Natalie L. Rasgon, MD
Department of Psychiatry and Behavioral
Sciences, Stanford University School of
Medicine, Palo Alto, Calif.

Rita Rein, CA
Department of Psychiatry and Behavioral
Sciences, Stanford University School of
Medicine, Palo Alto, Calif.

Akhil Shenoy, MD
Assistant Professor of Psychiatry, Icahn
School of Medicine at Mount Sinai,
New York, N.Y.

Robert L. Sheridan, MD
Harvard Medical School, Boston, Mass.

Sergio Starkstein, MD, PhD, FRANZCP
Professor of Psychiatry, Department of
Psychiatry, The University of Western
Australia, Perth, Western Australia

Frederick J. Stoddard, Jr., MD
Harvard Medical School, Boston, Mass.

James J. Strain, MD
Professor of Psychiatry, Professor of
Medical Education, Master Teacher,
Icahn School of Medicine at Mount Sinai,
New York, N.Y.

Jay J. Strain, MD
Assistant Professor of Surgery, Thomas
Jefferson School of Medicine, Einstein
Healthcare Network, Philadelphia, Pa.

Peter Tyrer, MD
Professor of Psychiatry, Imperial College,
London, England

Gary H. Wynn, MD
Department of Psychiatry, Uniformed
Services University of the Health Sciences,
Bethesda, Md.

Depression as a Systemic Illness

1

The Biological Basis of Depression
Insights from Animal Models

Eric J. Nestler

INTRODUCTION

Depression, like all psychiatric syndromes, is defined solely on the basis of behavioral abnormalities. We still lack today any biological measure—e.g., brain imaging, genetic, peripheral blood finding—that forms part of the diagnosis of depression. Depression is a highly heterogeneous syndrome, probably comprising numerous disease states and pathophysiological mechanisms. It also exhibits broad overlap with several other psychiatric syndromes, including anxiety disorders and post-traumatic stress disorder (PTSD). There is no clear biological distinction across these several diagnoses, and they are highly comorbid. In fact, in war-torn regions of the world, roughly one-third of individuals who seek psychiatric treatment are diagnosed with depression, another third with PTSD, and the final third with anxiety disorders.[1] Roughly 35% of the risk for depression is genetic, yet it has been extremely difficult to identify individual genes that pose that risk, with few genes reaching genome-wide significance in studies to date.[2] Finally, virtually all of today's antidepressant medications are based on discoveries made through serendipity over six decades ago and target the brain's monoamine pathways.[3] Sixty years later, we have arguably not introduced a single antidepressant medication with a novel mechanism of action, although ketamine (which targets glutamatergic pathways) is now undergoing clinical evaluation and shows considerable promise.[4]

How do we overcome these fundamental obstacles in depression research to better understand its biological underpinnings and to develop more effective treatments? By analogy with all other fields of medicine, animal models are an essential component of this effort. However, there are several fundamental limitations for animal models of depression (and for all psychiatric disorders, for that matter) that have dramatically hindered progress.[5] Many of the core symptoms of depression (e.g., guilt, ruminations, suicidality) are inherently inaccessible in animals. The absence of known strong genetic factors with high penetrance means that studies are performed on genetically normal animals that lack the heritable component seen in humans. Consequently, the field has focused on stress responses, with the rationale that adverse life events are a strong risk factor for depression.[6] Over the past several decades, we have learned a great deal about how rodents respond to acute or chronic stress. However, we still have a very limited understanding of which of those mechanisms, or other mechanisms, mediate the many forms of depression—and related syndromic outcomes of stress; namely, anxiety and PTSD—seen in humans.

Here we briefly summarize the range of animal models used in the depression field and what has been learned about depression from them. We highlight new experimental approaches that have dramatically advanced efforts to use animal models to delineate the neural circuits and molecular abnormalities that control depression-related behavioral abnormalities in animals.

ANIMAL MODELS OF DEPRESSION

Animal studies in depression can be divided into acute assays versus chronic stress models (Table 1.1). The former are seen as useful screens of the behavioral state of an animal, while the latter might replicate aspects of adaptive or maladaptive responses to stress in humans. An important consideration is the evaluation of the behavioral state of an animal, not only by whether it replicates the human syndrome of depression (or anxiety or PTSD), but also by whether it recapitulates domains of behavioral abnormalities seen across these diagnoses. This latter approach fits well with the RDoC (research domain criteria) approach to evaluating human syndromes, which looks beyond syndromes to specific behavioral impairments that track onto an established neural circuitry.[7]

The validity of an animal model is often described in three ways.[5] *Construct* or *etiological validity* refers to the degree to which the animal model recapitulates the causes of the human syndrome. *Face validity* refers to the degree to which the animal model recapitulates the core symptoms of the human syndrome. *Pharmacological validity* refers to the degree to which drugs that are effective in treating the animal model prove to be efficacious in humans. As our introduction indicated, all three levels of validity are a challenge for depression. We do not yet know what causes human depression (causative genetic or non-genetic factors), hence, complete construct validity is impossible. We know that chronic stress can increase the risk for depression in some individuals, although most individuals maintain normal functioning in the face of such stress. Thus, most chronic stress models in rodents are limited because they cannot perfectly distinguish adaptive vs. maladaptive responses to the stress. Face validity of animal depression models is limited by the focus on only the symptoms (e.g., anhedonia, sleep

Table 1.1 Examples of Behavioral Procedures in Rodents Used to Study Depression[a]

Chronic Stress Models	Acute Stress Assays	Phenotypic Screens
Chronic social defeat stress	Forced swim test	Sucrose preference
Maternal separation	Tail suspension test	Intracranial self-stimulation
Chronic variable stress	Novelty-suppressed feeding	Fear conditioning
Social isolation	Learned helplessness	Other cognitive tests
Chronic restraint stress		Other tests of natural reward

[a]The table does not list a large range of assays used to study anxiety-like behavior in rodents.

disturbances, social impairments, metabolic disturbances, etc.) that can be measured in animals. Pharmacological validation has almost completely failed, since it has not been possible—despite 60 years of research—to validate a non–monoamine-based antidepressant medication in humans. Finally, all chronic stress models in rodents produce mixed symptoms of depression- and anxiety-related behavioral abnormalities. Of course this reflects the mixed patterns seen in humans as well. Ultimately, a better understanding of which human syndrome is modeled by a given animal procedure will require a better delineation of that human syndrome.

Acute Stress and Phenotypic Assays

Acute stress and phenotypic assays are the most widely used in the field. Most, such as the forced swim test, tail suspension test, learned helplessness, and novelty-suppressed feeding, assess an animal's response to an acute stress. Other acute assays, such as the sucrose preference test and fear conditioning, are useful in assessing aspects of an animal's behavioral state. While these assays are very useful as screens, they cannot be viewed as animal models of depression since they lack construct and face validity. Another assay used to assess an animal's behavioral state is intracranial self-stimulation, which measures the degree to which an animal will work (e.g., press a lever) to deliver electrical current into the brain's reward circuitry.[8]

Chronic Stress Assays

The two best-validated chronic stress models are chronic social defeat stress and maternal separation. In the former model, a mouse is exposed repeatedly to a more aggressive, dominant mouse, typically over a course of 10 days. This induces a range of depression- and anxiety-related behavioral abnormalities.[9,10] Social defeat is unique, compared to other chronic stress models in adult rodents, in several respects. First, only about two-thirds of mice subjected to the stress develop this range of symptoms and are referred to as "susceptible." The remaining one-third avoid the depression-like symptoms and are referred to as "resilient."[11] Thus, social defeat stress makes it possible to distinguish between maladaptive responses to stress (seen in susceptible mice) and adaptive responses to stress (seen in resilient mice). Moreover, because the resilient mice display equal levels of anxiety-like behaviors, the models also make it possible to differentiate "depression" from "anxiety," as best as can be inferred from rodents. Additionally, unlike all other chronic stress models in adult rodents, where the behavioral abnormalities rapidly revert to normal within days after the last stress, a subset of the behavioral abnormalities induced by social defeat stress is permanent.[9,11,12] This makes it possible to establish pharmacological validity for social defeat stress: standard antidepressants reverse the long-lasting behavioral abnormalities only after repeated (weeks) administration.[8,12] The model also shows responses to ketamine, but not anxiolytic agents.[8,13,14] An original weakness of the social defeat model was that it was developed in male mice only, although recent advances have extended the approach to females as well.[15]

Maternal separation also shows considerable validation. We know that early life stress is a strong risk factor for depression in humans.[6] Mice and rats removed from their mothers during early life show lifelong increases in susceptibility to subsequent stressful events later in life.[16-19] Again, the paradigm produces a mixture of depression- and anxiety-like behavioral features. Chronic variable stress, also referred to as "chronic mild stress" or "chronic unpredictable stress," exposes rodents to different physical stresses each day (e.g., restraint, foot shock, cold temperatures, forced swimming, etc.). After repeated exposures, rats and mice succumb and display a range of depression- and anxiety-like symptoms.[20-22] A useful feature of chronic variable stress is that females are more susceptible than males,[21] which recapitulates the roughly twofold greater incidence of depression in woman and girls. A weakness of the procedure—as with repeated restraint or foot-shock stress as well—is that only physical stresses are employed, in contrast to the fact that the stress diathesis in human depression usually involves psychological and social forms of stress. Another weakness of the model is that the behavioral symptoms only persist a few days after the last stress, which means that antidepressant drugs can be studied for their ability to prevent deleterious outcomes but not reverse them post-stress.

NEUROBIOLOGY OF DEPRESSION

Over the past several decades, animal models of depression and acute behavioral assays have revealed a substantial amount of information about how the brain responds to stress. This work has defined brain regions and their circuits that control mood under normal conditions as well as responses to acute or chronic stress. The work has also defined numerous theories for cellular and molecular mechanisms of depression, which define clear steps forward in the development of improved treatments for the syndrome. While the molecular and cellular abnormalities defined in animal models have been replicated to an increasing degree in depressed humans examined at autopsy, the major gap in the field remains the lack of clinical validation of the therapeutic potential of these approaches. Following are brief summaries of some of the major advances in understanding depression, with a focus on the novel experimental approaches used.

Neural Circuitry

Work in rodents has largely confirmed decades-old hypotheses from studies of humans sustaining traumatic brain injury or stroke, and since confirmed by brain imaging approaches, that broad circuits in forebrain are in important in mood regulation (Figure 1.1).[23-25] These regions include several areas of prefrontal cortex, hippocampus, amygdala, nucleus accumbens, septal nuclei, and thalamus, among others. These regions display many reciprocal connections and function as a highly integrated circuit. Nevertheless, each region appears to mediate partly distinct functions: the prefrontal cortex regions are important for executive control, behavioral flexibility, impulsivity, and compulsivity; the hippocampus mediates declarative memory but functions more broadly in controlling emotions; the amygdala is important for associative memories for rewarding and aversive stimuli; the nucleus accumbens controls motor and probably emotional responses to rewarding and aversive stimuli; the septal nuclei also regulate responses to rewarding and aversive stimuli; and the thalamus integrates sensory information with cortical and subcortical regions.[26] Each of these regions is innervated

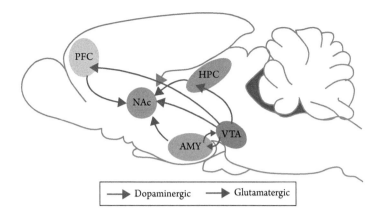

Figure 1.1 Brain regions involved in regulating mood. Depicted are the major components of the limbic-reward circuitry: dopaminergic neurons (*green*) project from the ventral tegmental area (VTA) to nucleus accumbens (NAc), prefrontal cortex (PFC), amygdala (AMY), and hippocampus (HPC), among several other regions. The NAc receives excitatory glutamatergic innervation (*red*) from the HPC, PFC, and AMY. From Bagot RC, Labonté B, Peña CJ, Nestler EJ (2014) Epigenetic signaling in psychiatric disorders: stress and depression. Dialogues Clin Neurosci 16:281-295.

by brainstem monoaminergic neurons, including dopamine, serotonin, and norepinephrine. Presumably, innervation by the latter two explains the actions of today's antidepressants, virtually all of which act via serotonergic and/or noradrenergic mechanisms.[3]

Recent work in animal models has taken advantage of optogenetic and DREADD (designer receptors activated by designer drug) tools, which make it possible to control the activity of specific circuits in the brain in awake-behaving animals. In optogenetics, a bacterial ion channel or pump that is activated by light is expressed—either with a viral vector or transgenically—in a given neuronal cell type. Light is then directed into a targeted brain region via an implanted optic fiber. By delivering light pulses at precise frequencies, it is possible to control the frequency (e.g., low frequency vs. high frequency) and pattern (e.g., tonic firing vs. phasic firing) of activity of the targeted circuit.[27] DREADDs are synthetic G protein-coupled receptors that link to an excitatory effector (e.g., Gq) or an inhibitory one (e.g., Gi). They can be activated upon systemic delivery of clozapine-N-oxide, which has minimal effects on endogenously expressed receptors.[28] Both approaches have strengths and weaknesses.

With these tools, it has been possible, for example, to demonstrate a crucial role for dopaminergic neurons in the midbrain ventral tegmental area in controlling responses to acute and to different types of chronic stress.[29,30] Interestingly, projections of these neurons to nucleus accumbens have a very different effect compared to projections to prefrontal cortex. Likewise, stimulation of the two different subtypes of projection neurons from nucleus accumbens, termed *D1-type* and *D2-type medium spiny neurons* based on the predominant type of dopamine receptor expressed, exert opposite effects on stress responses,[31] as do inputs to nucleus accumbens neurons from prefrontal cortex vs. hippocampus.[32] Related approaches have confirmed the importance of serotoninergic neurons in the midbrain dorsal raphe, and their reciprocal connections to prefrontal cortex, in mediating antidepressant-like responses,[33] as well as defined the neural circuitry involved in fear- and anxiety-related behaviors.[34,35]

These approaches are providing transformationally greater delineation of the neural circuits in the brain that control depression-related behavioral abnormalities than was possible in earlier research. This work is thereby essential for RDoC-oriented studies of diverse stress- and mood-related syndromes in humans. These advances are also informing the mechanism of action and identification of novel sites for deep brain stimulation, an experimental treatment for severe depression.[36] As well, given that ketamine is thought to produce its rapid antidepressant effects via glutamatergic mechanisms,[4,22,37-39] optogenetics and DREADDs should help define the mechanism of action of this novel therapeutic.

Transcriptomics

Technical innovations in our ability to map genome-wide changes in gene expression in the brain have provided further advances in our understanding of the pathophysiology of depression. RNA-sequencing (RNA-seq) makes it possible to quantify all RNA products expressed by the genome within a given brain region or even within a single cell type within that brain region. Since a majority of all RNAs expressed in a cell are non-coding (i.e., they serve regulatory functions), earlier microarray studies missed a substantial portion of expressed genes. Likewise, RNA-seq provides quantification of all splice variants encoded in a given gene, something not possible with microarrays.

We are now seeing for the first time large scale RNA-seq studies of several brain regions implicated in depression from a wide range of animal models.[40-43] It is likely that the coming years will bring still further RNA-seq characterization of animal models focused on individual cell types (neuronal as well as non-neuronal—astroglia, microglia, oligodendrocytes, endothelial cells), as well as RNA-seq of single cells in depression models. Early work in the latter area is revealing far greater heterogeneity within a given cell type thought to be largely homogeneous with earlier methods.[e.g., 44,45]

Work to date is already defining several interesting principles of stress responses in animal models. Each chronic stress model seems to regulate a largely distinct set of genes associated with the induction of similar depression-related behavioral abnormalities.[21 vs. 43] By overlaying such data on RNA-seq findings of depressed vs. control human brain—work that is now beginning to appear—it should be possible to provide a molecular validation of animal models, something heretofore not possible. Our early impression is that each chronic stress model in a rodent recapitulates a largely different subset of gene expression abnormalities seen in human depression, which is consistent with the notion that each model recapitulates a different aspect or subset of the very broad pathology subsumed under depression and related syndromes. In a related vein, RNA-seq profiling of animal models and depressed human brain will help guide efforts aimed at identifying specific genetic variations that contribute to the heritable risk for depression.

Studies of chronic social defeat stress, which enables the distinction between animals that are susceptible to chronic stress from those that are resilient (see the preceding discussion), have demonstrated that, to a great extent, resilience is the more plastic state, associated with regulation of far more genes across multiple brain regions compared with susceptibility.[11,43] These findings have raised the interesting perspective that, in addition to developing ways to prevent the deleterious effects of stress, another approach in anti-depressant drug discovery is to induce mechanisms of natural resilience in individuals who are inherently more susceptible. An interesting observation is the prominence of regulated genes that control gene transcription, including transcription factors and a host of proteins that control the epigenetic state of a gene and thereby its transcription.[46] As just some examples, the transcription factors ΔFosB and ß-catenin have been shown to promote resilience when acting within the nucleus accumbens.[13,47,48] Similar pro-resilience effects are seen upon inhibition of HDACs (histone deacetylases) or activation of certain histone methyltransferases (e.g., G9a) in this and certain other brain regions.[49-51]

Studies of chronic variable stress, which captures the greater susceptibility of females to chronic stress compared with males, are defining some of the molecular determinants of that greater susceptibility. As just one example, female mice express higher levels of DNMT3a (DNA methyltransferase 3a) in nucleus accumbens at baseline and show a greater induction of the enzyme in response to chronic stress.[21] Depressed humans likewise show higher levels of DNMT3a in nucleus accumbens at autopsy, an abnormality partially reversed with antidepressant medication. DNMT3a is an example of an epigenetic enzyme that controls gene activity via methylating cytosine nucleosides within the gene's sequence. Overexpressing DNMT3a in this brain region, by use of viral vectors, makes males as susceptible as females, while knocking out DNMT3a in nucleus accumbens makes females as resilient as males. Knocking out DNMT3a also shifts the pattern of gene expression—assessed by RNA-seq—in female nucleus accumbens closer to that seen in males.[21]

Related approaches are providing insight into the mechanisms of action of antidepressant treatments. This is important because, while we know the acute actions of most antidepressants (e.g., an SSRI [selective serotonin reuptake inhibitor] antagonizes the serotonin transporter), the changes that these sustained acute actions induce in brain with chronic treatment, and are required for the drugs' therapeutic efficacy, are not definitively known. Recent RNA-seq studies have demonstrated largely different gene expression changes induced across the range of forebrain regions implicated in depression.[14] They have also demonstrated that chronic antidepressant treatment is associated—in all brain regions—with the reversal of a subset of gene expression changes associated with susceptibility, induction of a subset of gene expression changes associated with resilience, as well as the regulation of a distinct cohort of genes not affected by chronic stress per se. Comparisons of these effects between chronic imipramine (a standard antidepressant that acts by antagonizing serotonin and norepinephrine transporters) and acute ketamine (an experimental rapidly acting antidepressant that is thought to act on glutamatergic synapses) shows largely distinct gene expression changes across several forebrain regions (Figure 1.2). The induction of genes affected in natural resilience is also seen at the chromatin level.[52] This type of work is providing an ever more comprehensive template of genes that could be targeted for novel therapeutics.

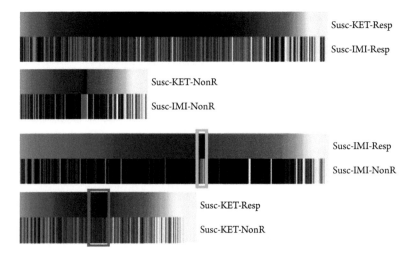

Figure 1.2 Transcriptomic profiles of imipramine (IMI) vs. ketamine (KET) responders (Resp) vs. non-responders (NonR) in nucleus accumbens. Male mice were subjected to chronic social defeat stress. Susceptible (Susc) mice were treated for 2 wk with saline or IMI or 13 d saline + 1 d KET. Roughly 50% of mice treated with IMI or KET responded behaviorally; the other half were treatment resistant. Top two heatmaps: note the largely different sets of genes affected in IMI vs. KET Resp (top) and NonR (bottom). Bottom two heatmaps: note IMI NonR generally fail to show regulation of genes seen in IMI Resp. This was less apparent in KET NonR vs. Resp. Interestingly, NonR is characterized by a small number of gene expression changes not seen in Resp (turquoise and purpose rectangles); these changes might actively oppose Resp. Several other interesting patterns were observed in this large dataset. From Bagot et al. (2016b).

Of course, transcriptional regulation is one of several ways in which cells and circuits respond to acute and chronic stress. Regulation of RNA processing, stability, and translation into protein, and of protein processing, stability, and intracellular trafficking, also play crucial roles in cellular adaptations. As tools are developed to allow the comprehensive analysis of these post-transcriptional mechanisms, it will be important to apply them to depression models.

Cellular and Molecular Mechanisms

The combination of the advanced circuit and molecular approaches just described is refining earlier hypotheses of the molecular and cellular basis of depression, as well as revealing fundamentally novel hypotheses. The reviewer is referred to recent reviews for more detailed descriptions of these mechanisms; a brief overview only is provided here.

It has long been known that a subset of patients with depression display hyperactivity of the *hypothalamic-pituitary-adrenal (HPA) axis*.[53-55] This knowledge led to the consideration of corticotropin releasing factor-1 (CRF1) antagonists as antidepressants. There is evidence that glucocorticoid receptor antagonists might show some efficacy in treatment, particularly of severe depression. However, more recent research has demonstrated the complexity of the HPA axis's role in depression and related syndromes. First, a subset of depressed patients display hypoactivity of the HPA axis, and a majority show no detectable derangement at all. Second, it is likely that activation of the HPA axis is a normal, adaptive part of the stress response that helps individual cope positively with stress. By contrast, sustained activation of the HPA axis, as occurs with chronic stress, has deleterious consequences in certain individuals, but this means that far more precise ways of intervening with the HPA axis are required to mine therapeutic activity in subsets of patients that show distinct abnormalities in axis function.

The neurotrophic hypothesis of depression proposes that prolonged exposure to stress, in vulnerable individuals, induces deleterious changes in neuronal morphology and function, effects mediated in part via alterations in several neurotrophic (nerve growth) factors.[56] A corollary of this hypothesis is that prolonged treatment with monoamine-based antidepressants is required in order to reverse such trophic effects. The neurotrophic factor best implicated in depression and antidepressant action is BDNF (brain-derived neurotrophic factor), the expression of which is suppressed in hippocampus and prefrontal cortex by chronic stress, effects reversed with chronic monoamine-based antidepressants or with acute ketamine. However, BDNF's role in depression is complicated by the fact that, while induction of BDNF exerts antidepressant-like effects in hippocampus and prefrontal cortex, it exerts depression-like effects in nucleus accumbens.[26] BDNF is just one of a large number of neurotrophic factors that has been shown to control chronic stress responses in laboratory animals. A key challenge in this line of research has been to develop ways of advancing these discoveries into the clinic. Thus, growth factors are proteins and do not cross the blood–brain barrier, and it has been difficult to generate small-molecule agonists or antagonists of growth factors to test their antidepressant potential in humans.

There is growing evidence for the involvement of immune mechanisms in depression.[57] First, a subset of depressed humans shows evidence of an inflammatory state based on elevated levels of certain pro-inflammatory cytokines (e.g., interleukin-6 [IL6], tumor necrosis factor-α) in their peripheral blood. Similar findings have been reported for susceptible mice after exposure to chronic stress.[58] Moreover, blockade of IL6 peripherally exerts a pro-resilient effect in mice, while transplantation of bone marrow from susceptible mice makes recipient mice more inherently susceptible, an effect not seen with IL6 knockout donor mice.[57] Findings such as these immediately raise the possibility of testing whether antibodies directed against IL6 or other cytokines, now used clinically in the treatment of a range of rheumatological diseases, show antidepressant efficacy in the depressed patients who display a hyperinflammatory state. An important related question is, how do peripheral cytokines influence depression-related behavioral outcomes? Presumably, peripheral cytokines enter the brain to control neuronal responses to act on areas of brain largely outside the blood–brain barrier to generate signals that then influence the rest of the brain. A related question is the extent to which the actions of the cytokines, and their centrally generated signals, act directly on neurons or indirectly by first influencing the host of non-neuronal cells present within the brain. As just one example, there has been increasing interest in resident microglial cells in the brain in controlling stress responses.[57] As additional information is obtained delineating the cellular and molecular circuitry controlled by cytokines, it should be possible to generate increasingly precise treatments to target abnormalities documented in subsets of depressed patients.

FUTURE DIRECTIONS

We have learned a vast amount about the brain over the past several decades. We have also learned a great deal about how the brain adapts vs. maladapts to chronic stress, in many cases validating such molecular and cellular adaptations in the brains of depressed humans at autopsy. Despite these advances, however, we have not significantly advanced the treatment of depression, which today relies on the same mechanisms of action of antidepressants that were discovered by serendipity sixty years ago. We believe that key challenges in clinical research, beyond the limitations inherent in animal research, are also among the major determinants for this failure in drug discovery efforts. It is far more difficult to perform small, exploratory clinical studies than it was a few decades ago. Due largely to regulatory burdens, pharmaceutical companies are far less willing today to share molecules with novel mechanisms of action with academic colleagues to explore their potential antidepressant efficacy. Likewise, the vast majority of academic centers do not have the funding or know-how to generate tool compounds—with novel mechanisms—and gain regulatory clearance to study their activity in humans. This is a gap that the National Institutes of Health has tried to overcome, but it has not yet succeeded. The failure of many antidepressant clinical studies also relates to difficulties with such trials. Unlike decades ago, when such clinical studies tested patients with uncomplicated depression, today's trials by necessity focus on individuals who do not adequately respond to any of the broad range of monoamine-based treatments currently available. Consequently, many patients who participate in antidepressant trials today have more severe cases of depression that are complicated with many comorbid pathologies.

Advances in the basic neurobiology of depression are providing a rich range of potential molecular targets for antidepressant therapeutics. We need to find a way to fund medicinal chemistry efforts through which tool compounds against these targets can be developed and then tested in small, exploratory clinical studies. The success of such studies is likely to be enhanced by focusing on subsets of the broad depression syndrome based on biological measurements, whether genetic risk factors, brain imaging findings, and a range of abnormalities (e.g., cytokines, RNA or protein expression profiles) in peripheral blood or cerebrospinal fluid (CSF). We believe that such capabilities will at long last jump-start drug discovery efforts in depression and bring much-needed relief to the roughly half of all depressed patients who do not respond fully to today's treatments.

REFERENCES

1. Kashdan TB, Morina N, Priebe S. Post-traumatic stress disorder, social anxiety disorder, and depression in survivors of the Kosovo war: experiential avoidance as a contributor to distress and quality of life. *J Anxiety Disord*. 2009;23:185–196.
2. Major Depressive Disorder Working Group of the Psychiatric GWAS Consortium, Ripke S, Wray NR, Lewis CM, et al. A mega-analysis of genome-wide association studies for major depressive disorder. *Mol Psychiatry*. 2013;18:497–511.
3. Berton O, Nestler EJ. New approaches to antidepressant drug discovery: beyond mono-amines. *Nature Rev Neurosci*. 2006;7:137–151.

4. Murrough JW, Charney DS. Is there anything really novel on the antidepressant horizon? *Curr Psychiatry Rep.* 2012;14:643–649.

5. Nestler EJ, Hyman SE. Animal models of neuropsychiatric disorders. *Nature Neurosci.* 2010;13:1161–1169.

6. Scott KM, McLaughlin KA, Smith DAR, Ellis PM. Childhood maltreatment and DSM-IV adult mental disorders: comparison of prospective and retrospective findings. *Br J Psychiatry.* 2012;200:469–775.

7. Cuthbert BN. Research domain criteria: toward future psychiatric nosologies. *Dialogues Clin Neurosci.* 2015;17:89–97.

8. Berton O, McClung CA, DiLeone RJ, et al. Essential role of BDNF in the mesolimbic dopamine pathway in social defeat stress. *Science.* 2006;311:864–868.

9. Golden SA, Covington HE 3rd, Berton O, Russo SJ. A standardized protocol for repeated social defeat stress in mice. *Nature Protoc.* 2011;6:1183–1191.

10. Krishnan V, Han MH, Graham DL, et al. Molecular adaptations underlying susceptibility and resistance to social defeat in brain reward regions. *Cell.* 2007;131:391–404.

11. Chuang JC, Krishnan V, Yu HG, et al. A beta3-adrenergic-leptin-melanocortin circuit regulates behavioral and metabolic changes induced by chronic stress. *Biol Psychiatry.* 2010;67:1075–1082.

12. Tsankova NM, Berton O, Renthal W, Kumar A, Neve RL, Nestler EJ. Sustained hippocampal chromatin regulation in hippocampus in a mouse model of depression and antidepressant action. *Nature Neurosci.* 2006;9:519–525.

13. Donahue RJ, Muschamp JW, Russo SJ, Nestler EJ, Carlezon WA Jr. Effects of striatal ΔFosB overexpression and ketamine on social defeat stress-induced anhedonia in mice. *Biol Psychiatry.* 2014;76:550–558.

14. Bagot TC, Cates HM, Purushothaman I, et al. Ketamine and imipramine reverse transcriptional signatures of susceptibility and induce resilience-specific gene expression profiles. *Biol Psychiatry.* 2017;81:285–295.

15. Russo SJ, Takahashi A, Zhang HX, et al. Establishment of repeated social defeat stress model in female mice. *Soc Neurosci Abs.* 2016;170:14.

16. Turecki G, Meaney MJ. Effects of the social environment and stress on glucocorticoid receptor gene methylation: A systematic review. *Biol Psychiatry.* 2016;79:87–96.

17. Kundakovic M, Champagne FA. Early-life experience, epigenetics, and the developing brain. *Neuropsychopharmacology.* 2015;40:141–153.

18. Molet J, Maras PM, Avishai-Eliner S, Baram TZ. Naturalistic rodent models of chronic early-life stress. *Dev Psychobiol.* 2014;56:1675–1688.

19. Franklin TB, Russig H, Weiss IC, et al. Epigenetic transmission of the impact of early stress across generations. *Biol Psychiatry.* 2010;68:408–415.

20. Hill MN, Hellemans KG, Verma P, Gorzalka BB, Weinberg J. Neurobiology of chronic mild stress: parallels to major depression. *Neurosci Biobehav Rev.* 2012;36:2085–3117.

21. Hodes GE, Pfau ML, Purushothaman I, et al. Sex differences in nucleus accumbens transcriptome profiles associated with susceptibility versus resilience to subchronic variable stress. *J Neurosci.* 2015;35:16362–16376.

22. Li N, Lee B, Liu RJ, et al. mTOR-dependent synapse formation underlies the rapid antidepressant effects of NMDA antagonists. *Science.* 2010;329:959–964.

23. Price JL, Drevets WC. Neurocircuitry of mood disorders. *Neuropsychopharmacology.* 2010;35:192–216.

24. Dunlop BW, Mayberg HS. Neuroimaging-based biomarkers for treatment selection in major depressive disorder. *Dialogues Clin Neurosci.* 2014;16:479–490.

25. Epstein J, Pan H, Kocsis JH, et al. Lack of ventral striatal response to positive stimuli in depressed versus normal subjects. *Am J Psychiatry*. 2006;163:1784–1790.
26. Russo SJ, Nestler EJ. The brain reward circuitry in mood disorders. *Nat Rev Neurosci*. 2013;14:609–625.
27. Rajasethupathy P, Ferenczi E, Deisseroth K. Targeting neural circuits. *Cell*. 2016;165:524–534.
28. Sternson SM, Roth BL. Chemogenetic tools to interrogate brain functions. *Annu Rev Neurosci*. 2014;37:387–407.
29. Chaudhury D, Walsh JJ, Friedman AK, et al. Rapid regulation of depression-related behaviours by control of midbrain dopamine neurons. *Nature*. 2013;493:532–536.
30. Tye KM, Mirzabekov JJ, Warden MR, et al. Dopamine neurons modulate neural encoding and expression of depression-related behaviour. *Nature*. 2013;493:537–541.
31. Francis TC, Chandra R, Friend DM, et al. Nucleus accumbens medium spiny neuron subtypes mediate depression-related outcomes to social defeat stress. *Biol Psychiatry*. 2015;77:212–222.
32. Bagot RC, Parise EM, Peña CJ, et al. Ventral hippocampal afferents to the nucleus accumbens regulate susceptibility to depression. *Nat Commun*. 2015;6:7062.
33. Warden MR, Selimbeyoglu A, Mirzabekov JJ, et al. A prefrontal cortex-brainstem neuronal projection that controls response to behavioural challenge. *Nature*. 2012;492:428–432.
34. Tovote P, Fadok JP, Lüthi A. Neuronal circuits for fear and anxiety. *Nat Rev Neurosci*. 2015;16:317–331.
35. Tye KM, Prakash R, Kim SY, et al. Amygdala circuitry mediating reversible and bidirectional control of anxiety. *Nature*. 2011;471:358–362.
36. Holtzheimer PE, Mayberg HS. Deep brain stimulation for psychiatric disorders. *Annu Rev*. 2011;34:289–307.
37. Kavalali ET, Monteggia LM. How does ketamine elicit a rapid antidepressant response? *Curr Opin Pharmacol*. 2015;20:35–39.
38. Gerhard DM, Wohleb ES, Duman RS. Emerging treatment mechanisms for depression: focus on glutamate and synaptic plasticity. *Drug Discov Today*. 2016;21:454–464.
39. Zanos P, Moaddel R, Morris PJ, et al. NMDAR inhibition-independent antidepressant actions of ketamine metabolites. *Nature*. 2016;533:481–486.
40. Andrus BM, Blizinsky K, Vedell PT, et al. Gene expression patterns in the hippocampus and amygdala of endogenous depression and chronic stress models. *Mol Psychiatry*. 2012;17:49–61.
41. Malki K, Tosto M.G, Jumabhoy I, et al. Integrative mouse and human mRNA studies using WGCNA nominates novel candidate genes involved in the pathogenesis of major depressive disorder. *Pharmacogenomics*. 2013;14:1979–1990.
42. Chang LC, Jamain S, Lin CW, Rujescu D, Tseng GC, Sibille E. A conserved BDNF, glutamate- and GABA-enriched gene module related to human depression identified by coexpression meta-analysis and DNA variant genome-wide association studies. *PloS One*. 2014;9:e90980.
43. Bagot RC, Cates HM, Purushothaman I, et al. Circuit-wide transcriptional profiling reveals brain region-specific gene networks regulating depression susceptibility. *Neuron*. 2016;90:969–983.
44. Mo A, Mukamel EA, Davis FP, et al. Epigenomic signatures of neuronal diversity in the mammalian brain. *Neuron*. 2015;86:1369–1384.

45. Okaty BW, Freret ME, Rood BD, et al. Multi-scale molecular deconstruction of the serotonin neuron system. *Neuron.* 2015;88:774–791.
46. Peña CJ, Bagot RC, Labonté B, Nestler EJ. Epigenetic signaling in psychiatric disorders. *J Mol Biol.* 2014;426:3389–3412.
47. Nestler EJ. ΔFosB: a transcriptional regulator of stress and antidepressant responses. *Eur J Pharmacol.* 2015;753:66–72.
48. Dias C, Feng J, Sun H, et al. β-catenin mediates stress resilience through Dicer1/microRNA regulation. *Nature.* 2014;516:51–55.
49. Covington HE III, Maze I, LaPlant QC, et al. Antidepressant actions of HDAC inhibitors. *J Neurosci.* 2009;29:11451–11460.
50. Covington HE, Maze I, Sun HS, et al. A role for repressive histone methylation in cocaine-induced vulnerability to stress. *Neuron.* 2011;71:656–670.
51. Covington HE 3rd, Maze I, Vialou V, Nestler EJ. Antidepressant action of HDAC inhibition in the prefrontal cortex. *Neuroscience.* 2015;298:329–335.
52. Wilkinson MB, Xiao GH, Kumar A, et al. Imipramine treatment and resiliency exhibit similar chromatin regulation in a key brain reward region. *J Neurosci.* 2009;29:7820–7832.
53. McEwen BS, Gray JD, Nasca C. 60 years of neuroendocrinology: Redefining neuroendocrinology: stress, sex and cognitive and emotional regulation. *J Endocrinol.* 2015;226:T67–T83.
54. Mehta D, Binder EB. Gene × environment vulnerability factors for PTSD: the HPA-axis. *Neuropharmacology.* 2012;62:654–662.
55. Schatzberg AF. Anna-Monika Award Lecture, DGPPN Kongress, 2013: The role of the hypothalamic-pituitary-adrenal (HPA) axis in the pathogenesis of psychotic major depression. *World J Biol Psychiatry.* 2015;16:2–11.
56. Duman RS, Monteggia LM. A neurotrophic model for stress-related mood disorders. *Biol Psychiatry.* 2006;59:1116–1127.
57. Hodes GE, Pfau ML, Leboeuf M, et al. Individual differences in the peripheral immune system promote resilience versus susceptibility to social stress. *Proc Natl Acad Sci USA.* 2014;111:16136–16141.
58. Hodes GE, Kana V, Menard C, Merad M, Russo SJ. Neuroimmune mechanisms of depression. *Nat Neurosci.* 2015;18:1386–1393.

2

The Brain and Body on Stress
Allostatic Load and Mechanisms for Depression and Dementia

Bruce S. McEwen and Natalie L. Rasgon

INTRODUCTION

The brain and body are in continuous communication through the neuroendocrine, autonomic, metabolic, and immune systems. Depression and other mental health disorders involve not only dysregulation of neuronal architecture and function, but also systemic physiological dysregulation. Moreover, medications used to treat mental health disorders affect systemic physiology. The two chapter authors are, respectively, a basic scientist, neuroendocrinologist, and neuroscientist; and a clinician-researcher trained in both obstetrics/gynecology and psychiatry, whose paths have converged. Thus this is a story not only about physical disease and mental health but also about the importance of collaboration in directions, translation, and reverse-translation.

Allostatic load is a concept that has evolved to describe the consequences, over time, of dysregulation of brain–body communication by life experiences and health-related behaviors that lead not only to systemic pathophysiology but also to brain changes that underlie psychiatric disorders. This review outlines the basic principles of brain–body communication and the plasticity and vulnerability of the brain and underlying cellular and molecular mechanisms, including actions of sex as well as stress hormones and sex differences. It then describes some examples of how this information from clinical observations and animal models has led to discoveries about the human brain involving systemic hormones and their effects upon brain plasticity and vulnerability. These effects interact and accumulate over the life course to impair mood and cause systemic as well as brain pathophysiology. Comorbidity and multi-morbidity of disorders is very common, and early life adversity increases their frequency (Tomasdottir et al. 2015). The hippocampal formation figures prominently in this story, and it was also the brain structure outside of the hypothalamus to be recognized as a target for glucocorticoids and stress (McEwen et al. 2015b). It is also the hippocampus that figures now in insulin resistance, cognitive impairment, depression, and Alzheimer's disease and which prominently via the "glucocorticoid cascade hypothesis" (Sapolsky et al. 1986) also figures in development of the concept of allostatic load, which begins this story.

A MODERN VIEW OF BRAIN–BODY INTERACTIONS

Allostasis and Allostatic Load/Overload

The brain is a plastic and vulnerable organ that not only controls neuroendocrine, autonomic, immune, and metabolic functions, but also responds to signals from the body, including steroid and metabolic hormones, that alter its architecture and function (McEwen 1998, McEwen & Stellar 1993) (Figure 2.1). There are two sides to this story: on one hand, the body responds to almost any event or challenge, whether or not we call it "stress," by releasing chemical mediators. For example, catecholamines increase heart rate and blood pressure—to promote coping with the situation; on the other hand, chronic elevation of these same mediators—e.g., chronically increased heart rate and blood pressure—produce a chronic wear and tear on the cardiovascular system that can result, over time, in disorders such as strokes and heart attacks. For this reason, the term "allostasis" was introduced by Sterling and Eyer (Sterling & Eyer 1988) to refer to the active process by which the body responds to daily events and maintains homeostasis (*allostasis* literally means "achieving stability through change"). Because chronically increased allostasis can lead to disease, we introduced the term *allostatic load* to refer to the wear and tear that results either from too much stress or from the inefficient management of allostasis, such as not turning off the response when it is no longer needed (McEwen 1998). Other forms of allostatic load involve not turning on an adequate response in the first place, or not habituating to the recurrence of the same stressor and thus dampening the allostatic response. The term "allostatic overload" was introduced to highlight a more

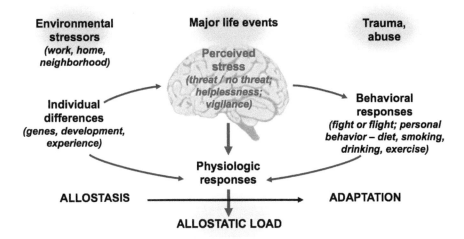

Figure 2.1 Central role of the brain in allostasis and the behavioral and physiological response to stressors, overuse and dysregulation of which lead to allostatic load and overload. From (McEwen 1998) by permission.

severe form of cumulative change that led to disease and death (McEwen & Wingfield 2003), along with distinctions between two types of allostatic load and overload: Type 1, in the natural world, in which the search for adequate nutrition dominates; and Type 2, where calories are adequate or in excess, and psychosocial stressors dominate.

Protection via allostasis and wear-and-tear on the body and brain through allostatic load/overload are the two contrasting sides of the physiology involved in defending the body against the challenges of daily life. Besides adrenalin and noradrenalin, there are many mediators that participate in allostasis, and they are linked in a network of regulation that is non-linear, meaning that each mediator has the ability to regulate the activity of the other mediators, sometimes in a biphasic manner (McEwen 2006) (Figure 2.2). Glucocorticoids produced by the adrenal cortex in response to adrenocorticotropic hormone (ACTH) from the pituitary gland is the other major "stress hormone." Pro- and anti-inflammatory cytokines are produced by many cells in the body, and they regulate each other and are in turn regulated by glucocorticoids and catecholamines. Whereas catecholamines can increase proinflammatory cytokine production, glucocorticoids are known to inhibit this production. Yet there are exceptions—proinflammatory effects of glucocorticoids that depend on dose and cell or tissue type (Dinkel et al. 2003, Frank et al. 2012). The parasympathetic nervous system also plays an important regulatory role in this non-linear network of allostasis, since it generally opposes the sympathetic nervous system and, for example, slows the heart and also has anti-inflammatory effects (Borovikova et al. 2000, Sloan et al. 2007).

What this non-linearity means is that when any one mediator is increased or decreased, there are compensatory changes in the other mediators that depend on time course and level of change of each of the mediators. Unfortunately, we cannot measure all components of this system simultaneously, and we must therefore rely on measurements of only a few of them in any one study. Yet the non-linearity must be kept in mind when we interpret the results.

A good example of the biphasic actions of stress—that is, "protection vs. damage"—is in the immune system, in which an acute stressor activates an acquired immune response via

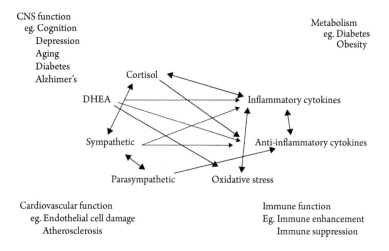

Figure 2.2 The network of allostasis in which multiple mediators of adaptation interact with each other non-linearly and simultaneously affect organs and systems throughout the body.

mediation by catecholamines and glucocorticoids and locally produced immune mediators; yet a chronic exposure to the same stressor over several weeks has the opposite effect and results in immune suppression (Dhabhar 2009, Dhabhar et al. 2012). Acute stress-induced immune enhancement is good for enhancing immunization, fighting an infection, or repairing a wound, but it is deleterious to health for an autoimmune conditions such as psoriasis or Krohn's disease. On the other hand, immune suppression is good in the case of an autoimmune disorder and deleterious for fighting an infection or repairing a wound. In an immune-sensitive skin cancer, acute stress is effective in inhibiting tumor progression while chronic stress exacerbates progression (Dhabhar et al. 2010, Saul et al. 2005).

Key Role of the Brain

Stress is a major factor in psychiatric illnesses, and the brain is the key organ of the stress response because it determines what is threatening and therefore stressful, and also controls the behavioral and physiological responses (see Figure 2.1). There are enormous individual differences in the response to stress, based upon the experience of the individual early in life and in adult life. Positive or negative experiences in school, at work, or in romantic and family interpersonal relationships can bias an individual towards either a positive or negative response in a new situation.

Early-life experiences carry an even greater weight in terms of how an individual reacts to new situations. Early-life physical and sexual abuse carry with them a lifelong burden of behavioral and pathophysiological problems (Felitti et al. 1998). Cold and uncaring families produce long-lasting emotional problems in children (Repetti et al. 2002). Some of these effects are seen on brain structure and function and in the risk for later depression and post-traumatic stress disorder (PTSD; Shonkoff et al. 2009). One of the biological consequences of early-life adversity is the prolonged elevation in inflammatory cytokines as well as poor dental health, obesity, and elevated blood pressure in children and young adults (Danese & McEwen 2012). Harsh language is among the components of early-life adversity and has been shown to increase inflammatory markers (Miller & Chen 2010). Overall, early-life adversity increases comorbidity and multi-morbidity of systemic disorders and mental health disorders (Tomasdottir et al. 2015). And the physical environment makes a huge difference, with crowding, noise, and ugliness, along with physical danger, being major contributors to allostatic overload both during development and throughout adult life (Chang et al. 2009, Diez Roux & Mair 2010, Evans et al. 2005).

Epigenetics

Gene–environment interactions are key to how the brain develops and changes with experiences. *Epigenetics* now refers to events "above the genome" that regulate expression of genetic information without altering the DNA sequence. Besides the CpG[1] methylation described

---

[1] The CpG sites or CG sites are regions of DNA where a cytosine nucleotide is followed by a guanine nucleotide in the linear sequence of bases along its 5′ → 3′ direction. *CpG* is shorthand for *5′—C—phosphate—G—3′*, that is, cytosine and guanine separated by only one phosphate; phosphate links any two nucleosides together in DNA.

before, other mechanisms include histone modifications that repress or activate chromatin unfolding (Allfrey 1970) and the actions of non-coding RNAs (Mehler 2008), as well as transposons and retrotransposons (Griffiths & Hunter 2014) and RNA editing (Mehler & Mattick 2007). For prevention and treatment, it is important to focus on strategies that center around the use of targeted behavioral therapies, along with treatments, including pharmaceutical agents, that "open up windows of plasticity" in the brain and facilitate the efficacy of the behavioral interventions (McEwen 2012). This is because a major challenge throughout the life course is to find ways of redirecting future behavior and physiology in more positive and healthier directions (Halfon et al. 2014). In keeping with the original definition of epigenetics (Waddington 1942) as the emergence of characteristics not previously evident or even predictable from an earlier developmental stage (e.g., think about a fertilized frog or human egg, which look similar, but see what happens as each develops), we do not mean "reversibility" as in "rolling back the developmental clock" but rather as in "redirection."

Animal models have been useful in providing insights into behavioral and physiological mechanisms. Individual differences in their anxiety-like behaviors are evident (Cavigelli & McClintock 2003, Nasca et al. 2015). Early-life maternal care in rodents is a powerful determinant of lifelong emotional reactivity and stress hormone reactivity, and increases in both are associated with earlier cognitive decline and a shorter lifespan (Meaney et al. 1991). Effects of early maternal care are transmitted across generations by the subsequent behavior of the female offspring as they become mothers, and methylation of DNA on key genes appears to play a role in this epigenetic transmission (Francis et al. 1999, Meaney & Szyf 2005). Yet, the mother is not the sole determinant of the offspring's emotional and physical development, but rather modulates it by her behavior towards the offspring, particularly in the immediate aftermath of pups' experiences of novelty inside or outside of the home cage (Tang et al. 2014). Furthermore, in rodents, abuse of the young is associated with an attachment, rather than an avoidance, of the abusive mother, an effect that increases the chances that the pup can continue to obtain food and other support until weaning (Moriceau & Sullivan 2006). Moreover, other conditions that affect the rearing process can also affect emotionality in offspring. For example, uncertainty in the food supply for rhesus monkey mothers leads to increased emotionality in their offspring and possibly an earlier onset of obesity and diabetes (Coplan et al. 2001, Kaufman et al. 2007).

Besides the important role of the social and physical environment and experiences of individuals in the health outcomes, genetic factors also play an important role. Different alleles of commonly occurring genes determine how individuals will respond to experiences. For example, the short form of the serotonin transporter is associated with a number of conditions such as alcoholism, and individuals who have this allele are more vulnerable to respond to stressful experiences by developing depressive illness (Caspi et al. 2003, Spinelli et al. 2012). In childhood, individuals with an allele of the monoamine oxidase A gene are more vulnerable to abuse in childhood and more likely to themselves become abusers and show antisocial behaviors, compared to individuals with another commonly occurring allele (Caspi et al. 2002). Nevertheless, in a positive, nurturing environment, as formulated by Suomi and by Tom Boyce and colleagues (Boyce & Ellis 2005, Obradovic et al. 2010, Suomi 2006), these same alleles may lead to successful outcomes, which has led them to be called "reactive or context-sensitive alleles" rather than "bad genes."

BRAIN AS A TARGET OF STRESS

The fundamental discovery of the communication between hypothalamus and pituitary by Geoffrey Harris established the basis for understanding brain–body communication via the neuroendocrine system (Harris 1970). As originally conceived, and investigated productively with findings of releasing factors in the hypothalamus for pituitary hormones (e.g., Guillemin 1978, Schally et al. 1973, Vale et al. 1981), the field of neuroendocrinology has flourished. At the same time, steroid hormones were shown to bind to intracellular receptors that regulate gene expression in tissues such as the liver, or the prostate and uterus in the case of sex hormones (Jensen & Jacobson 1962). The focus of steroid hormone feedback to regulate neuroendocrine function was naturally upon the pituitary and the hypothalamus, and this work continues to uncover important aspects of neuroendocrine regulation (Meites 1992).

Hippocampus

The McEwen laboratory entered this field by serendipitously discovering adrenal steroids, and, later, estrogen receptors, in the hippocampal formation of the rat (Gerlach & McEwen 1972, Loy et al. 1988, McEwen & Plapinger 1970, McEwen et al. 1968, Milner et al. 2001), and we and others extended these findings to the infrahuman primate brain as well as to other regions of the brain involved in cognitive and emotional regulation (Gerlach et al. 1976). This has catalyzed studies that look at actions of hormonal feedback on the brain, not only to regulate hypothalamic functions, but also to influence neurological, cognitive, and emotional functions of the whole brain, with translation to the human brain in relation to aging, mood disorders, and the impact of the social environment. This chapter describes research in our and other laboratories that redefined neuroendocrinology as a field that also studies two-way brain–body communication via the neuroendocrine, autonomic, immune, and metabolic systems. This research has uncovered the remodeling of brain architecture mediated by hormones working with other cellular mediators. These actions occur via epigenetic mechanisms involving both genomic and non-genomic processes over the life course, and there is ongoing translation of the findings on animal models to the human condition, including the effects of adverse early-life experiences and the relationship of socioeconomic status and health through the development of the concept of allostatic load (McEwen and Stellar 1993; McEwen 1998).

By administering ^{3}H corticosterone into adrenalectomized rats, we discovered receptors for adrenal steroids in the hippocampal formation of the rat and, later, the rhesus monkey (Gerlach & McEwen 1972, Gerlach et al. 1976, McEwen & Plapinger 1970, McEwen et al. 1968; Figure 2.3). Other work revealed such receptors in the hippocampal equivalent in other species, including birds (Dickens et al. 2009, McEwen 1976). In retrospect, these findings broadened the perspective that glucocorticoids provided negative feedback control of the hypothalamic-pituitary-adrenal (HPA) axis to include actions of adrenal steroids on other brain functions such as memory and learning and control of mood and other aspects of behavior (McEwen 2010).

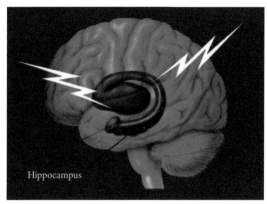

Contextual, episodic, spatial memory

Mood regulation – target of depression

Hippocampus
ATROPHIES in:
• Major depression
• Type 2 diabetes
• Post-traumatic
  stress disorder
• Cushing's disease

ALSO as a result of:
• Chronic stress
• Chronic jet lag
• Lack of exercise
• Chronic inflammation

Hippocampus

Figure 2.3 The hippocampus shrinks in mental health and systemic disorders and also in relation to chronic stress, jet lag and chronic systemic inflammation.

The hippocampus is one of the most sensitive and malleable regions of the brain and is also very important in cognitive function and mood regulation (McEwen et al. 2016). The dentate gyrus-CA3 system, which is delicately balanced anatomically and thus vulnerable to overstimulation, as in seizures, is believed to play a role in the memory of sequences of events, although long-term storage of memory occurs in other brain regions (Lisman 1999). Moreover, the anterior part of the hippocampus has strong connections to the amygdala and prefrontal cortex and is a nexus of vulnerability to depression. But because the hippocampal dentate gyrus-CornuAmonis3 (DG-CA3) system is so delicately balanced in its function and vulnerability to damage, there is also adaptive structural plasticity, in that new neurons continue to be produced in the dentate gyrus throughout adult life (Cameron et al. 1998), and CA3 pyramidal cells undergo a reversible remodeling of their dendrites in conditions such as hibernation and chronic stress (Magarinos et al. 2006, McEwen 1999). The role of this plasticity may be to protect against permanent damage. As a result, the hippocampus undergoes a number of adaptive changes in response to acute and chronic stress via a host of cellular and molecular mechanisms (McEwen et al. 2015a), and it also shows positive effects of regular physical activity on hippocampal volume and memory (Erickson et al. 2011) (Figures 2.3 and 2.4).

Prefrontal Cortex and Amygdala

Repeated stress also causes changes in other brain regions such as the prefrontal cortex and amygdala. Repeated stress causes dendritic shortening in the medial prefrontal cortex (McEwen & Morrison 2013) but produces dendritic growth in neurons in amygdala, as well as in orbitofrontal cortex. Excitatory amino acids and brain-derived neurotrophic factor (BDNF) are involved (Chattarji et al. 2015, Lakshminarasimhan & Chattarji 2012, McEwen & Morrison 2013).

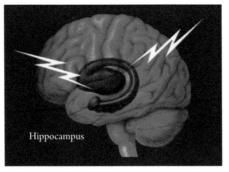

Hippocampus *INCREASES* in size with:
• Regular exercise
• Intense learning
• Anti-depressant treatment

Figure 2.4 The hippocampus increases in volume with regular exercise, intense learning and certain antidepressant treatments, of which physical activity is one of the most effective.

Contrasting Effects

Acute stress induces spine synapses in hippocampal CA1 region of hippocampus, and both acute and chronic stress also increase spine synapse formation in amygdala; but chronic stress decreases it in hippocampus. Moreover, chronic stress for 21 days or longer impairs hippocampal-dependent cognitive function and enhances amygdala-dependent unlearned fear and fear conditioning, which are consistent with the opposite effects of stress on hippocampal and amygdala structure (Chattarji et al. 2015). Chronic stress also increases aggression between animals living in the same cage, and this probably reflects another aspect of hyperactivity of the amygdala (Wood et al. 2008). Behavioral correlates of remodeling in the prefrontal cortex include impairment in attention set shifting, possibly reflecting structural remodeling in the medial prefrontal cortex (McEwen & Morrison 2013).

Sex Differences

Subtle sex differences exist for many of these functions that are developmentally programmed by hormones and by not-yet-precisely-defined genetic factors, including the mitochondrial genome. These sex differences and responses to sex hormones in brain regions, and upon functions not previously regarded as subject to such differences, indicate that we are entering a new era in our ability to understand and appreciate the variety of gender-related behaviors and brain functions.

Indeed, animal models of stress effects on the brain show that females and males respond differently to acute and chronic stressors because of developmental factors involving both epigenetic effects of hormones along with genes in the sex chromosomes themselves (McCarthy & Arnold 2011). Sex differences in the brain are subtle but widespread (cite Milner/McEwen in press), yet males and females do many things equally well. In human subjects, taking tests on empathy, men and women do equally well, but the brain activation patterns during the tests show different brain regions are activated (Derntl et al. 2010). This is reminiscent of an animal model study in which, despite no overall sex differences in fear-conditioning freezing behavior, the neural processes underlying successful or failed extinction maintenance are sex-specific (Gruene et al. 2014). Given other work showing sex differences in stress-induced structural plasticity in prefrontal cortex projections to amygdala and other cortical areas (Shansky et al. 2010), these findings are relevant not only to sex differences in fear conditioning and extinction, but, according to Gruene et al., "also to exposure-based clinical therapies, which are similar in premise to fear extinction and which are primarily used to treat disorders that are more common in women than in men" (Gruene et al. 2014).

CELLULAR AND MOLECULAR MECHANISMS

Glucocorticoid Hormone Actions

The brain is the central organ involved in perceiving and adapting to social and physical stressors via multiple interacting mediators, from the cell surface, to the cytoskeleton, to epigenetic regulation and non-genomic mechanisms. A key result of stress is structural remodeling of neural architecture, which may be a sign of successful adaptation, whereas persistence of these changes when stress ends indicates failed resilience. Excitatory amino acids and glucocorticoids play key roles in these processes, along with a growing list of extra- and intracellular mediators that includes endocannabinoids and BDNF. The result is a continually changing pattern of gene expression mediated by epigenetic mechanisms involving histone modifications and CpG methylation and hydroxymethylation, as well as by the activity of retrotransposons that may alter genomic stability. Elucidation of the underlying mechanisms of plasticity and vulnerability of the brain provides a basis for understanding the efficacy of interventions for anxiety and depressive disorders as well as age-related cognitive decline (McEwen et al. 2015a, McEwen et al. 2016).

Sex Hormones' Actions

Sex hormones act throughout the entire brain of both males and females via both genomic and non-genomic receptors. Sex hormones can act through many cellular and molecular processes that alter structure and function of neural systems and influence behavior, as well as providing neuroprotection (McEwen & Milner 2007). Within neurons, sex hormone receptors are found in nuclei and are also located near membranes where they are associated with presynaptic terminals, mitochondria, spine apparatus, and post-synaptic densities. Sex hormone receptors also are found in glial cells. Hormonal regulation of a variety of signaling pathways as well as direct and indirect effects upon gene expression induce spine synapses, up- or down-regulate and alter the distribution of neurotransmitter receptors, regulate neuropeptide expression and cholinergic and Gamma Amino Butyric Acid (GABA) activity, as well as govern calcium sequestration and oxidative stress. Many neural and behavioral functions are affected, including mood, cognitive function, blood pressure regulation, motor coordination, pain, and opioid sensitivity (McEwen & Milner 2007).

SYSTEMIC HORMONES AS CONTRIBUTORS TO BRAIN DISORDERS

Recognition that hormones play an important role in modulating brain structure and function has opened the way to showing how circulating hormones contribute to brain disorders when their normal functions to promote adaptation go awry. Regarding glucocorticoids, Cushing's disease is a prominent example. In Cushing's disease, there are depressive symptoms along with a smaller hippocampus and memory problems that can be relieved by surgical correction of the hypercortisolemia (Murphy 1991, Starkman & Schteingart 1981). Both major depression and Cushing's disease are associated with chronic elevation of cortisol that results in gradual loss of minerals from bone and contributes to abdominal obesity. In major depressive illness, as well as in Cushing's disease, the duration of the illness, and not the age of the subjects, predicts a progressive reduction in volume of the hippocampus, determined by structural magnetic resonance imaging (MRI; MacQueen et al. 2003, Sheline et al. 1999, Starkman et al. 1992).

The hippocampus figures prominently, as there is a variety of other anxiety-related disorders, such as PTSD (Pitman 2001, Vythilingam et al. 2002) and borderline personality disorder (Driessen et al. 2000), in which atrophy of the hippocampus has been reported, suggesting that this is a common process reflecting chronic imbalance in the activity of adaptive systems, such as the HPA axis, but also including endogenous neurotransmitters, such as glutamate. Inflammation is also a factor related to many disorders of modern life, and elevation of IL6 has been linked to reduced hippocampal volume (Marsland et al. 2008) as well as to poor sleep (Friedman et al. 2005).

Although there is little evidence regarding the effects of ordinary life stressors on brain structure, there are indications from functional imaging of individuals undergoing ordinary stressors, such as counting backwards, that there are lasting changes in neural activity (Wang et al. 2005), and a 20-year history of chronic perceived stress has been linked in a cross-sectional study to smaller hippocampal volume (Gianaros et al. 2007). Moreover, jet-lag and lack of adequate recovery are reported to lead to a smaller temporal lobe, memory impairment, and dysregulated and elevated cortisol (Cho 2001).

Brain regions besides the hippocampus, particularly the amygdala and prefrontal cortex, show altered patterns of activity in positron emission tomography (PET) and fMRI and also demonstrate changes in volume with recurrent depression: decreased volume of hippocampus and prefrontal cortex and amygdala (Drevets et al. 1997, Sheline 2003, Sheline et al. 1998, Sheline et al. 1999). Interestingly, however, amygdala volume has been reported to increase in the first episode of depression, whereas hippocampal volume is not decreased (Frodl et al. 2003, MacQueen et al. 2008). It has been known for some time that stress hormones, such as cortisol, are involved in psychopathology, reflecting emotional arousal and psychic disorganization rather than the specific disorder per se (Sachar et al. 1973). But there is more than cortisol affecting the brain, and, in particular, metabolic hormones have many effects that alter systemic physiology and mental health.

GLUCOSE REGULATION, COGNITION, INSULIN RESISTANCE, DEMENTIA, AND THE HIPPOCAMPUS

The hippocampus is very sensitive to energy availability, as shown by its vulnerability to damage from stroke and seizures; it is also affected by systemic insulin resistance, although insulin resistance in the brain can be induced in the absence of systemic insulin resistance and significantly affects cognitive function (Grillo et al. 2015), as will be elaborated in this section of the chapter. Elucidation of the many facets of these relationships further illustrates the importance of the brain–body interactions in brain health and systemic illness, including the role of metabolic hormones and differences in their actions in brain and body.

Involvement of Metabolic Hormones and Glucose Availability in Normal Cognitive Function

An important factor for hippocampal structure and function is glucose regulation; realization of this has led to insights about the ability of metabolic hormones such as insulin, leptin, ghrelin, and Insulin-like growth factor 1 (IGF-1) to enter and regulate hippocampal health and function (McEwen, 2007) (Figure 2.5). When the hippocampus is activated by a cognitive task, it needs glucose (McNay et al. 2000),

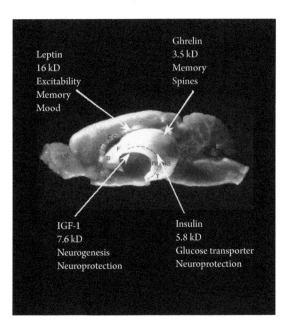

Figure 2.5 Four peptide/protein hormones, insulin- like growth factor I (IGF-I), insulin, ghrelin, and leptin, are able to enter the brain and affect structural remodeling or other functions in the hippocampus. A transport process is involved, and specific receptors are expressed in hippocampus as well as in other brain regions. Molecular sizes are indicated for each hormone in kilodaltons. From (McEwen 2007) by permission.

and this changes with aging (Gold 1987) (McNay & Gold 2001). Consistent with Sapolsky's glucocorticoid endangerment hypothesis (Sapolsky 1992), cortisol inhibits glucose uptake in the healthy aging brain as a way of preventing damaging glycation of proteins by excess glucose (Reagan et al. 2000).

Besides glucocorticoids and excitatory amino acids, a number of protein hormones have been shown to affect the hippocampus. The hippocampus has receptors for IGF-1 and insulin, and it responds to circulating insulin to translocate glucose transporters to cell membranes (Dore et al. 1997, Piroli et al. 2007b). Circulating IGF-1 is a key mediator of the ability of physical activity to increase neurogenesis in the dentate gyrus of the hippocampal formation (Aberg et al. 2000, Carro et al. 2001). IGF-1 is taken up into brain via a transport system different from that which transports insulin, although there is some overlap (Banks et al. 2012, Pulford & Ishii 2001, Yu et al. 2006). IGF-1 is a member of the growth hormone family, and growth hormone is implicated in cognitive function and mood regulation (Donahue et al. 2006, Nyberg 2000).

Growth hormone is expressed in the hippocampus where it is upregulated by acute stress and also, in females, by estradiol (Donahue et al. 2006). Interestingly, although growth hormone mRNA is expressed in hippocampus (Donahue et al. 2002), growth hormone also enters the brain in small amounts from the circulation, although not by a specific transport system (Pan et al. 2005). Furthermore, circulating ghrelin, a pro-appetitive hormone, has been shown to increase synapse formation in hippocampal pyramidal neurons and to improve hippocampal-dependent memory (Diano et al. 2006). Ghrelin is transported into brain via a saturable system (Banks et al. 2002), and receptors for ghrelin are expressed in hippocampus, as well as in other regions of the brain (Zigman et al. 2006).

Another metabolic hormone, leptin, has been found to exert antidepressant effects when infused directly into the hippocampus (Lu et al. 2006). Leptin is transported into the brain, and both glucose and insulin mediate the ability of fasting to increase leptin transport into the brain (Kastin & Akerstrom 2001). Leptin receptors are found in hippocampus, among other brain regions, and leptin has actions in hippocampus, via excitatory amino acid receptors, that reduce the probability of seizures and enhance aspects of cognitive function (Harvey et al. 2005).

Polycystic Ovary Syndrome (PCOS), Insulin Resistance, and Psychiatric Disorders

A remarkable example of dysregulation of brain–body communication is that polycystic ovarian syndrome (PCOS)—the most common source of infertility among reproductive-aged women—is associated with increased levels of major depression, bipolar illness, and schizophrenia (Barry et al. 2011, Rassi et al. 2010). PCOS is a complex neuroendocrine disorder with insulin resistance (IR) at its core. Hyperandrogenism is another core component of PCOS, and may in part be a sequel of the IR (Tsilchorozidou et al. 2004). Androgens in particular, and sex hormones in general, may be involved in PCOS effects on brain function and behavior in view of the widespread presence in the brain of sex hormone receptors, as described earlier in this chapter, although the exact nature of those influences is not clear. Once again, many of the findings focus on the hippocampus.

Insulin Resistance and Depression

A key feature of PCOS is insulin resistance, and this finding has triggered a broader investigation of insulin resistance in both men and women and its possible role in depression. Moreover, depression is often associated with insulin resistance and metabolic syndrome in some individuals, and treatment with a Peroxisome proliferator-activated receptor gamma (PPAR-γ or PPARG) agent, pioglitazone, showed improvement in depressive symptoms, but only in subjects with insulin resistance (Lin et al. 2015).

Insulin Resistance in Hippocampus and Hypothalamus

What is the nature of the insulin resistance in the brain? When hypothalamic insulin receptors were depleted by a locally applied antisense, systemic features of diabetes appeared, and there was also increased depressive- and anxiety-like behavior, along with a depletion of BDNF in the hippocampus and hypothalamus (Grillo et al. 2011). Indeed, a short-term corticosterone treatment causes not only systemic insulin resistance, but also insulin resistance in the hippocampus, reflected by decreased glucose transporter type 4 (GLUT-4) levels and reduced insulin-stimulated insulin receptor phosphorylation (Piroli et al. 2007). Moreover, the systemic metabolic state plays a role in the brain, in that fatty Zucker rats have poorer hippocampal-dependent memory than lean Zucker rats, as well as impaired translocation of an insulin-dependent glucose transporter to hippocampal membranes (Winocur et al. 2005). Moreover, a diet rich in fat has been shown to impair hippocampal-dependent memory (Winocur & Greenwood 1999), and a combination of a high fat diet and a three-week predator exposure causes retraction of dendrites in the CA3 hippocampus, even though neither treatment alone had this effect (Baran et al. 2005). Indeed, systemic metabolism, particularly triglycerides and leptin resistance in the hippocampus, has turned out to be very important, as a mild food-restriction paradigm both prevented and reversed the obesity phenotype in the rats in which hypothalamic insulin receptors had been inactivated by antisense (Grillo et al. 2014). Both of these paradigms restored long-term potentiation (LTP) in the CA1 region and reversed the decreases in the phosphorylated/total ratio of GluA1 Ser845 α-amino-3-hydroxy-5-methyl-4-isoxazolepropionic acid receptor (AMPA) receptor subunit expression observed in the hippocampus of insulin receptor antisense lentivirus (hypo-IRAS) rats. Because regulation of the GluA1 Ser845 AMPA receptor subunit phosphorylation is a key feature of leptin action, the impairment of insulin action in hypo-IRAS rats is mediated through the impairment of hippocampal leptin activity (Grillo et al. 2014).

However, while glucose uptake is important, and impaired leptin signaling by elevated triglycerides can impair insulin action, it is not the dominant feature of insulin action and insulin resistance in the hippocampus (Fadel & Reagan 2016). Antisense inactivation of hippocampal insulin receptors produced impaired long-term potentiation and hippocampal-dependent learning without any systemic metabolic disturbance (Grillo et al. 2015). While antisense inactivation of insulin receptors is not a likely mechanism in pathophysiology, it has been shown that excessive stimulation of N-methyl-D-aspartate (NMDA) receptors by glutamate and sustained calcium influx stimulates the activity of tyrosine phosphatases on insulin receptors and attenuates insulin signal transduction (De Felice et al. 2014).

Another process that may be involved in brain insulin resistance is the active transport of IGF-1 into the brain, which is activated by neural activity (Nishijima et al. 2010); impairment of this has not yet been demonstrated in insulin resistance, but the requirement of neural activity may be one of the reasons that exercise is beneficial for cognitive function and against insulin resistance. In that connection, the activity-induced break-down of glycogen and transport of lactate into neurons is essential for long-term memory formation. Disrupting the expression of the neuronal lactate transporter Monocarboxylate transporter 2 (MCT2) leads to failure of long-term memory and amnesia; in particular, glycogenolysis and astrocytic lactate transporters are also critical for the molecular changes required for memory formation, including the induction of phospho-cAMP response element binding (CREB), activity-regulated cytoskeleton-associated protein (Arc), and phospho-cofilin (Suzuki et al. 2011). Further studies of this process are needed in relation to hippocampal insulin resistance.

Pharmacological Treatment and Systemic Consequences

The insulin resistance story illustrates another important consequence of brain–body interactions of the type discussed in this chapter. There are consequences of pharmacological treatment with medications such as valproic acid, antipsychotic drugs, and SSRIs used to treat bipolar disorder, major depression, and schizophrenia; namely, the disruption of systemic functions involving weight gain and sexual dysfunction (Kenna et al. 2009). Some antipsychotic drugs are known to promote weight gain along with other disturbances of the neuroendocrine system (Leucht et al. 2013), and SSRIs produce sexual dysfunction (Taylor et al. 2013). The story for PCOS, insulin resistance, and bipolar disorder, however, illustrates the difficulty of separating cause from effect. Indeed, it was in women using valproate for bipolar disorder that PCOS was first detected, and both insulin resistance and glucocorticoid resistance and the resulting overproduction of mineralocorticoids and androgens in PCOS may be causal factors for bipolar disorder (reviewed in Jiang et al. 2009). Yet, for bipolar illness in women, there is evidence for hyperlipidemia and insulin resistance even before treatment with valproate (Stemmle et al. 2009), and the overlap between PCOS and bipolar illness suggests an overlapping genetic basis and resulting endophenotype (Jiang et al. 2009) in which endocrine dysregulation plays a significant role.

Insulin Resistance, the Human Hippocampus, and the Risk of Dementia

Metabolic factors involving glucose regulation and insulin resistance play a role in hippocampal volume change in the human hippocampus in mild cognitive impairment (MCI) with aging (Convit et al. 2003, Rasgon et al. 2001). Poor glucose regulation is associated with smaller hippocampal volume and poorer memory function in individuals in their 60s and 70s who have MCI (McIntyre et al. 2010), and both MCI and type 2, as well as type 1, diabetes are recognized as risk factors for depression and dementia, as will now be described (de Leon et al. 2001, Haan 2006, Ott et al. 1996, Rasgon et al. 2001).

Within the life-course perspective of epigenetic effects of a progression of lifetime experiences and health-related behaviors operating on different genotypes, there is growing evidence for a relationship between insulin resistance and the risk of cognitive decline and dementia (Rasgon & Jarvik 2004, Rasgon et al. 2011). Hippocampal shrinkage is reported in women with insulin resistance who are at risk of Alzheimer's disease (Rasgon et al. 2011), and in men as well as women with type 2 diabetes (Gold et al. 2007). Hippocampal shrinkage is an index of early Alzheimer's disease (de Leon et al. 2004, Hampel et al. 2008). We have seen that elevated glucocorticoid levels can also shut off glucose and endanger the survival of hippocampal neurons (Sapolsky 1992). The normal physiological regulation apparently does not happen in the Alzheimer brain in which input and output of the hippocampus is damaged (de Leon et al. 1997, DeLeon et al. 1988).

An oxidative stress and inflammatory cascade has been suggested as a pathway from insulin resistance to Alzheimer's pathology (Gold et al. 2013, Manolopoulos et al. 2010), representing an example of an allostatic overload, Possible interventions include hormone therapy, particularly unopposed estrogen (Rasgon et al. 2014), and PPARγ•agonists such as pioglitazone (Gold et al. 2013, Lin et al. 2015), along with lifestyle changes leading to increased physical activity. Given the occurrence of obesity and type 2 diabetes already in adolescent youth (Yau et al. 2012), early-life intervention is imperative wherever possible to redirect the progression of the allostatic load towards a healthier path.

CONCLUSION

Neuroscientists, including those in psychiatry, have in the past treated the brain largely in isolation from the rest of the body, while, conversely, the disciplines of endocrinology and general medicine have viewed the body largely without regard to the influence of higher brain centers above the hypothalamus and pituitary gland. But now there is greater recognition of brain–body interactions affecting the limbic and cognitive systems of brain, with consequences of the influence for systemic physiology and disease and vice versa, and resulting multi-morbidity, based upon the types of information summarized in this chapter.

REFERENCES

Aberg MAI, Aberg ND, Hedbacker H, Oscarsson J, Eriksson PS. Peripheral infusion of IGF-1 selectively induces neurogenesis in the adult rat hippocampus. *J Neurosci.* 2000;20:2896–2903.

Allfrey VG. Changes in chromosomal proteins at times of gene activation. *Fed Proc.* 1970;29:1447–1460.

Banks WA, Owen JB, Erickson MA. Insulin in the brain: there and back again. *Pharmacol Ther.* 2012;136:82–93.

Banks WA, Tschop M, Robinson SM, Heiman ML. Extent and direction of ghrelin transport across the blood-brain barrier is determined by its unique primary structure. *J Pharmacol Exper Therapeut.* 2002;302:822–827.

Baran SE, Campbell AM, Kleen JK, et al. Combination of high fat diet and chronic stress retracts hippocampal dendrites. *NeuroReport* 2005;16:39–43.

Barry JA, Kuczmierczyk AR, Hardiman PJ. Anxiety and depression in polycystic ovary syndrome: a systematic review and meta-analysis. *Hum Reprod.* 2011;26:2442–2451.

Borovikova LV, Ivanova S, Zhang M, et al. Vagus nerve stimulation attenuates the systemic inflammatory response to endotoxin. *Nature*. 2000;405:458–462.

Boyce WT, Ellis BJ. Biological sensitivity to context: I. An evolutionary-developmental theory of the origins and functions of stress reactivity. *Dev Psychopathol*. 2005;17:271–301.

Cameron HA, Tanapat P, Gould E. Adrenal steroids and N-methyl-D-aspartate receptor activation regulate neurogenesis in the dentate gyrus of adult rats through a common pathway. *Neuroscience*. 1998;82:349–354.

Carro E, Trejo JL, Busiguina S, Torres-Aleman I. Circulating insulin-like growth factor 1 mediates the protective effects of physical exercise against brain insults of different etiology and anatomy. *J Neurosci*. 2001;21:5678–5684.

Caspi A, McClay J, Moffitt TE, et al. Role of genotype in the cycle of violence in maltreated children. *Science*. 2002;297:851–854.

Caspi A, Sugden K, Moffitt TE, et al. Influence of life stress on depression: moderation by a polymorphism in the 5-HTT gene. *Science*. 2003;301:386–389.

Cavigelli SA, McClintock MK. Fear of novelty in infant rats predicts adult corticosterone dynamics and an early death. *Proc Natl Acad Sci USA*. 2003;100:16131–16136.

Chang VW, Hillier AE, Mehta NK. Neighborhood racial isolation, disorder and obesity. *Social Forces*. 2009;87:2063–2092.

Chattarji S, Tomar A, Suvrathan A, Ghosh S, Rahman MM. Neighborhood matters: divergent patterns of stress-induced plasticity across the brain. *Nat Neurosci*. 2015;18:1364–1375.

Cho K. Chronic "jet lag" produces temporal lobe atrophy and spatial cognitive deficits. *Nature Neurosci*. 2001;4:567–568.

Convit A, Wolf OT, Tarshish C, de Leon MJ. Reduced glucose tolerance is associated with poor memory performance and hippocampal atrophy among normal elderly. *Proc Natl Acad Sci USA*. 2003;100:2019–2022.

Coplan JD, Smith ELP, Altemus M, et al. Variable foraging demand rearing: sustained elevations in cisternal cerebrospinal fluid corticotropin-releasing factor concentrations in adult primates. *Biol Psychiatry* 2001;50:200–204.

Danese A, McEwen BS. Adverse childhood experiences, allostasis, allostatic load, and age-related disease. *Physiol Behav*. 2012;106:29–39.

De Felice FG, Lourenco MV, Ferreira ST. How does brain insulin resistance develop in Alzheimer's disease? *Alzheimers Dement*. 2014;10:S26–S32.

de Leon MJ, Convit A, Wolf OT, et al. Prediction of cognitive decline in normal elderly subjects with 2-[^{18}F]yfluoro-2-deoxy-D-glucose/positron-emission tomography (FDG/PET). *Proc Natl Acad Sci USA*. 2001;98:10966–10971.

de Leon MJ, DeSanti S, Zinkowski R, et al. MRI and CSF studies in the early diagnosis of Alzheimer's disease. *J Intern Med*. 2004;256:205–223.

de Leon MJ, McRae T, Rusinek H, et al. Cortisol reduces hippocampal glucose metabolism in normal elderly, but not in Alzheimer's disease. *J Clin Endocrinol Metabol*. 1997;82:3251–3259.

DeLeon MJ, McRae T, Tsai J, et al. Abnormal cortisol response in Alzheimer's disease linked to hippocampal atrophy. *Lancet*. 1988;2(8607):391–392.

Derntl B, Finkelmeyer A, Eickhoff S, et al. Multidimensional assessment of empathic abilities: neural correlates and gender differences. *Psychoneuroendocrinology*. 2010;35:67–82.

Dhabhar FS. Enhancing versus suppressive effects of stress on immune function: implications for immunoprotection and immunopathology. *Neuroimmunomodulation*. 2009;16:300–317.

Dhabhar FS, Malarkey WB, Neri E, McEwen BS. Stress-induced redistribution of immune cells—from barracks to boulevards to battlefields: a tale of three hormones—Curt Richter Award winner. *Psychoneuroendocrinology.* 2012;37:1345–1368.

Dhabhar FS, Saul AN, Daugherty C, Holmes TH, Bouley DM, Oberyszyn TM. Short-term stress enhances cellular immunity and increases early resistance to squamous cell carcinoma. *Brain Behav Immun.* 2010;24:127–137.

Diano S, Farr SA, Benoit SC, et al. Ghrelin controls hippocampal spine synapse density and memory performance. *Nature Neurosci.* 2006;9:381–388.

Dickens M, Romero LM, Cyr NE, Dunn IC, Meddle SL. Chronic stress alters glucocorticoid receptor and mineralocorticoid receptor mRNA expression in the European starling (*Sturnus vulgaris*) brain. *J Neuroendocrinol.* 2009;21:832–840.

Diez Roux AV, Mair C. Neighborhoods and health. *Ann NY Acad Sci.* 2010;1186:125–145.

Dinkel K, MacPherson A, Sapolsky RM. Novel glucocorticoid effects on acute inflammation in the CNS. *J Neurochem.* 2003;84:705–716.

Donahue CP, Jensen RV, Ochiishi T, et al. Transcriptional profiling reveals regulated genes in the hippocampus during memory formation. *Hippocampus.* 2002;12:821–833.

Donahue CP, Kosik KS, Shors TJ. Growth hormone is produced within the hippocampus where it responds to age, sex, and stress. *Proc Natl Acad Sci USA.* 2006;103:6031–6036.

Dore S, Kar S, Rowe W, Quirion R. Distribution and levels of [^{125}I]IGF-I, [^{125}I]IGF-II and [^{125}I]insulin receptor binding sites in the hippocampus of aged memory-unimpaired and -impaired rats. *Neuroscience.* 1997;80:1033–1040.

Drevets WC, Price JL, Simpson Jr JR, et al. Subgenual prefrontal cortex abnormalities in mood disorders. *Nature.* 1997;386:824–827.

Driessen M, Hermann J, Stahl K, et al. Magnetic resonance imaging volumes of the hippocampus and the amygdala in women with borderline personality disorder and early traumatization. *Arch Gen Psychiatry.* 2000;57:1115–1122.

Erickson KI, Voss MW, Prakash RS, et al. Exercise training increases size of hippocampus and improves memory. *Proc Natl Acad Sci USA.* 2011;108:3017–3022.

Evans GW, Gonnella C, Marcynyszyn LA, Gentile L, Salpekar N. The role of chaos in poverty and children's socioemotional adjustment. *Psychol Sci.* 2005;16:560–565.

Fadel JR, Reagan LP. Stop signs in hippocampal insulin signaling: the role of insulin resistance in structural, functional and behavioral deficits. *Curr Opin Behav Sci.* 2016;9:47–54.

Felitti VJ, Anda RF, Nordenberg D, et al. Relationship of childhood abuse and household dysfunction to many of the leading causes of death in adults. The Adverse Childhood Experiences (ACE) study. *Am J Prev Med.* 1998;14:245–258.

Francis D, Diorio J, Liu D, Meaney MJ. Nongenomic transmission across generations of maternal behavior and stress responses in the rat. *Science.* 1999;286:1155–1158.

Frank MG, Thompson BM, Watkins LR, Maier SF. Glucocorticoids mediate stress-induced priming of microglial pro-inflammatory responses. *Brain Behav Immun.* 2012;26:337–345.

Friedman EM, Hayney MS, Love GD, et al. Social relationships, sleep quality, and interleukin-6 in aging women. *Proc Natl Acad Sci USA.* 2005;102:18757–18762.

Frodl T, Meisenzahl EM, Zetzsche T, et al. Larger amygdala volumes in first depressive episode as compared to recurrent major depression and healthy control subjects. *Biol Psychiatry.* 2003;53:338–344.

Gerlach J, McEwen BS. Rat brain binds adrenal steroid hormone: radioautography of hippocampus with corticosterone. *Science.* 1972;175:1133–1136.

Gerlach J, McEwen BS, Pfaff DW, et al. Cells in regions of rhesus monkey brain and pituitary retain radioactive estradiol, corticosterone and cortisol differently. *Brain Res.* 1976;103:603–612.

Gianaros PJ, Jennings JR, Sheu LK, Greer PJ, Kuller LH, Matthews KA. Prospective reports of chronic life stress predict decreased grey matter volume in the hippocampus. *NeuroImage.* 2007;35:795–803.

Gold PE. Sweet memories. *Am Scientist.* 1987;75:151–155.

Gold PW, Licinio J, Pavlatou MG. Pathological parainflammation and endoplasmic reticulum stress in depression: potential translational targets through the CNS insulin, klotho and PPAR-gamma systems. *Mol Psychiatry.* 2013;18:154–165.

Gold SM, Dziobek I, Sweat V, et al. Hippocampal damage and memory impairments as possible early brain complications of type 2 diabetes. *Diabetologia.* 2007;50:711–719.

Griffiths BB, Hunter RG. Neuroepigenetics of stress. *Neuroscience.* 2014;275:420–435.

Grillo CA, Mulder P, Macht VA, et al. Dietary restriction reverses obesity-induced anhedonia. *Physiol Behav.* 2014;128:126–132.

Grillo CA, Piroli GG, Junor L, et al. Obesity/hyperleptinemic phenotype impairs structural and functional plasticity in the rat hippocampus. *Physiol Behav.* 2011;105:138–144.

Grillo CA, Piroli GG, Lawrence RC, et al. Hippocampal insulin resistance impairs spatial learning and synaptic plasticity. *Diabetes.* 2015;64:3927–3936.

Gruene TM, Roberts E, Thomas V, Ronzio A, Shansky RM. Sex-specific neuroanatomical correlates of fear expression in prefrontal-amygdala circuits. *Biol Psychiatry.* 2015;78:186–193.

Guillemin R. Peptides in the brain: the new endocrinology of the neuron. *Science.* 1978;202:390–402.

Haan MN. Therapy insight: type 2 diabetes mellitus and the risk of late-onset Alzheimer's disease. *Nature Clin Pract Neurol.* 2006;2:159–166.

Halfon N, Larson K, Lu M, Tullis E, Russ S. Lifecourse health development: past, present and future. *Matern Child Health J.* 2014;18:344–365.

Hampel H, Burger K, Teipel SJ, Bokde AL, Zetterberg H, Blennow K. Core candidate neurochemical and imaging biomarkers of Alzheimer's disease. *Alzheimers Dement.* 2008;4:38–48.

Harris GW. Effects of the nervous system on the pituitary-adrenal activity. *Prog Brain Res.*1970;32:86–88.

Harvey J, Shanley LJ, O'Malley D, Irving AJ. Leptin: a potential cognitive enhancer? *Biochem Soc Trans.* 2005;33:1029–1032.

Jensen E, Jacobson H. Basic guides to the mechanism of estrogen action. *Rec Prog Horm Res.* 1962;18:387–408.

Jiang B, Kenna HA, Rasgon NL. Genetic overlap between polycystic ovary syndrome and bipolar disorder: the endophenotype hypothesis. *Med Hypotheses.* 2009;73:996–1004.

Kastin AJ, Akerstrom V. Glucose and insulin increase the transport of leptin through the blood-brain barrier in normal mice but not in streptozotocin-diabetic mice. *Neuroendocrinology.* 2001;73:237–242.

Kaufman D, Banerji MA, Shorman I, et al. Early-life stress and the development of obesity and insulin resistance in juvenile bonnet macaques. *Diabetes.* 2007;56:1–5.

Kenna HA, Jiang B, Rasgon NL. Reproductive and metabolic abnormalities associated with bipolar disorder and its treatment. *Harv Rev Psychiatry.* 2009;17:138–146.

Lakshminarasimhan H, Chattarji S. Stress leads to contrasting effects on the levels of brain derived neurotrophic factor in the hippocampus and amygdala. *PLoS One.* 2012;7:e30481.

Leucht S, Cipriani A, Spineli L, et al. Comparative efficacy and tolerability of 15 antipsychotic drugs in schizophrenia: a multiple-treatments meta-analysis. *Lancet*. 2013;382:951–962.

Lin KW, Wroolie TE, Robakis T, Rasgon NL. Adjuvant pioglitazone for unremitted depression: clinical correlates of treatment response. *Psychiatry Res*. 2015;230:846–852.

Lisman JE. Relating hippocampal circuitry to function: recall of memory sequences by reciprocal dentate-CA3 interactions. *Neuron*. 1999;22:233–242.

Loy R, Gerlach J, McEwen BS. Autoradiographic localization of estradiol-binding neurons in rat hippocampal formation and entorhinal cortex. *Dev Brain Res*. 1988;39:245–251.

Lu X-Y, Kim CS, Frazer A, Zhang W. Leptin: A potential novel antidepressant. *Proc Natl Acad Sci USA*. 2006;103:1593–1598.

MacQueen GM, Campbell S, McEwen BS, et al. Course of illness, hippocampal function, and hippocampal volume in major depression. *Proc Natl Acad Sci USA*. 2003;100:1387–1392.

MacQueen GM, Yucel K, Taylor VH, Macdonald K, Joffe R. Posterior hippocampal volumes are associated with remission rates in patients with major depressive disorder. *Biol Psychiatry*. 2008;64(10):880–883.

Magarinos AM, McEwen BS, Saboureau M, Pevet P. Rapid and reversible changes in intrahippocampal connectivity during the course of hibernation in European hamsters. *Proc Natl Acad Sci USA*. 2006;103:18775–18780.

Manolopoulos KN, Klotz LO, Korsten P, Bornstein SR, Barthel A. Linking Alzheimer's disease to insulin resistance: the FoxO response to oxidative stress. *Mol Psychiatry*. 2010;15:1046–1052.

Marsland AL, Gianaros PJ, Abramowitch SM, Manuck SB, Hariri AR. Interleukin-6 covaries inversely with hippocampal grey matter volume in middle-aged adults. *Biol Psychiatry*. 2008;64:484–490.

McCarthy MM, Arnold AP. Reframing sexual differentiation of the brain. *Nat Neurosci*. 2011;14:677–683.

McEwen BS.. Steroid hormone receptors in developing and mature brain tissue. In: *Neurotransmitters, hormones and receptors: novel approaches*, ed. S Snyder, BS McEwen. Washington, DC: Society of Neuroscience; 1976:50–66

McEwen BS. Protective and damaging effects of stress mediators. *NEJM*. 1998;338:171–179.

McEwen BS. Stress and hippocampal plasticity. *Annu Rev Neurosci*. 1999;22:105–122.

McEwen BS. Protective and damaging effects of stress mediators: central role of the brain. *Dial Clin Neurosci Stress*. 2006;8:367–381.

McEwen BS. Physiology and neurobiology of stress and adaptation: Central role of the brain. *Physiol Rev*. 2007;87:873–904.

McEwen BS. Stress, sex, and neural adaptation to a changing environment: mechanisms of neuronal remodeling. *Ann NY Acad Sci*. 2010;1204(Suppl):E38–E59.

McEwen BS. Brain on stress: how the social environment gets under the skin. *Proc Natl Acad Sci USA*. 2012;109(Suppl 2):17180–17185.

McEwen BS, Bowles NP, Gray JD, et al. Mechanisms of stress in the brain. *Nat Neurosci*. 2015a;18:1353–1363.

McEwen BS, Gray JD, Nasca C. 60 years of neuroendocrinology: redefining neuroendocrinology: stress, sex and cognitive and emotional regulation. *J Endocrinol*. 2015b;226:T67–T83.

McEwen BS, Milner TA. Hippocampal formation: shedding light on the influence of sex and stress on the brain. *Brain Res Rev*. 2007;55:343–355.

McEwen, B.S., Milner, T.A. Review understanding the broad influence of sex hormones and sex differences in the brain. *J. Neurosci. Res*. 2017; 95,24–39.

McEwen BS, Morrison JH. The brain on stress: vulnerability and plasticity of the prefrontal cortex over the life course. *Neuron.* 2013;79:16–29.

McEwen BS, Nasca C, Gray JD. Stress effects on neuronal structure: hippocampus, amygdala, and prefrontal cortex. *Neuropsychopharmacology.* 2016;41:3–23.

McEwen BS, Plapinger L. Association of corticosterone-1,23H with macromolecules extracted from brain cell nuclei. *Nature.* 1970;226:263–264.

McEwen BS, Stellar E. Stress and the individual. Mechanisms leading to disease. *Arch Intern Med.* 1993;153:2093–2101.

McEwen BS, Weiss J, Schwartz L. Selective retention of corticosterone by limbic structures in rat brain. *Nature.* 1968;220:911–912.

McEwen BS, Wingfield JC. The concept of allostasis in biology and biomedicine. *Horm Behav.* 2003;43:2–15.

McIntyre RS, Kenna HA, Nguyen HT, et al. Brain volume abnormalities and neurocognitive deficits in diabetes mellitus: points of pathophysiological commonality with mood disorders? *Advance Ther.* 2010;27:63–80.

McNay EC, Fries TM, Gold PE. Decreases in rat extracellular hippocampal glucose concentration associated with cognitive demand during a spatial task. *Proc Natl Acad Sci USA.* 2000;97:2881–2885.

McNay EC, Gold PE. Age-related differences in hippocampal extracellular fluid glucose concentration during behavioral testing and following systemic glucose administration. *J Gerontol.* 2001;56A:B66–B71.

Meaney M, Aitken D, Bhatnagar S, Sapolsky R. Postnatal handling attenuates certain neuroendocrine, anatomical and cognitive dysfunctions associated with aging in female rats. *Neurobiol Aging.* 1991;12:31–38.

Meaney MJ, Szyf M. Environmental programming of stress responses through DNA methylation: life at the interface between a dynamic environment and a fixed genome. *Dialog Clin Neurosci.* 2005;7:103–123.

Mehler MF. Epigenetic principles and mechanisms underlying nervous system functions in health and disease. *Prog Neurobiol.* 2008;86:305–341.

Mehler MF, Mattick JS. Noncoding RNAs and RNA editing in brain development, functional diversification, and neurological disease. *Physiol Rev.* 2007;87:799–823.

Meites J. Short history of neuroendocrinology and the International Society of Neuroendocrinology. *Neuroendocrinology.* 1992;56:1–10.

Miller GE, Chen E. Harsh family climate in early life presages the emergence of a proinflammatory phenotype in adolescence. *Psychol Sci.* 2010;21:848–856.

Milner TA, McEwen BS, Hayashi S, Li CJ, Reagen L, Alves SE. Ultrastructural evidence that hippocampal alpha estrogen receptors are located at extranuclear sites. *J Comp Neurol.* 2001;429:355–371.

Moriceau S, Sullivan R. Maternal presence serves as a switch between learning fear and attraction in infancy. *Nature Neurosci.* 2006;8:1004–1006.

Murphy BEP. Treatment of major depression with steroid suppressive drugs. *J Steroid Biochem Mol Biol.* 1991;39:239–244.

Nasca C, Bigio B, Zelli D, Nicoletti F, McEwen BS. Mind the gap: glucocorticoids modulate hippocampal glutamate tone underlying individual differences in stress susceptibility. *Mol Psychiatry.* 2015;20:755–763.

Nishijima T, Piriz J, Duflot S, et al. Neuronal activity drives localized blood-brain-barrier transport of serum insulin-like growth factor-I into the CNS. *Neuron.* 2010;67:834–846.

Nyberg F. Growth hormone in the brain: characteristics of specific brain targets for the hormone and their functional significance. *Front Neuroendocrin.* 2000;21:330–348.

Obradovic J, Bush NR, Stamperdahl J, Adler NE, Boyce WT. Biological sensitivity to context: the interactive effects of stress reactivity and family adversity on socioemotional behavior and school readiness. *Child Dev.* 2010;81:270–289.

Ott A, Stolk RP, Hofman A, van Harskamp F, Grobbee DE, Breteler MMB. Association of diabetes mellitus and dementia: the Rotterdam study. *Diabetologia.* 1996;39:1392–1397.

Pan W, Yu Y, Cain CM, Nyberg F, Couraud PO, Kastin AJ. Permeation of growth hormone across the blood-brain barrier. *Endocrinology.* 2005;146:4898–4904.

Piroli GG, Grillo CA, Reznikov LR, et al. Corticosterone impairs insulin-stimulated translocation of GLUT4 in the rat hippocampus. *Neuroendocrinology* 2007;85:71–80.

Pitman RK. Hippocampal diminution in PTSD: more (or less?) than meets the eye. *Hippocampus.* 2001;11:73–74.

Pulford BE, Ishii DN. Uptake of circulating insulin-like growth factors (IGFs) into cerebrospinal fluid appears to be independent of the IGF receptors as well as IGF-binding proteins. *Endocrinology.* 2001;142:213–220.

Rasgon N, Jarvik GP, Jarvik L. Affective disorders and Alzheimer disease: a missing-link hypothesis. *Am J Geriatr Psychiatry.* 2001;9:444–445.

Rasgon N, Jarvik L. Insulin resistance, affective disorders, and Alzheimer's disease: review and hypothesis. *J Gerontol.* 2004;59A: 178–183.

Rasgon NL, Geist CL, Kenna HA, Wroolie TE, Williams KE, Silverman DH. Prospective randomized trial to assess effects of continuing hormone therapy on cerebral function in postmenopausal women at risk for dementia. *PLoS One.* 2014;9:e89095.

Rasgon NL, Kenna HA, Wroolie TE, et al. Insulin resistance and hippocampal volume in women at risk for Alzheimer's disease. *Neurobiol Aging.* 2011;32:1942–1948.

Rassi A, Veras AB, dos Reis M, et al. Prevalence of psychiatric disorders in patients with polycystic ovary syndrome. *Comp Psychiatry.* 2010;51:599–602.

Reagan LP, Magarinos AM, Yee DK, et al. Oxidative stress and HNE conjugation of GLUT3 are increased in the hippocampus of diabetic rats subjected to stress. *Brain Res.* 2000;862:292–300.

Repetti RL, Taylor SE, Seeman TE. Risky families: family social environments and the mental and physical health of offspirng. *Psychol Bull.* 2002;128:330–366.

Sachar EJ, Hellman L, Roffwarg HP, Halpern FS, Fukushima DK, Gallagher TF. Disrupted 24-hour patterns of cortisol secretion in psychotic depression. *Arch Gen Psychiatry.* 1973;28:19–24.

Sapolsky R. Stress, the aging brain and the mechanisms of neuron death. *Cambridge MIT Press.* 1992;1:423.

Sapolsky RM, Krey LC, McEwen BS. The neuroendocrinology of stress and aging: the glucocorticoid cascade hypothesis. *Endocr Rev.* 1986;7:284–301.

Saul AN, Oberyszyn TM, Daugherty C, et al. Chronic stress and susceptibility to skin cancer. *J Natl Cancer Inst.* 2005;97:1760–1767.

Schally AV, Arimura A, Kastin AJ. Hypothalamic regulatory hormones. *Science.* 1973;179:341–350.

Shansky RM, Hamo C, Hof PR, Lou W, McEwen BS, Morrison JH. Estrogen promotes stress sensitivity in a prefrontal cortex-amygdala pathway. *Cereb Cortex.* 2010;20:2560–2567.

Sheline YI. Neuroimaging studies of mood disorder effects on the brain. *Biol Psychiatry.* 2003;54:338–352.

Sheline YI, Gado MH, Price JL. Amygdala core nuclei volumes are decreased in recurrent major depression. *NeuroReport*. 1998;9:2023–2028.

Sheline YI, Sanghavi M, Mintun MA, Gado MH. Depression duration but not age predicts hippocampal volume loss in medically healthy women with recurrent major depression. *J Neurosci*. 1999;19:5034–5043.

Shonkoff JP, Boyce WT, McEwen BS. Neuroscience, molecular biology, and the childhood roots of health disparities. *JAMA*. 2009;301:2252–2259.

Sloan RP, McCreath H, Tracey KJ, Sidney S, Liu K, Seeman T. RR interval variability is inversely related to inflammatory markers: the CARDIA study. *Mol Med*. 2007;13:178–184.

Spinelli S, Schwandt ML, Lindell SG, et al. The serotonin transporter gene linked polymorphic region is associated with the behavioral response to repeated stress exposure in infant rhesus macaques. *Dev Psychopathol*. 2012;24:157–165.

Starkman MN, Gebarski SS, Berent S, Schteingart DE. Hippocampal formation volume, memory dysfunction, and cortisol levels in partiens with Cushing's syndrome. *Biol Psychiatry*. 1992;32:756–765.

Starkman MN, Schteingart DE. Neuropsychiatric manifestations of patients with Cushing's syndrome. *Arch Intern Med*. 1981;141:215–219.

Stemmle PG, Kenna HA, Wang PW, Hill SJ, Ketter TA, Rasgon NL. Insulin resistance and hyperlipidemia in women with bipolar disorder. *J Psychiatr Res*. 2009;43:341–343.

Sterling P, Eyer J. Allostasis: a new paradigm to explain arousal pathology. In: *Handbook of life stress, cognition and health*, ed. S Fisher, J Reason. New York: John Wiley & Sons; 1988:629–649.

Suomi SJ. Risk, resilience, and gene x environment interactions in rhesus monkeys. *Ann NY Acad Sci*. 2006;1094:52–62.

Suzuki A, Stern SA, Bozdagi O, et al. Astrocyte-neuron lactate transport is required for long-term memory formation. *Cell*. 2011;144:810–823.

Tang AC, Reeb-Sutherland BC, Romeo RD, McEwen BS. On the causes of early life experience effects: evaluating the role of Mom. *Front Neuroendocrinol*. 2014;35:245–251.

Taylor MJ, Rudkin L, Bullemor-Day P, Lubin J, Chukwujekwu C, Hawton K. Strategies for managing sexual dysfunction induced by antidepressant medication. *Cochrane Database Syst Rev*. 2013;5: CD003382.

Tomasdottir MO, Sigurdsson JA, Petursson H, et al. Self reported childhood difficulties, adult multimorbidity and allostatic load: a cross-sectional analysis of the Norwegian HUNT study. *PLoS One*. 2015;10:e0130591.

Tsilchorozidou T, Overton C, Conway GS. The pathophysiology of polycystic ovary syndrome. *Clin Endocrinol*. 2004;60:1–17.

Vale W, Spiess J, Rivier C, Rivier J. Characterization of a 41-residue ovine hypothalamic peptide that stimulates secretion of corticotropin and beta-endorphin. *Science*. 1981;213:1394–1397.

Vythilingam M, Heim C, Newport J, et al. Childhood trauma associated with smaller hippocampal volume in women with major depression. *Am J Psychiatry*. 2002;159:2072–2080.

Waddington CH. The epigenotype. *Endeavour*. 1942;1:18–20.

Wang J, Rao H, Wetmore GS, et al. Perfusion functional MRI reveals cerebral blood flow pattern under psychological stress. *Proc Natl Acad Sci USA*. 2005;102:17804–17809.

Winocur G, Greenwood CE. The effects of high fat diets and environment influences on cognitive performance in rats. *Behav Brain Res*. 1999;101:153–161.

Winocur G, Piroli GG, Grillo C, et al. Memory impairment in obese Zucker rats: an investigation of cognitive function in an animal model of insulin resistance and obesity. *Behav Neurosci.* 2005;119:1389–1395.

Wood GE, Norris EH, Waters E, Stoldt JT, McEwen BS. Chronic immobilization stress alters aspects of emotionality and associative learning in the rat. *Behav Neurosci.* 2008;122:282–292.

Yau PL, Castro MG, Tagani A, Tsui WH, Convit A. Obesity and metabolic syndrome and functional and structural brain impairments in adolescence. *Pediatrics.* 2012;130:e856–e864.

Yu Y, Kastin AJ, Pan W. Reciprocal interactions of insulin and insulin-like growth factor I in receptor-mediated transport across the blood-brain barrier. *Endocrinology.* 2006;147:2611–2615.

Zigman JM, Jones JE, Lee CE, Saper CB, Elmquist JK. Expression of ghrelin receptor mRNA in the rat and the mouse brain. *J Comp Neurol.* 2006;494:528–548.

3

Depression as a Recurrent, Progressive Illness
Need for Long-Term Prevention

Robert M. Post

INTRODUCTION

Depression is a recurrent, progressive illness, which tends to run a more difficult course with each new episode. This is the case for both unipolar major depression and for depressions occurring in the context of bipolar disorder (depressions along with hypomanic or manic episodes). Many different elements of these affective illnesses show evidence of illness progression, especially if the depressions are inadequately treated and prevented.

The aspects of recurrent depression that show evidence of illness progression include the following:

1. Episodes recur faster, with a shorter well-interval after each successive one;
2. Recurrent episodes require less precipitation by stressors (become more autonomous);
3. Medical and psychiatric comorbidities accumulate, including the likelihood of substance abuse;
4. Cognition deteriorates as a function of the number of previous episodes;
5. Prefrontal cortical neuroanatomical deficits increase;
6. Treatment refractoriness increases;
7. End-stage complications such as inadequate self-care and dementia may occur; and
8. Loss of one or more decades of life expectancy occurs, more from cardiovascular disease than from suicide.

There are two different types of mechanisms involved in these manifestations of illness progression. One is the nonspecific wear and tear that comes with inflammation, hypothalamic pituitary adrenal (HPA) overactivity, oxidative stress, and the like, which have already been introduced in the earlier chapters of Nestler and McEwen in this book and will be explicated in further detail in later chapters as well.

The second type of mechanism is more specific and is the major theme of this chapter. It is the increasing reactivity or sensitization that occurs upon recurrence of: depressive episodes (episode sensitization), stressors (stress sensitization), and bouts of substance abuse typified by stimulants such as cocaine (psychomotor stimulant-induced behavioral sensitization). Not only does each of these three types of sensitization show more pathological behavioral reactivity upon repetition, but each shows cross-sensitization to the other two, resulting in a positive feedback cycle and downward spiral of illness deterioration.

Each of these three types of sensitization necessarily has a memory component to it, since the increases in pathological behaviors upon recurrence of episodes, stressors, or bouts of substance abuse depend on some memory trace of the prior experience. As in normal memory, epigenetic mechanisms appear to be critical mediators of each type of sensitization, and blockade of epigenetic processes will inhibit each type of sensitization.

The therapeutic implications of these three types of sensitization that drive illness progression are clear and indicate the importance of preventing episodes, modulating stressors, and avoiding, or treating, substance abuse. This preventive therapeutic approach would have multiple benefits. It would minimize the sensitization and cross-sensitization effects driving illness progression and their associated epigenetic alterations. Hypothetically, it would also minimize the secondary or nonspecific effects of stressors, episodes, and abused substances on inflammation, glucocorticoids, and oxidative stress, as well as the neurochemical and neuroanatomical changes that emerge as a function of the number or duration of prior episodes.

The major theme of this volume and the evidence presented supporting it—that depression is a systemic disease—further enhance the imperative of employing consistent long-term prophylaxis to prevent recurrent depression and sensitization effects. However, this admonition about the necessity of long-term prevention of depressive episodes is neither universally taught nor adequately employed in clinical practice. Having a history of multiple prior depressive episodes not only places an individual at increased risk of more rapid recurrences, but is among the strongest predictors of treatment refractoriness and cognitive dysfunction. Thus, consistent, effective, long-term prophylaxis not only reduces clinical symptoms and dysfunction, but it helps prevent illness deterioration and the development of treatment refractoriness.

As such, this conception of illness progression and the processes driving it should reinforce the already existent guidelines of most academic and research organizations and societies. That is, after the experience of two or three prior episodes of unipolar depression, one should recommend lifelong prophylaxis with antidepressants, and after one or two prior episodes of bipolar disorder, lifelong pharmacological management with lithium, mood-stabilizing anticonvulsants, or atypical antipsychotics is also recommended. Similar recommendations about lifetime treatment for high blood pressure, cholesterol, or blood sugar are widely practiced and readily accepted, and treatment of recurrent depression and bipolar disorder should have the same type of cachet and support.

EPISODE AND STRESS SENSITIZATION

More than 100 years ago, Emil Kraepelin[1] described the fundamental elements of episode and stress sensitization. Successive recurrent episodes tended to occur faster; i.e., with a shorter well-interval. Initial episodes, he saw, were often precipitated by psychosocial stress, but with multiple recurrences, they became more sensitive to triggering by stressors, and in addition could begin to occur more autonomously with lesser amounts of stressors necessary (Figure 3.1). Kraepelin indicated that with further episodes, more minor stressors and then the mere anticipation of stressors might be sufficient to precipitate episodes, and then, ultimately, episodes would begin to occur spontaneously without any obvious triggers at all. The process of transition from to triggered to spontaneous episodes suggests what is now thought of as a type of learning or conditioning, and is modelled by kindling as discussed below.

Thus Kraepelin emphasized that the episodes tended to occur more rapidly (what we refer to as "episode sensitization") and become more sensitive to stressors where initial stress might be insufficient to trigger an episode, but with further stressors, episodes would occur more readily and regularly (stress sensitization) and then progress to the point that full-blown stressors were no longer required.

Over the past century, more systematic evidence in support of Kraepelin's observations has been forthcoming. Post[2] reviewed the clinical literature and found considerable support for both types of sensitization—episode acceleration and increased sensitivity to stressors. He also compared the process of evolution of multiple triggered episodes to those occurring spontaneously as analogous to what occurs in amygdala kindling, described by Goddard et al.[3] In kindling of the amygdala, initially subthreshold, once-daily electrical stimulation for 1 second eventually results in the development of full-blown major motor seizures, but with sufficient numbers of triggered seizures, seizures

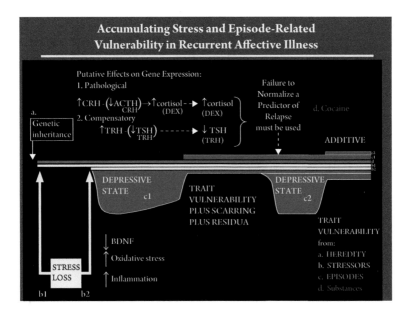

Figure 3.1 Constant Vulnerability from Genetic: Accumulating Vulnerability from Stressors, Mood Episodes, and Substance Abuse.

also begin to occur spontaneously without the need for any stimulation of the amygdala at all (Figure 3.2). The kindling model is a behaviorally and biochemically non-homologous one for the evolution of the recurrent affective disorders, but the phases of illness evolution bear some similarity to those seen in depression and bipolar disorder, particularly the early, increasing reactivity in kindling acquisition, the recurrent full-blown triggered episodes in mid-phase, and then the transition to spontaneous episodes.

Subsequent analyses and reviews have further supported propositions of both episode and stress sensitization. Kessing et al.[4,5] reviewed the enormous literature on episode acceleration as a function of the number of prior episodes for both unipolar and bipolar depression. Using new statistical methods, he found in 20,350 patients from the Danish Case Registry, that for "women with unipolar disorder and for all kinds of patients with bipolar disorder, the rate of recurrence was affected by the number of prior episodes even when the effect was adjusted for individual frailty toward recurrence."[5]

Kendler et al.[6,7] presented data in support of the kindling-like evolution of episodes from precipitated to spontaneous. He found that over the first five to seven episodes of depression, psychosocial stressors appeared to be involved in the triggering of depressions, but with more recurrences, there was less involvement of stressors.

Slavich et al.[8] found a similar progression from triggered to spontaneous, with the transition happening after about five episodes. Stroud et al.[9] and Treadway et al.[10] also have data consistent with sensitization model and the effects of a greater number of episodes on anatomical changes in hippocampus and prefrontal cortex, as reviewed by Post et al.[11]

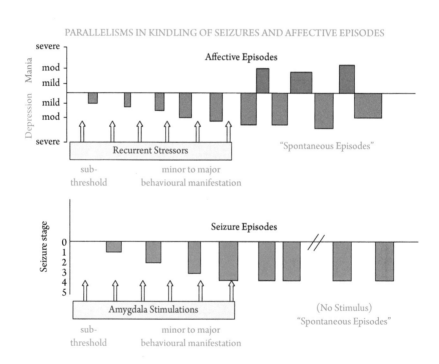

Figure 3.2 Episode Progression in the Mood Disorders vs Kindling of Amygdala Seizures.

Early life adversity may sensitize the individual to later stressors in adulthood precipitating a full-blown depression, while those without the childhood stressors do not appear as vulnerable to the stressors later in life.[12–14] The literature suggests that there also may be gene–environmental interactions; for example, those with the short form of the serotonin transporter may be particularly susceptible.[12,13]

STRESSOR SENSITIZATION AND ACCUMULATION IN BIPOLAR DISORDER

In bipolar disorder, there appear to be both stress sensitization and stressor accumulation. With sufficient numbers of triggered recurrent episodes, the progression to spontaneity is readily apparent. Many patients begin to cycle with increasing rapidity through several stages.[15] "Rapid cycling" is usually quantified as four or more episodes/year; "ultra-rapid cycling" as four or more episodes/month; and "ultra-ultra rapid (or ultradian) cycling" as multiple switches between depression and mania within a single day on four or more days/week. With these latter kinds of ultra-rapid recurrences, it is difficult to conceptualize that stresses would be driving these increasingly rapid and chaotic mood and behavioral fluctuations. In addition to this conventional view of stress sensitization progressing to autonomy, there also appears to be stressor accumulation in patients with bipolar disorder.

Those with adversity in childhood (verbal, physical, or sexual abuse) have an earlier onset of their bipolar disorder than those without these stressors.[16,17] In addition, those who experience stressors early in life experience more stressors both in the year prior to the first and prior to the latest episode experienced prior to their network entry at average age 40.[18]

PRECLINICAL MODELS OF SENSITIZATION TO MOOD EPISODES, STRESSORS, AND SUBSTANCES OF ABUSE: EPIGENETIC MECHANISMS

As described by Nestler, one of the better models of depression is that induced by defeat stress.[19,20] Interestingly, it takes several exposures to the larger, more aggressive animal before the full range of depressive-like behaviors in the rodent becomes manifest. These anxiety-like behaviors, social avoidance, and endocrine and neurochemical abnormalities emerge after repeated experiences and are accompanied by decreases in brain-derived neurotrophic factor (BDNF) in the hippocampus and increases in BDNF in the nucleus accumbens.[21,22] If either of these opposing changes in BDNF is prevented, the depressive-like behaviors do not occur. As described by Nestler et al., these changes in BDNF appear to be a byproduct of a multitude of environmentally induced epigenetic changes.

Epigenetic changes involve chemical modifications such as DNA methylation, histone acetylation and methylation, and micro-RNA (miRNA), which do not affect inherited gene sequences, but alter the ease in which genes are turned on or off. Typically, although not uniformly, DNA and histone methylation are repressive, while histone acetylation activates gene expression. There is great complexity to these effects, and DNA and histone modification interact with each other and a multitude of transcription factors. Some of these changes (epigenetic marks) are malleable, and others are lasting and lifelong.

Roth et al.[23] found that neonatal adversity in the first 10 days of a rat pup's life decreased BDNF in its prefrontal cortex and altered its behavior in a lifelong fashion. This was associated with methylation of the promoter for BDNF, and if this methylation was inhibited by the methyl transferase inhibitor zebularine, the BDNF decrements and behavioral alterations did not occur.

Similarly, cocaine-induced behavioral sensitization (which involves increases in motor activity and stereotypy in response to repetition of the same dose[24] and often involves a conditioned or context-dependent component) is associated with increases in BDNF in the nucleus accumbens, and sensitization is also prevented by the administration of zebularine.[25] Thus, there appears to be an epigenetic-based memory-like component to each type of sensitization, and the increases in BDNF in the accumbens and decreases in BDNF in the hippocampus in each type suggest some overlapping or potential mechanisms in common. Moreover, Krishnan et al.[26] reported that in autopsy specimens, individuals dying with a depression diagnosis also showed the same increases in BDNF in the nucleus accumbens and decreases in BDNF in the hippocampus compared to controls, further suggesting homology with changes in the defeat stress model of depression.

Besides the BDNF changes, which are necessary and sufficient to produce depressive-like behavior in the defeat stress model,[21,22] Hodes et al.[27] have shown that interleukin-6 (Il-6) produced from white blood cells is a critical component. If Il-6 production or actions are blocked, the depressive behaviors of defeat stress do not occur, presenting the possibility that depressive proclivity could reside not only in the mind, but also in one's lymphocytes. If blocking Il-6 and other inflammatory cytokines, such as tumor necrosis factor alpha (TNF-alpha),[28,29] in human depression proves to be therapeutically valuable, this would further help clinch depression as a systemic illness not only in its consequences, but also as part of its etiology.

BASIC SCIENCE AND CLINICAL EVIDENCE OF CROSS-SENSITIZATION

Early on, Antelman[30] showed that stress-sensitized animals show increased reactivity to stimulants and vice versa, suggesting cross-sensitization by acute stressors and stimulants. Both animals and humans who experience stressful experiences early in life are also more prone to develop and sustain stimulant self-administration and addiction.[31-33] Affective episodes and stimulant use also appear to engender new stressors, and stressors can precipitate the occurrence of new mood episodes as well as relapses to substance abuse, further suggesting a potential positive feedback cycle of progressive and accelerating dyscontrol of all three types of sensitization[24] (Figure 3.3).

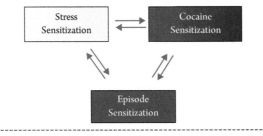

Repetition of each Increases Responsivity to Itself and the Two Others

Figure 3.3 Sensitization and Cross Sensitization to Stress, Mood Episodes, and Bouts of Substance Abuse in the Recurrent Affective Disorders.

N-ACETYLCYSTEINE: EFFECTIVE IN DEPRESSION AND MULTIPLE HABITS AND ADDICTIONS

Not only does the phenomenon of cross-sensitization among stressors, episodes, and bouts of substance abuse suggest some neurobiological mechanisms in common (such as the BDNF changes), it also suggests that some drugs could have therapeutic effects in each type of sensitization. Double-blind placebo-controlled data support the view that N-acetylcysteine (NAC) has therapeutic value in depressed patients[34,35] and in a variety of substance abuse disorders, including cocaine, alcohol, and marijuana in adolescents.[24,36] Kalivas and associates[37] found that cocaine reinstatement in rodents was associated with marked increase in glutamate in the nucleus accumbens upon a signal that cocaine might again be available. He reasoned that if this increase in excitatory neurotransmitter signal could be inhibited, cocaine reinstatement would be lessened, and this is what he found. NAC increases the number of glial glutamate transporters that help clear synaptic glutamate. The data on cocaine in rodents inspired clinical trials in humans, and NAC proved helpful in this and many other clinical conditions and addictions, as summarized in Box 3.1.

What many of the conditions in Box 3.1 have in common is an apparent over-active habit memory system (which is unconscious and encoded in the striatum) as opposed to the conscious representational memory system (encoded in the medial temporal lobe—amygdala and hippocampus).[38] In this fashion, it could be considered that defeat stressed animals and depressed patients over-learn depressive responses to stress, and addicted individuals over-learn and increase their responsiveness to and craving for drugs of abuse, as suggested by the increases in BDNF in the nucleus accumbens in each instance.

NAC not only decreases the magnitude of synaptic glutamate in the accumbens, but it reverses many of the cocaine-induced physiological and neuroanatomical changes. NAC reverses the cocaine-related loss of long term potentiation (LTP) and long term depression (LTD) in the cortex–accumbens pathway and restores the normal size of dendritic spines on the accumbens medium spiny neurons.

Box 3.1 N-Acetylcysteine (NAC)**: Positive effects on mood, addictions, and compulsions—Is this related to dampening of glutamate signaling in the striatal habit memory system?

I. Affective and Cognitive Symptoms
   A. Bipolar depression[34]
   B. Unipolar depression[104]
   C. Schizophrenia, especially negative symptoms[35]
   D. Autism (stereotypy and irritability; adjunctive risperidone)[105–107 (a)]
II. Addictions
   A. Cocaine craving[108–110]
   B. Amphetamine craving[111]
   C. Gambling urges[112,113]
   D. Marijuana[114] (Gray 2012)
   E. Nicotine[113,115,116 (b)]
III. Compulsions
   A. Trichotillomania[117]
   B. Obsessive-compulsive disorder (OCD) (as an adjunct to SSRI), especially obsessive symptoms[118 108]

** NAC: Placebo controlled trials; typical maximum doses: 500 mg capsules, two caps twice daily
(a) To 2700 mg/day
(b) Mayo Clinic used 2500 mg/day

NAC is the therapeutic ingredient in Mucomyst, used for acetaminophen (Tylenol) overdoses, as it is an antioxidant and glutathione precursor. NAC in 500 mg and 600 mg capsules can be bought over the counter in health food stores, and because of its broad spectrum of clinical effects in many syndromes involving pathological increases in the striatal habit memory system and its safety, it is highly recommended for current clinical use.

FUTURE EPIGENETIC TARGETED THERAPEUTICS

In contrast, the epigenetic-driven mechanisms of each type of sensitization may ultimately be amenable to direct manipulation with drugs targeting these changes, but so far, only valproate, a histone deacetylase inhibitor, is available in this category of drugs. Valproate's effects in addictions are not well studied, although it is clearly effective in mania. It is also reported to enhance to extinction learning by specifically increasing a BDNF promoter subtype involved in extinction learning.[39] Drugs targeting different aspects of epigenetic procession are already being used in the therapy of some cancers where the idea is not to kill pathological cells, but to return them to more normal functioning. The hope would be that more direct reversal of some of the epigenetic changes underlying stress, episode, and cocaine-induced sensitization would lead to more durable and perhaps permanent reversal of some of the vulnerability to the syndromes associated with sensitization.

A direct epigenetic approach could be of considerable clinical value, as current therapies of unipolar depression require ongoing antidepressant (AD) administration to maintain long-term response.[40] ADs reduce the rate of relapse into a new episode by about 75% compared to placebo, the statistical significance of which is astronomical.[41] If first-generation tricyclic antidepressants or second-generation antidepressants are discontinued, relapses occur at a high rate with placebo substitution.[40-43] About 50% of patients relapse in the first year off ADs; about 75% by the second year off; and about 85% by the third year off.[15]

This need for sustained treatment would make sense from the data in the defeat stress model where defeat stress is associated with a trimethylation of histone H3K27 suppressing BDNF in the hippocampus, but ADs that reverse the defeat stress behaviors and the BDNF decreases (by other pathways), do not reverse the H3K27me3 mark, which appears to mediate the underlying vulnerability to depression.[26] If related epigenetic depression-vulnerability markers in humans were found and directly reversed, one might ultimately have a situation more akin to a cure where continuous treatment would not be necessary. Obviously, this futuristic view would necessarily be based on the assumption that the vulnerability was based on environmentally mediated and not genetically induced alterations.

MORE PSYCHIATRIC ILLNESS IN OFFSPRING AND PROGENITORS OF BIPOLAR PATIENTS FROM THE U.S. THAN EUROPE

The view that sensitization and cross-sensitization to stressors, mood episodes, and bouts of substance abuse can all drive illness progression in the recurrent affective disorders provides a unique perspective on circumstances in the United States compared to the Netherlands and Germany (abbreviated here as "Europe"). Each type of sensitization appears more common and more virulent in the U.S. than in Europe.[18] Compared to bipolar patients from Europe, those from the U.S. experience more stressors in childhood, at illness onset, and before the latest episode[16]; more episodes and rapid cycling; and more alcohol and substance abuse. In addition they also have more of two other poor prognosis factors—early onset of their bipolar disorder and an anxiety disorder comorbidity[44] (Table 3.1).

While these factors probably have an epigenetic basis, those from the U.S. also are associated with more genetic/familial vulnerability.[17,18] The U.S. patients' parents and grandparents also have more illness in the form of depression, bipolar disorder, suicide attempts, alcohol and substance abuse, and "other" illness compared to those of the Europeans (Table 3.2). Familial loading for psychiatric illness is related to early onset bipolar disorder[45,46] and to greater amounts of illness in the patient's offspring.[47] Compared to the Europeans, the offspring of U.S. patients with bipolar illness also have more depression, bipolar disorder, suicide attempts, substance abuse, and "other" illness,

Table 3.1 United States vs. Europe: Illness and Adversity

MORE ILLNESS, ADVERSITY IN THE U.S. THAN IN EUROPE

	US (N = 676)	EUROPE (N = 292)
ANXIETY DISORDER	46.6%	28.1%
ALCOHOL ABUSE	33.1%	14.7%
SUBSTANCE ABUSE	38.3%	17.8%
RAPID CYCLING	74.1%	41.5%
>20 EPISODES	59.0%	23.3%
Hospitalizations	Fewer	More
PROSPECTIVE		
NON-RESPONDERS	51.7%	31.1%

indicating that four generations of those from the U.S. have more illness than those from Europe.[47]

A COHORT EFFECT DRIVING EARLIER AGES OF ONSET OF DEPRESSIVE DISORDERS

In addition to the increased risk for childhood-onset mood and behavioral disorders based on greater genetic and psychosocial stress vulnerability factors, another largely unrecognized trend is driving an increased incidence and an earlier age of onset of both depression and bipolar disorder, what is referred to as a "secular time trend," a cohort or generational effect. Considerable evidence supports the proposition that each birth cohort since the early 1900s has had an earlier age of onset of these two mood

Table 3.2 Four Generations of Those from the United States with More Illness Than Those from The Netherlands and Germany

	IV.	III.	II.		I.
	Great-grandparents	Grandparents	Patients with bipolar disorder	Spouses	Offspring
Depression	***	***	N.A.	***	***
Bipolar	***	***	N.A.	—	***
Suicide attempt	**	**	***	*	ns
Alcohol	**	*	***	—	**
Drugs	*	*	**	—	***
"Other"	***	**	((***))	***	***

* = p < . 05; ** = p < .01; *** = p < .001 more of this illness in the U.S. than in Europe; N.A. = not applicable; ns = not significant; (( )) = an anxiety disorder comorbidity.
Compared to Europeans, patients with bipolar disorder (II) from the U.S. also had more poor prognosis factors, including more numerous onsets of bipolar disorder in childhood; abuse in childhood; 20 or more episodes; rapid cycling; and treatment refractoriness (all p < .001).

disorders.[48-51] In addition, there appears to be a cohort effect for attention-deficit hyper-activity disorder (ADHD) and substance abuse disorders. There may also be a generational effect for childhood adversity, such that multiple genetic and environmental factors are combining to drive several mood and behavioral disorders to onsets earlier in children's lives.

The epigenetic effects based on maternal or paternal behavior are now well described and accepted.[23,52-55] However, new data indicate that effects of some parental experiences can also be transmitted transgenerationally in the absence of behavioral contact with the parent. The phenomenon is best demonstrated in the offspring of male rats who experience stressors or substances of abuse during their adulthood and then mate with a naïve female, but have no contact with the rat pups.[56-64] Yet the rat pups retain some behavioral alterations based on the paternal stressors or exposure to drugs. The effects have been documented based on epigenetic marks carried in sperm and include alterations in DNA methylation, histone modifications, and microRNA.[65] These data, to the extent they are further validated in humans, suggest transgenerational transmission of vulnerability to illness based on three mechanisms: genetics, traditional epigenetics, and epigenetic effects carried in the sexual gametes. The relative contribution of the latter epigenetic effects is not likely to be as great as that from genetics and traditional epigenetics.

THE DOUBLE LIABILITY OF EARLY ONSET MOOD DISORDERS

This greater illness burden in the United States is largely unrecognized and under-appreciated, but it has enormous implications for clinical therapeutics and health care policy. Early onset of both depression and bipolar illness runs a more difficult course[66,67] than adult onset illness and is associated with much longer delay to first treatment.[67] Delay to first treatment is itself a poor prognosis factor and is associated with more time and severity of depression as an adult.[67] In the United States, more than one quarter of patients had onset of illness before age 13, and two thirds before age 19.[18,66] This contrasts with the Europeans, where only one third had onsets before age 19.

Thus, in the United States, bipolar disorder in well-diagnosed adults is an illness of childhood and adolescent onset, and those with childhood onsets fare even more poorly than those with adolescent onsets.[67,68] Early onset illness is more likely to be associated with two other poor-prognosis factors—an anxiety disorder comorbidity and a substance abuse disorder—as well as more mood episodes, rapid cycling, suicide attempts, and treatment refractoriness as an adult (Figure 3.4).

Geller et al.[69,70] followed those with childhood onsets of their bipolar disorder for eight years and found that than they remained ill some two-thirds of the time, but also that some 37% of the patients never received any of the consensus-recommended treatments for bipolar disorder, such as lithium, an anticonvulsant mood stabilizer (such as valproate or carbamazepine), or an atypical antipsychotic. Those who did receive lithium did best and had more time in remission. These data suggest that earlier and more effective intervention might have yielded a more benign course of illness.

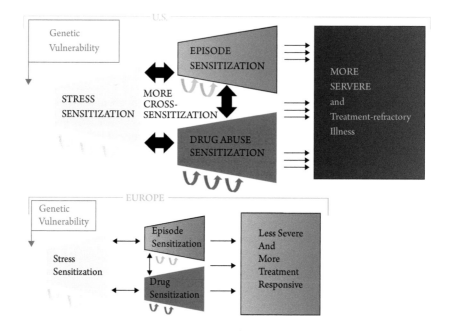

Fig 3.4 Early onset mood disorders in the US vs in Europe.

EARLY MULTIMODAL INTERVENTION CHANGES THE COURSE OF BIPOLAR DISORDER

The assumption based on the Geller et al.[70] study about more effective treatment intervention being associated with a less severe course of illness, has now been documented in a controlled clinical trial. Kessing et al.[71] randomized patients in Denmark with a first hospitalization for mania to two years either in a specialty clinic with multimodal treatment, or treatment as usual (TAU). Those who received the clinic treatment (which included psychotherapy, pharmacotherapy, illness education, and symptom monitoring and recognition) had many fewer relapses than those in TAU. After the two years were over, all returned to TAU, but over the next four years, the patients who had been previously randomized to specialty clinics continued to do well, while those who had had TAU from the outset continued to deteriorate and relapse at a much higher rate.

These data of Kessing et al.[71] make it eminently clear that early, excellent treatment can change the long-term course of illness from a severe relapsing one into a much more benign one. The same would appear to very much be the case for recurrent unipolar disorder, but such a randomized trial has not as yet been conducted. The health care situation in the United States is not currently geared to routinely make this type of intervention described by Kessing et al. widely available, and it is leaving successive generations of U.S. patients at high risk of a poor long-term outcome and multiple difficulties that are associated with poorly treated illness (Figure 3.5). These include dysfunction and disability, social and educational deficiency, medical and psychiatric comorbidities, cognitive

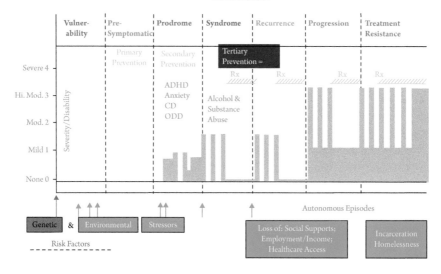

Figure 3.5 Greater Genetic and Environmental (Epigenetic) Vulnerability in the United States than in the Netherlands and Germany.

dysfunction, and early demise and loss of years of a decade or two of life expectancy, more from cardiovascular disease than from suicide.[72,73]

Cognitive dysfunction as a function of the number of previous episodes deserves special recognition. Kessing and Anderson[74] showed that the experience of two either unipolar or bipolar depressions was associated with the general population rate of dementia in older individuals. However, the occurrence of four episodes resulted in a doubling of the rate of dementia in old age. Other data indicate that depression is also one of the major risk factors for mild cognitive impairment (MCI) progressing to full-blown Alzheimer's disease. These data together provide further evidence of depression interacting with the progression of neurological dysfunction, and also suggest the importance of making this information more widely known to patients and the medical community in further supporting the recommendations for long-term prophylaxis of the mood disorders.

There are some suggestive data that lithium could decrease the incidence of dementia in old age,[74-76] or that even in small doses (150 mg/day), it could slow the decline in MCI over a one-year study compared to placebo.[76] Lithium increases BDNF and B-cell lymphoma 2 (BCL-2) and hippocampal and cortical volume, as well as directly increasing telomere length via its increases in telomerase activity.[77]

OFFSPRING OF PATIENTS WITH MOOD DISORDERS ARE AT HIGH RISK FOR MANY PSYCHIATRIC ILLNESSES

The recent data of Axelson et al.[78] crystalize the problem of risk of illness to the offspring of a bipolar parent. Upon a 6.7-year follow up, 74% of the offspring received a major psychiatric diagnosis of at least one of the common illnesses of childhood. About 20% were diagnosed with a bipolar spectrum disorder, but even more with anxiety, depression, ADHD, disruptive behavioral disorder, or a substance abuse disorder. Moreover, 80% of the offspring of a parent with unipolar depression upon 20-year follow-up received a similar range of psychiatric diagnoses.[79]

These data, replicated in the meta-analysis of Rasic et al.,[80] indicate that increased illness awareness and recognition in the offspring of a parent with a mood disorder, especially in the United States, is a good place to start in attempting to reverse some of the trend for poor illness-recognition and delayed or inadequate treatment. Having primary care physicians and adult psychiatrists ask all parents with a mood disorder about how their children are faring is indicated. Parents can help physicians with early recognition by joining the Child Network, which allows them to rate their child's symptoms of depression, anxiety, ADHD, oppositional behavior, and mania on a weekly basis on a secure website. Finding informed consent information and joining the Network can be done at www.bipolarnews.org (click on *Child Network*). The ratings can be printed out longitudinally for easy recognition of symptom course, need for treatment, and effectiveness of any given. Physicians actively asking for such a record would also enhance participation and access to the type of information about multiple common childhood disorders beyond depression and bipolar disorder, such as anxiety disorder, ADHD, and oppositional syndromes such as oppositional defiant disorder and disruptive mood disorder.

Effective treatment of a mother with a depressive disorder has also been shown to reduce the likelihood that her offspring will develop a psychiatric illness. Wickramaratne et al.[81] found that the mothers whose depression was treated to remission had children with fewer psychiatric problems than those who were treated but whose depression did not remit. So attention to the treatment of depression in the whole family unit is also of considerable import.

EARLY INTERVENTIONS: PSYCHOTHERAPY AND PHARMACOTHERAPY

Such a screening and longitudinal follow-up device as the Child Network can help with illness recognition in very young children (aged 2–12), so that evaluation and treatment can proceed as necessary, either directly by the physician or upon referral. Psychotherapeutic intervention is highly effective for many early syndromes. Miklowitz et al.[82] reported that children randomized to family-focused treatment (FFT), which emphasizes illness education and enhanced communication within the family, was much more effective than TAU for children with depression, bipolar-not otherwise specified (BP-NOS), or cyclothymia who had a family member with bipolar disorder. Fristad et al.[83] report similarly good results with their multi-family oriented therapy, as do West et al.[84] with their RAINBOW therapy, and the preventive effect of psychotherapy for anxiety disorders in children at high risk[85] is well documented.

EFFECT OF CHILDHOOD TOXIC STRESS
ON MEDICAL AND PSYCHIATRIC ILLNESS
IN ADULTHOOD

Shonkoff and Gardner[86] make the case that pediatricians and other primary care providers (PCPs) should become the guardians of children's medical and psychiatric health. They review the data of Filleti et al.[87] and Anda et al.[88] that childhood adversity is a major cause of poor medical health in adulthood. Childhood adversity seen in a general medical practice is associated with obesity, cancer, stroke, chronic obstructive pulmonary disorder (COPD), diabetes, fractures, hepatitis, asthma, headaches, pulmonary disease, and autoimmune disorders, in addition to overall worse health, functional disability, increased numbers of doctors' office visits, obstetrical and gynecological problems, somatization, and premature mortality.

Similarly, in our cohort of patients with bipolar disorder, a history of childhood adversity was associated not only with an earlier onset and more adverse course of bipolar disorder, but with a great many medical conditions as well.[16,17,89] The total childhood adversity score was related to the total number of medical comorbidities a patient had, as well as an increased incidence of 11 specific medical conditions. These included asthma, arthritis, allergies, chronic fatigue syndrome, chronic menstrual irregularities, fibromyalgia, head injury (without loss of consciousness), hypertension, hypotension, irritable bowel syndrome, and migraine headaches.

Consistent with our findings of a greater amount of psychosocial adversity in childhood in bipolar patients from the United States compared to Europe, multiple medical conditions were also more prevalent in the U.S. than Europe.[45] These included significantly more allergies, arthritis, asthma, fibromyalgia, head injury (without loss of consciousness), hyperglycemia, irritable bowel syndrome, migraine headaches, and seizures. There was a striking doubling of the rate of obesity in the United States (33.2%) vs. Europe (15.4%), while the rate of overweight was quite similar (30.3% vs. 33.3%).[89]

While one might wonder about the poor mental health of children in the United States compared to Germany or the Netherlands, it should be noted that this situation is not exclusive to children's health, but may extend to adult health in general as well. Banks et al.[90] reported that American white males over age 55 were much sicker over a vast number of medical illnesses than those from the British Isles, even after smoking status, weight, socioeconomic status, and health care access were accounted for. They concluded that the Americans were sicker than the British. We conclude that children from the United States are at high risk for psychiatric illness, and that this deserves serious attempts at better intervention and prevention.

CHILDHOOD ONSET BIPOLAR DISORDER IS
ALREADY ASSOCIATED WITH MEDICAL PROBLEMS

Our data on excess medical illness in adult patients from the United States compared to Europe converge with the prospective data of Jerrell et al.[91] that even young children with bipolar illness (aged 13–17) already have a variety of medical comorbidities, many of which would put them a high risk for subsequent cardiovascular disorder. These included obesity, type II diabetes, dyslipidemia, endocrine disorder, organic brain disorder, migraine, epilepsy, asthma, and even early cardiovascular disease.

These data were further supplemented by Goldstein et al.,[92] who found evidence of vascular endothelial cell wall abnormalities in youngsters with bipolar disorder. Goldstein and Young[93] reviewed the literature indicating considerable support for multiple correlates of cardiovascular disease, including decreases in BDNF and increases in inflammatory marker such as Il-1, Il-6, TNF-alpha, and corticotropin releasing hormone (CRH). They also found evidence of increases in Il-6 and CRP that correlated with the degree of patient's cognitive impairment.[94]

Shonkoff and Gardner[86] not only link childhood adversity (abuse and neglect, what they label as "toxic stress") to the diverse medical problems in adulthood noted here, but also depression, learning and behavioral disorders, and poor mental well-being. The common element of toxic stress in childhood setting off both depression and a vast array of medical disorders further makes the case for the systematic interrelationships of depression and a wide array of systemic illnesses.

STRESS AND DEPRESSIVE EPISODES SHORTEN TELOMERES

In addition to the multiple endocrine, inflammatory, neurotrophic factor, and oxidative stress pathways as potential mediators of this link, effects of childhood stress on telomere length deserve special attention.[95,96] An increased percentage of short telomeres is associated with a large variety of medical and psychiatric illnesses, as well as premature aging. An increased number of depressive episodes has also been associated with telomere shortening,[97,98] suggesting another potential mechanism for illness progression, medical comorbidities, and premature loss of life expectancy.

While toxic stress, implacable anger, and mood episodes are associated with telomere shortening, a good diet, exercise, mindfulness/meditation, and a positive and altruistic outlook on life are associated with preserved telomere length. As noted, lithium also directly increases telomere length by increasing telomerase activity.[77] Hudziak et al.[99] recommend universal teaching of music, mindfulness, and exercise, each of which has been shown to increase children's gray or white matter brain development. He recommends these for all school children, and then enhanced use of these and related techniques in those at high risk for illness and in those who are already symptomatic.

PRESCRIBE WELLNESS; TREAT AND REFER THOSE WITH PRODROMAL SYMPTOMS OR FULL-BLOWN ILLNESS

Recommending a good diet, a regimen of exercise and good sleep hygiene, and mindfulness for parents to instill in their young children may be a good place to start for any

Table 3.3 Study Preventive Strategies for Those at Very High Risk as a Function of the Risks of the Treatment Intervention

Prevention Types I, II, III:

I Primary	II Secondary	III Tertiary
Good Diet	Psychotherapy	Lithium (Li)
Exercise	N-acetylcysteine	Li + VPA
Omega-3-	Omega-3	+LTG
Fatty Acids	Fatty Acids	+OXC/CBZ
Mindfulness	Minocycline	AA ± CBZ
----------	E-M power	VPA
NO RISK	----------	OXC/CBZ
	LOW RISK Rx	LTG

		HIGHER RISK Rx

Rx = treatment; VPA = valproic acid; LTG = lamotrigine; OXC = oxcarbmazepine; CBZ = carbamazepine.

child, and particularly for one at high risk because their parent has a mood disorder. After psychotherapy, safe and well-tolerated interventions have priority over stronger evidence-based medicines for very young children with difficult mood and behavioral symptoms (Table 3.3). Thus, although only a modicum of data support their use in children, one might consider omega-3-fatty acids,[100] n-acetylcysteine, vitamin D_3, and the like in relationship to their benign side-effect profiles.[101]

With more major illness, more conventional agents may need to be explored, including antidepressants for unipolar depression, and mood stabilizers (lithium, lamotrigine, valproate, and carbamazepine) and atypical antipsychotics for bipolar disorder.[70,102] Treating these full-syndrome illnesses early and well may prevent the adverse prognosis that typically is associated with childhood compared to adult onset depression and bipolar disorder.[66,67]

DIFFERENTIATING ADHD FROM BIPOLAR DISORDER

For pediatricians and PCPs, making the distinction between the very common syndrome of ADHD and the less common and less appreciated bipolar disorder in young children is of considerable import, as the two syndromes very often co-occur in very young children and require different therapeutics. ADHD responds well to stimulants, but bipolar disorder in the context of comorbid ADHD requires mood stabilization first, and then small doses of stimulants for whatever residual ADHD symptoms may remain. Tips that the presentation may be one of bipolar disorder include the presence of decreased need for sleep, inappropriate mood elevation and euphoria, severe aggression, homicidal or suicidal ideation, hypersexuality, and evidence of psychosis such as hallucinations or delusions, as well as an overall more severe and complex symptom presentation.[103]

CHANGING THE PERNICIOUS COURSE OF MOOD DISORDERS WITH EARLY INTERVENTION

Pediatricians, internists, and PCPs have changed the course of diabetes in youngsters and adults with comprehensive care and better self- and provider-monitoring, yielding much healthier lives and greater longevity. Such an outcome is within the grasp of those with depression and bipolar disorder, but it will take the same kind of concerted, lifelong, multimodal health care as is given to diabetics. Monitoring one's mood and behavior (at www.bipolarnews.org [click on *Child Network*] or MyMoodMonitor; WhatsMyM3), as well as inflammatory markers and other predictors of clinical responsiveness, should become as routine as measuring one's glucose, blood pressure, or cholesterol.

Appreciating depression and bipolar disorder as recurrent, potentially progressive illnesses intimately intertwined with systemic abnormalities and medical comorbidities as revealed in this volume should help change the approaches to these psychiatric illnesses in the direction of earlier and more concerted intervention and prevention. These recurrent mood disorders are not "mental" illnesses in the older, pejorative conceptualization of being ephemeral, evanescent, abstract, unreal, "all in one's mind or imagination," but are medical illness of brain and body needing great respect for their potentially serious and lethal consequences.

REFERENCES

1. Kraepelin E. *Manic-depressive insanity and paranoia.* Edinburgh, UK: Livingstone; 1921.
2. Post RM. Transduction of psychosocial stress into the neurobiology of recurrent affective disorder. *Am J Psychiatry.* Aug 1992;149(8):999–1010.
3. Goddard GV, McIntyre DC, Leech CK. A permanent change in brain function resulting from daily electrical stimulation. *Exper Neurol.* Nov 1969;25(3):295–330.
4. Kessing LV, Mortensen PB, Bolwig TG. Clinical definitions of sensitisation in affective disorder: a case register study of prevalence and prediction. *J Affect Disord.* Jan 1998;47(1–3):31–39.
5. Kessing LV, Olsen EW, Andersen PK. Recurrence in affective disorder: analyses with frailty models. *Am J Epidemiol.* Mar 1 1999;149(5):404–411.
6. Kendler KS, Thornton LM, Gardner CO. Stressful life events and previous episodes in the etiology of major depression in women: an evaluation of the "kindling" hypothesis. *Am J Psychiatry.* Aug 2000;157(8):1243–1251.
7. Kendler KS, Thornton LM, Gardner CO. Genetic risk, number of previous depressive episodes, and stressful life events in predicting onset of major depression. *Am J Psychiatry.* Apr 2001;158(4):582–586.
8. Slavich GM, Monroe SM, Gotlib IH. Early parental loss and depression history: associations with recent life stress in major depressive disorder. *J Psychiatr Res.* Sep 2011;45(9):1146–1152.
9. Stroud CB, Davila J, Hammen C, Vrshek-Schallhorn S. Severe and nonsevere events in first onsets versus recurrences of depression: evidence for stress sensitization. *J Abnorm Psychol.* Feb 2011;120(1):142–154.
10. Treadway MT, Waskom ML, Dillon DG, et al. Illness progression, recent stress, and morphometry of hippocampal subfields and medial prefrontal cortex in major depression. *Biol Psychiatry.* Feb 1 2015;77(3):285–294.

11. Post RM, Fleming J, Kapczinski F. Neurobiological correlates of illness progression in the recurrent affective disorders. *J Psychiatr Res.* May 2012;46(5):561–573.
12. Caspi A, Sugden K, Moffitt TE, et al. Influence of life stress on depression: moderation by a polymorphism in the 5-HTT gene. *Science.* Jul 18 2003;301(5631):386–389.
13. Risch N, Herrell R, Lehner T, et al. Interaction between the serotonin transporter gene (5-HTTLPR), stressful life events, and risk of depression: a meta-analysis. *JAMA.* Jun 17 2009;301(23):2462–2471.
14. Rutter M. Biological implications of gene-environment interaction. *J Abnorm Child Psych.* Oct 2008;36(7):969–975.
15. Post RM, Leverich GS. *Treatment of bipolar illness: a casebook for clinicians and patients.* New York: Norton; 2008.
16. Post RM, Altshuler L, Leverich G, et al. More stressors prior to and during the course of bipolar illness in patients from the United States compared with the Netherlands and Germany. *Psychiatry Res.* Dec 30 2013;210(3):880–886.
17. Post RM, Altshuler LL, Kupka R, et al. Verbal abuse, like physical and sexual abuse, in childhood is associated with an earlier onset and more difficult course of bipolar disorder. *Bipolar Disord.* May 2015;17(3):323–330.
18. Post RM, Leverich GS, Kupka R, et al. Increased parental history of bipolar disorder in the United States: association with early age of onset. *Acta Psychiatr Scand.* May 2014;129(5):375–382.
19. Covington HE 3rd, Miczek KA. Intense cocaine self-administration after episodic social defeat stress, but not after aggressive behavior: dissociation from corticosterone activation. *Psychopharmacology.* Dec 2005;183(3):331–340.
20. Miczek KA. Aggressive and social stress responses in genetically modified mice: from horizontal to vertical strategy. *Psychopharmacology.* Nov 1999;147(1):17–19.
21. Tsankova NM, Berton O, Renthal W, Kumar A, Neve RL, Nestler EJ. Sustained hippocampal chromatin regulation in a mouse model of depression and antidepressant action. *Nat Neurosci.* Apr 2006;9(4):519–525.
22. Berton O, McClung CA, Dileone RJ, et al. Essential role of BDNF in the mesolimbic dopamine pathway in social defeat stress. *Science.* Feb 10 2006;311(5762):864–868.
23. Roth TL, Lubin FD, Funk AJ, Sweatt JD. Lasting epigenetic influence of early-life adversity on the BDNF gene. *Biol Psychiatry.* May 1 2009;65(9):760–769.
24. Post RM, Kalivas P. Bipolar disorder and substance abuse: pathological and therapeutic implications of their comorbidity and cross sensitization. *Br J Psychiatry.* 2013;202:172–176.
25. Anier K, Malinovskaja K, Aonurm-Helm A, Zharkovsky A, Kalda A. DNA methylation regulates cocaine-induced behavioral sensitization in mice. *Neuropsychopharmacology.* Nov 2010;35(12):2450–2461.
26. Krishnan V, Han MH, Graham DL, et al. Molecular adaptations underlying susceptibility and resistance to social defeat in brain reward regions. *Cell.* Oct 19 2007;131(2):391–404.
27. Hodes GE, Pfau ML, Leboeuf M, et al. Individual differences in the peripheral immune system promote resilience versus susceptibility to social stress. *Proc Natl Acad Sci U S A.* Nov 11 2014;111(45):16136–16141.
28. Raison CL, Rutherford RE, Woolwine BJ, et al. A randomized controlled trial of the tumor necrosis factor antagonist infliximab for treatment-resistant depression: the role of baseline inflammatory biomarkers. *JAMA Psychiatry.* Jan 2013;70(1):31–41.
29. Maes M, Anderson G, Kubera M, Berk M. Targeting classical IL-6 signalling or IL-6 trans-signalling in depression? *Expert Opin Ther Targets.* May 2014;18(5):495–512.

30. Antelman SM. *Stressor-induced sensitization to subsequent stress: implications for the development and treatment of clinical disorders.* Caldwell, NJ: Telford Press; 1988.

31. Kalivas PW, Stewart J. Dopamine transmission in the initiation and expression of drug- and stress-induced sensitization of motor activity. *Brain Res.* Sep–Dec 1991;16(3):223–244.

32. Kalivas PW, Volkow ND. The neural basis of addiction: a pathology of motivation and choice. *Am J Psychiatry.* Aug 2005;162(8):1403–1413.

33. Post R, Post S. Molecular and cellular developmental vulnerabilities to the onset of affective disorders in children and adolescents: some implications for therapeutics. In: Steiner H, ed. *Handbook of mental health interventions in children and adolescents.* San Francisco: Jossey-Bass; 2004:140–192.

34. Berk M, Copolov DL, Dean O, et al. N-acetyl cysteine for depressive symptoms in bipolar disorder—a double-blind randomized placebo-controlled trial. *Biol Psychiatry.* Sep 15 2008;64(6):468–475.

35. Berk M, Copolov D, Dean O, et al. N-acetyl cysteine as a glutathione precursor for schizophrenia—a double-blind, randomized, placebo-controlled trial. *Biol Psychiatry.* Sep 1 2008;64(5):361–368.

36. Berk M, Malhi GS, Gray LJ, Dean OM. The promise of N-acetylcysteine in neuropsychiatry. *Trend Pharmacol Sci.* Mar 2013;34(3):167–177.

37. Kalivas PW, Lalumiere RT, Knackstedt L, Shen H. Glutamate transmission in addiction. *Neuropharmacology.* 2009;56(Suppl 1):169–173.

38. Mishkin M, Appenzeller T. The anatomy of memory. *Sci Am.* Jun 1987;256(6):80–89.

39. Bredy TW, Barad M. The histone deacetylase inhibitor valproic acid enhances acquisition, extinction, and reconsolidation of conditioned fear. *Learn Mem.* Jan 2008;15(1):39–45.

40. Geddes JR, Carney SM, Davies C, et al. Relapse prevention with antidepressant drug treatment in depressive disorders: a systematic review. *Lancet.* Feb 22 2003;361(9358):653–661.

41. Davis JM. Overview: maintenance therapy in psychiatry: II. affective disorders. *Am J Psychiatry.* Jan 1976;133(1):1–13.

42. Hansen R, Gaynes B, Thieda P, et al. Meta-analysis of major depressive disorder relapse and recurrence with second-generation antidepressants. *Psychiatr Serv.* Oct 2008;59(10):1121–1130.

43. Williams N, Simpson AN, Simpson K, Nahas Z. Relapse rates with long-term antidepressant drug therapy: a meta-analysis. *Hum Psychopharmacol.* Jul 2009;24(5):401–408.

44. Post RM, Altshuler L, Kupka R, et al. More pernicious course of bipolar disorder in the United States than in many European countries: implications for policy and treatment. *J Affect Disord.* May 2014;160:27–33.

45. Post RM, Leverich GS, Kupka R, et al. Increases in multiple psychiatric disorders in parents and grandparents of patients with bipolar disorder from the USA compared with The Netherlands and Germany. *Psychiatr Genet.* Oct 2015;25(5):194–200.

46. Post RM, Altshuler L, Kupka R, et al. Multigenerational positive family history of psychiatric disorders is associated with a poor prognosis in bipolar disorder. *J Neuropsychiatry Clin Neurosci.* Fall 2015;27(4):304–310.

47. Post RM, Altshuler LL, Kupka R, et al. More illness in offspring of bipolar patients from the U.S. compared to Europe. *J Affect Disord.* Feb 2016;191:180–186.

48. Lange KJ, McInnis MG. Studies of anticipation in bipolar affective disorder. *CNS Spectrums.* Mar 2002;7(3):196–202.

49. Kessler RC, Angermeyer M, Anthony JC, et al. Lifetime prevalence and age-of-onset distributions of mental disorders in the World Health Organization's World Mental Health Survey Initiative. *World Psychiatry.* Oct 2007;6(3):168–176.

50. Chengappa KN, Kupfer DJ, Frank E, et al. Relationship of birth cohort and early age at onset of illness in a bipolar disorder case registry. *Am J Psychiatry.* Sep 2003;160(9):1636–1642.
51. da Silva Magalhaes PV, Gomes FA, Kunz M, Kapczinski F. Birth-cohort and dual diagnosis effects on age-at-onset in Brazilian patients with bipolar I disorder. *Acta Psychiatr Scand.* Dec 2009;120(6):492–495.
52. Champagne F, Meaney MJ. Like mother, like daughter: evidence for non-genomic transmission of parental behavior and stress responsivity. *Prog Brain Res.* 2001;133:287–302.
53. Weaver IC, Cervoni N, Champagne FA, et al. Epigenetic programming by maternal behavior. *Nat Neurosci.* Aug 2004;7(8):847–854.
54. Plotsky PM, Thrivikraman KV, Nemeroff CB, Caldji C, Sharma S, Meaney MJ. Long-term consequences of neonatal rearing on central corticotropin-releasing factor systems in adult male rat offspring. *Neuropsychopharmacology.* Dec 2005;30(12):2192–2204.
55. McGowan PO, Sasaki A, D'Alessio AC, et al. Epigenetic regulation of the glucocorticoid receptor in human brain associates with childhood abuse. *Nat Neurosci.* Mar 2009;12(3):342–348.
56. Dias BG, Ressler KJ. Parental olfactory experience influences behavior and neural structure in subsequent generations. *Nat Neurosci.* Jan 2014;17(1):89–96.
57. Vassoler FM, Byrnes EM, Pierce RC. The impact of exposure to addictive drugs on future generations: physiological and behavioral effects. *Neuropharmacology.* Jan 2014;76 Pt B:269–275.
58. Govorko D, Bekdash RA, Zhang C, Sarkar DK. Male germline transmits fetal alcohol adverse effect on hypothalamic proopiomelanocortin gene across generations. *Biol Psychiatry.* Sep 1 2012;72(5):378–388.
59. Szutorisz H, DiNieri JA, Sweet E, et al. Parental THC exposure leads to compulsive heroin-seeking and altered striatal synaptic plasticity in the subsequent generation. *Neuropsychopharmacology.* May 2014;39(6):1315–1323.
60. Dietz DM, Nestler EJ. From father to offspring: paternal transmission of depressive-like behaviors. *Neuropsychopharmacology.* Jan 2012;37(1):311–312.
61. Byrnes JJ, Johnson NL, Schenk ME, Byrnes EM. Cannabinoid exposure in adolescent female rats induces transgenerational effects on morphine conditioned place preference in male offspring. *J Psychopharmacol.* Oct 2012;26(10):1348–1354.
62. Byrnes JJ, Johnson NL, Carini LM, Byrnes EM. Multigenerational effects of adolescent morphine exposure on dopamine D2 receptor function. *Psychopharmacology.* May 2013;227(2):263–272.
63. Gapp K, von Ziegler L, Tweedie-Cullen RY, Mansuy IM. Early life epigenetic programming and transmission of stress-induced traits in mammals: how and when can environmental factors influence traits and their transgenerational inheritance? *BioEssays.* May 2014;36(5):491–502.
64. Rodgers AB, Bale TL. Germ cell origins of posttraumatic stress disorder risk: the transgenerational impact of parental stress experience. *Biol Psychiatry.* Sep 1 2015;78(5):307–314.
65. Bale TL. Lifetime stress experience: transgenerational epigenetics and germ cell programming. *Dialogues Clin Neurosci.* Sep 2014;16(3):297–305.
66. Perlis RH, Miyahara S, Marangell LB, et al. Long-term implications of early onset in bipolar disorder: data from the first 1000 participants in the Systematic Treatment Enhancement Program for Bipolar Disorder (STEP-BD). *Biol Psychiatry.* May 1 2004;55(9):875–881.
67. Post RM, Leverich GS, Kupka RW, et al. Early-onset bipolar disorder and treatment delay are risk factors for poor outcome in adulthood. *J Clin Psychiatry.* Jul 2010;71(7):864–872.

68. Holtzman JN, Miller S, Hooshmand F, et al. Childhood- compared to adolescent-onset bipolar disorder has more statistically significant clinical correlates. *J Affect Disord.* Jul 1 2015;179:114–120.

69. Geller B, Tillman R, Bolhofner K, Zimerman B. Pharmacological and non-drug treatment of child bipolar I disorder during prospective eight-year follow-up. *Bipolar Disord.* Mar 2010;12(2):164–171.

70. Geller B, Luby JL, Joshi P, et al. A randomized controlled trial of risperidone, lithium, or divalproex sodium for initial treatment of bipolar I disorder, manic or mixed phase, in children and adolescents. *Arch Gen Psychiatry.* May 2012;69(5):515–528.

71. Kessing LV, Hansen HV, Hvenegaard A, et al. Treatment in a specialised out-patient mood disorder clinic v. standard out-patient treatment in the early course of bipolar disorder: randomised clinical trial. *Br J Psychiatry.* Mar 2013;202(3):212–219.

72. Colton CW, Manderscheid RW. Congruencies in increased mortality rates, years of potential life lost, and causes of death among public mental health clients in eight states. *PCD.* Apr 2006;3(2):A42.

73. Newcomer JW, Hennekens CH. Severe mental illness and risk of cardiovascular disease. *JAMA.* Oct 17 2007;298(15):1794–1796.

74. Kessing LV, Andersen PK. Does the risk of developing dementia increase with the number of episodes in patients with depressive disorder and in patients with bipolar disorder? *J Neurol Neurosurg Psychiatry.* Dec 2004;75(12):1662–1666.

75. Kessing LV, Sondergard L, Forman JL, Andersen PK. Lithium treatment and risk of dementia. *Arch Gen Psychiatry.* Nov 2008;65(11):1331–1335.

76. Forlenza OV, Diniz BS, Radanovic M, Santos FS, Talib LL, Gattaz WF. Disease-modifying properties of long-term lithium treatment for amnestic mild cognitive impairment: randomised controlled trial. *Br J Psychiatry.* May 2011;198(5):351–356.

77. Martinsson L, Wei Y, Xu D, et al. Long-term lithium treatment in bipolar disorder is associated with longer leukocyte telomeres. *Translat Psychiatry.* 2013;3:e261.

78. Axelson D, Goldstein B, Goldstein T, et al. Diagnostic precursors to bipolar disorder in offspring of parents with bipolar disorder: a longitudinal study. *Am J Psychiatry.* Jul 2015;172(7):638–646.

79. Weissman MM, Wickramaratne P, Nomura Y, Warner V, Pilowsky D, Verdeli H. Offspring of depressed parents: 20 years later. *Am J Psychiatry.* Jun 2006;163(6):1001–1008.

80. Rasic D, Hajek T, Alda M, Uher R. Risk of mental illness in offspring of parents with schizophrenia, bipolar disorder, and major depressive disorder: a meta-analysis of family high-risk studies. *Schizophr Bull.* Jan 2014;40(1):28–38.

81. Wickramaratne P, Gameroff MJ, Pilowsky DJ, et al. Children of depressed mothers 1 year after remission of maternal depression: findings from the STAR*D-Child study. *Am J Psychiatry.* Jun 2011;168(6):593–602.

82. Miklowitz DJ, George EL, Richards JA, Simoneau TL, Suddath RL. A randomized study of family-focused psychoeducation and pharmacotherapy in the outpatient management of bipolar disorder. *Arch Gen Psychiatry.* Sep 2003;60(9):904–912.

83. Fristad MA, Verducci JS, Walters K, Young ME. Impact of multifamily psychoeducational psychotherapy in treating children aged 8 to 12 years with mood disorders. *Arch Gen Psychiatry.* Sep 2009;66(9):1013–1021.

84. West AE, Jacobs RH, Westerholm R, et al. Child and family-focused cognitive-behavioral therapy for pediatric bipolar disorder: pilot study of group treatment format. *J Can Acad Child Adolesc Psychiatry.* Aug 2009;18(3):239–246.

85. Ginsburg GS, Drake KL, Tein JY, Teetsel R, Riddle MA. Preventing onset of anxiety disorders in offspring of anxious parents: a randomized controlled trial of a family-based intervention. *Am J Psychiatry.* Dec 2015;172(12):1207–1214.

86. Shonkoff JP, Garner AS. The lifelong effects of early childhood adversity and toxic stress. *Pediatrics.* Jan 2012;129(1):e232–e246.

87. Felitti VJ, Anda RF, Nordenberg D, et al. Relationship of childhood abuse and household dysfunction to many of the leading causes of death in adults. The Adverse Childhood Experiences (ACE) study. *Am J Prev Med.* May 1998;14(4):245–258.

88. Anda RF, Felitti VJ, Bremner JD, et al. The enduring effects of abuse and related adverse experiences in childhood. A convergence of evidence from neurobiology and epidemiology. *Eur Arch Psychiatry Clin Neurosci.* Apr 2006;256(3):174–186.

89. Post RM, Altshuler LL, Leverich GS, et al. More medical comorbidities in patients with bipolar disorder from the United States than from the Netherlands and Germany. *J Nerv Ment Dis.* Apr 2014;202(4):265–270.

90. Banks J, Marmot M, Oldfield Z, Smith JP. Disease and disadvantage in the United States and in England. *JAMA.* May 3 2006;295(17):2037–2045.

91. Jerrell JM, McIntyre RS, Tripathi A. A cohort study of the prevalence and impact of comorbid medical conditions in pediatric bipolar disorder. *J Clin Psychiatry.* Nov 2010;71(11):1518–1525.

92. Goldstein BI, Fagiolini A, Houck P, Kupfer DJ. Cardiovascular disease and hypertension among adults with bipolar I disorder in the United States. *Bipolar Disord.* Sep 2009;11(6):657–662.

93. Goldstein BI, Young LT. Toward clinically applicable biomarkers in bipolar disorder: focus on BDNF, inflammatory markers, and endothelial function. *Curr Psychiatry Rep.* Dec 2013;15(12):425.

94. Goldstein BI, Collinger KA, Lotrich F, et al. Preliminary findings regarding proinflammatory markers and brain-derived neurotrophic factor among adolescents with bipolar spectrum disorders. *J Child Adolesc Psychopharmacol.* Oct 2011;21(5):479–484.

95. Epel ES, Blackburn EH, Lin J, et al. Accelerated telomere shortening in response to life stress. *Proc Natl Acad Sci U S A.* Dec 7 2004;101(49):17312–17315.

96. Entringer S, Epel ES, Kumsta R, et al. Stress exposure in intrauterine life is associated with shorter telomere length in young adulthood. *Proc Natl Acad Sci U S A.* Aug 16 2011;108(33):E513–E518.

97. Elvsashagen T, Vera E, Boen E, et al. The load of short telomeres is increased and associated with lifetime number of depressive episodes in bipolar II disorder. *J Affect Disord.* Dec 2011;135(1–3):43–50.

98. Wolkowitz OM, Mellon SH, Epel ES, et al. Leukocyte telomere length in major depression: correlations with chronicity, inflammation and oxidative stress—preliminary findings. *PloS One.* 2011;6(3):e17837.

99. Hudziak JJ, Albaugh MD, Ducharme S, et al. Cortical thickness maturation and duration of music training: health-promoting activities shape brain development. *J Am Acad Child Adolesc Psychiatry.* Nov 2014;53(11):1153–1161, 1161 e1151–e1152.

100. Amminger GP, Schafer MR, Schlogelhofer M, Klier CM, McGorry PD. Longer-term outcome in the prevention of psychotic disorders by the Vienna omega-3 study. *Nat Commun.* 2015;6:7934.

101. Post RM, Chang K, Frye MA. Paradigm shift: preliminary clinical categorization of ultrahigh risk for childhood bipolar disorder to facilitate studies on prevention. *J Clin Psychiatry.* Feb 2013;74(2):167–169.

102. Kowatch RA, Fristad M, Birmaher B, Wagner KD, Findling RL, Hellander M. Treatment guidelines for children and adolescents with bipolar disorder. *J Am Acad Child Adolesc Psychiatry*. Mar 2005;44(3):213–235.

103. Post R, Findling R, Luckenbaugh D. Number, severity, and quality of symptoms discriminate early onset bipolar disorder from ADHD. *Psy Annals*. 2014d;44(9):416–422.

104. Berk M, Dean OM, Cotton SM, et al. Maintenance N-acetyl cysteine treatment for bipolar disorder: a double-blind randomized placebo controlled trial. *BMC Med*. 2012;10:91.

105. Hardan AY, Fung LK, Libove RA, et al. A randomized controlled pilot trial of oral N-acetylcysteine in children with autism. *Biol Psychiatry*. Jun 1 2012;71(11):956–961.

106. Nikoo M, Radnia H, Farokhnia M, Mohammadi MR, Akhondzadeh S. N-acetylcysteine as an adjunctive therapy to risperidone for treatment of irritability in autism: a randomized, double-blind, placebo-controlled clinical trial of efficacy and safety. *Clin Neuropharmacol*. Jan–Feb 2015;38(1):11–17.

107. Ghanizadeh A, Moghimi-Sarani E. A randomized double blind placebo controlled clinical trial of N-acetylcysteine added to risperidone for treating autistic disorders. *BMC Psychiatry*. 2013;13:196.

108. LaRowe SD, Mardikian P, Malcolm R, et al. Safety and tolerability of N-acetylcysteine in cocaine-dependent individuals. *Am J Addict*. Jan–Feb 2006;15(1):105–110.

109. Amen SL, Piacentine LB, Ahmad ME, et al. Repeated N-acetyl cysteine reduces cocaine seeking in rodents and craving in cocaine-dependent humans. *Neuropsychopharmacology*. Mar 2011;36(4):871–878.

110. Baker DA, McFarland K, Lake RW, Shen H, Toda S, Kalivas PW. N-acetyl cysteine-induced blockade of cocaine-induced reinstatement. *Ann NY Acad Sci*. Nov 2003;1003:349–351.

111. Grant JE, Odlaug BL, Kim SW. A double-blind, placebo-controlled study of N-acetyl cysteine plus naltrexone for methamphetamine dependence. *Eur Neuropsychopharmacol*. Nov 2010;20(11):823–828.

112. Grant JE, Kim SW, Odlaug BL. N-acetyl cysteine, a glutamate-modulating agent, in the treatment of pathological gambling: a pilot study. *Biol Psychiatry*. Sep 15 2007;62(6):652–657.

113. Grant JE, Odlaug BL, Chamberlain SR, et al. A randomized, placebo-controlled trial of N-acetylcysteine plus imaginal desensitization for nicotine-dependent pathological gamblers. *J Clin Psychiatry*. Jan 2014;75(1):39–45.

114. Gray KM, Carpenter MJ, Baker NL, et al. A double-blind randomized controlled trial of N-acetylcysteine in cannabis-dependent adolescents. *Am J Psychiatry*. Aug 2012;169(8):805–812.

115. Knackstedt LA, LaRowe S, Mardikian P, et al. The role of cystine-glutamate exchange in nicotine dependence in rats and humans. *Biol Psychiatry*. May 15 2009;65(10):841–845.

116. Schmaal L, Berk L, Hulstijn KP, Cousijn J, Wiers RW, van den Brink W. Efficacy of N-acetylcysteine in the treatment of nicotine dependence: a double-blind placebo-controlled pilot study. *Eur Addict Res*. 2011;17(4):211–216.

117. Grant JE, Odlaug BL, Kim SW. N-acetylcysteine, a glutamate modulator, in the treatment of trichotillomania: a double-blind, placebo-controlled study. *Arch Gen Psychiatry*. Jul 2009;66(7):756–763.

118. Lafleur DL, Pittenger C, Kelmendi B, et al. N-acetylcysteine augmentation in serotonin reuptake inhibitor refractory obsessive-compulsive disorder. *Psychopharmacology*. Jan 2006;184(2):254–256.

4

Biological Effects of Depression in Cardiac Illness

Nicole Mavrides and Charles Nemeroff

INTRODUCTION

Cardiovascular disease (CVD) is the cause of death of up to a third of American adults and is the leading cause of death in the developing world.[1] Coronary artery disease (CAD) is defined as ischemic symptoms associated with coronary angiographic evidence of 50% or more blockage in at least one major coronary artery, previous hospitalization for a myocardial infarction (MI), or angina.[2] Depression is defined by the DSM-5 (*Diagnostic and Statistical Manual of Mental Disorders, 5th Edition*) as the loss of interest or pleasure in daily activities for more than two weeks, representing a significant change from baseline, with impaired function. In addition, five of nine additional symptoms are required. Depression is extremely common in patients with CVD/CAD and has been associated with both poor functional and poor cardiovascular outcomes.[3] Depression and CVD have been linked, beginning with the seminal Maltzberg article in 1937, which demonstrated that patients with severe depression had a higher mortality than the general population, and moreover, that the surplus deaths were largely attributable to CVD.[4,5] The interface between psychiatry and cardiovascular disease is complex and bidirectional, including the effects of psychosocial factors and mood and anxiety disorders on the vascular system and the effects of CVD on the brain, psychological functions, and psychopathology.[1]

Over the past 20 years, there have been many studies that have examined the relationship between depression and CVD, and there is virtually universal agreement that depression is associated with an increased risk of the development of CAD, and that depression is a predictor of poor outcome (morbidity and mortality) in patients with cardiovascular disease.[6,7] Depression is a risk factor for CAD, angina, heart failure, MI, and mortality. It is linked to a poorer quality of life, and those with depression are two to three times less likely to adhere to medications and treatments, demonstrating higher readmission rates to hospitals and greater health service usage than patients who are not depressed.[6,8] Increasing recognition of the relationship between depression and CVD led the American Heart Association to recommend routine screening for depression in patients with CAD. Depression increases the risk of the development of CVD 1.5-fold;

patients with CVD and depression have a two- to three-fold increased risk of future cardiac events compared to cardiac patients without depression.[9]

Depression in cardiac disease is extremely common; up to 12–17% of hospitalized patients with CAD meet criteria for major depressive disorder.[10] Other psychological states that have been identified as contributing to the risk of CAD besides depression are anxiety, panic, anger, type A behavior patterns, stress, type D personality, and sleep disorders.[1] Environmental factors such as trauma and stress can affect adaptive responses, which can lead to depression and can affect the cardiovascular system negatively. Recently, studies have started to focus less on the association of depression and CVD and more on understanding the biology and pathophysiological processes that characterize depression in cardiac disease. Inflammation, heart rate variability, hypothalamic-pituitary-adrenal and hypothalamic-pituitary-thyroid axis function, platelet clotting abnormalities, as well as vascular calcification, oxidative stress, and genetic factors, all have been posited to play a role in mediating the increased risk of CAD in patients with depression.[4] In addition, the biological effects of childhood abuse and neglect, personality factors, and psychosocial factors can also potentially mediate the risk of CAD in depressive patients. This chapter will review the major epidemiological findings in patients with depression and cardiovascular disease, as well as discussing the pathophysiological and biological mechanisms that might explain the bidirectional association between the two conditions.

EPIDEMIOLOGY

Cardiovascular disease and depression are both extremely common and prevalent disorders. In one of the largest studies of psychiatric disorder prevalence rates in the United States, the National Comorbidity Study reported a lifetime prevalence of major depressive disorder (MDD) of 16.6%, higher in women than in men. In the United States, the lifetime risk of cardiovascular death by age 80 is 4.7–6.4% of those without cardiovascular risk factors, and 20.5–29.6% of the patients with two or more cardiac risk factors.[9,11] These risk factors include diabetes mellitus, smoking, total cholesterol level ≥180 mg/dl, and untreated blood pressure ≥120 mmHG systolic and ≥80 mmHg diastolic.[11–13] Depression is thought to increase the risk and at times accelerate the progression of some serious medical conditions, including cardiovascular disease, stroke, cancer, renal disease, and diabetes.[8] The prevalence of MDD in patients with CAD, including those with stable or unstable angina or MI, can be estimated as between 15–20%. In addition, another 30–45% of patients can have clinically significant depressive symptoms without meeting DSM-5 criteria for MDD.[6,12,13] The results from the majority of the published studies support an association between CAD and depression.

Holahan et al. studied 388 patients with depression compared to 404 controls over a 10-year period. They reported that the patients with depression had a two-thirds higher likelihood of developing a serious physical illness, including CAD, compared to controls.[14] Similarly, in the National Health Examination Follow-up Study, 2,832 adults between the ages of 45 and 77 years with no CVD history who demonstrated depressed mood and hopelessness had an increased risk of both fatal ischemic heart disease (risk ratio [RR] 1.5, 95% confidence interval [CI] 1.0–2.3) and nonfatal ischemic heart disease

(RR 1.5, 95% CI 1.11–4.06), even after controlling for other risk factors and demographics.[11,15] In a seminal study conducted in the early 1990s, Frasure-Smith and colleagues revealed that patients diagnosed with MDD after an MI had higher mortality rates than patients without MDD.[16] Similarly, the Stockholm Female Coronary Risk Study followed almost 300 women for five years and found that the women with two or more depressive symptoms had an increased risk (hazard ratio of 1.9) of future cardiac events, compared to those with one or no depressive symptoms.[17] A recent meta-analysis of 22 studies of post-MI patients found that post-MI depression was associated with a 2–2.5 increased risk of negative cardiovascular outcomes.[18]

Major depression was a significant predictor of subsequent development of both CAD (RR 2.12) and MI (RR 2.12) in the Johns Hopkins Precursor Study of male medical students who were followed for 40 years. The increase in risk persisted even when the depressive symptoms had occurred more than 10 years prior.[11,19] The Stockholm Heart Epidemiology Program (SHEEP) study evaluated the risk of MI among individuals hospitalized for depressive symptoms over a 26-year period. This case control study examined 1,799 patients and 2,339 controls and demonstrated a significantly increased risk (RR 2.3) for acute MI among patients who had been hospitalized for depression—even after controlling for cardiovascular risk factors.[20]

In the EPIC-Norfolk United Kingdom Prospective Cohort Study, patients with MDD were 2.7 times more likely to die from ischemic heart disease than were the participants who did not have depression. This was a very large study that included 8,261 men and 11,388 women without clinically relevant heart disease who were followed for 8.5 years to determine the effect of depression on mortality from ischemic heart disease.[21] The data from the Danish Psychiatric Central Research Register produced results that were fairly similar, showing a positive association between depression and acute MI (incidence rate ratio 1.16).[22] When reviewing the Women's Ischemia Syndrome Evaluation (WISE) study, it was seen that women with elevated depression scores or any prior treatment for depression (or both) had significantly increased rates of mortality and cardiovascular events (including congestive heart failure, stroke, unstable angina, MI, revascularization). This was significant even after adjusting for other risk factors related to cardiac disease.[23] In another study, by Frasure-Smith et al., depressive symptoms immediately after an MI were associated with a four- to six-fold amplification of risk of cardiac mortality six and 18 months after the MI.[24,25] In the National Health and Nutrition Examination Study (NHANES), depression was shown to increase the risk of death from ischemic heart disease in patients both with and without hypertension.[26] In the Baltimore Epidemiological Catchment Area Study, individuals with a history of manic or hypomanic episode (n = 58) had an almost three-fold increase in cardiovascular disease compared to those with no history of a mood disorder (n = 1,339). This study also demonstrated that a history of dysphoria and MDD could increase the risk of MI.[6,27]

Depression also appears to predict cardiac morbidity and mortality in other cardiac populations. At least three studies have found that pre–coronary artery bypass graft (CABG) depressive symptoms are associated with an increase in cardiac morbidity at six and 12 months follow-up. The evidence is vast in suggesting that depression is extremely prevalent in patients with congestive heart failure, atrial fibrillation, and those who have undergone a CABG, and moreover, that depression exerts a major adverse effect on morbidity and mortality.[28,29,30] Many mechanisms have attempted to explain the link between cardiovascular disease and depression; some are behavioral and some are physiological, as will be discussed in the following sections.

PHYSIOLOGICAL MECHANISMS OF DEPRESSION

The putative physiological mechanisms by which depression may contribute to increase CVD and particularly cardiac morbidity and mortality are several. It is likely that a combination of the mechanisms discussed next act in concert to make the connection between depression and cardiac disease.[11,31]

Inflammation

In the past 10–15 years, much research has been devoted to searching for the role of chronic inflammation in the pathogenesis of many chronic medical conditions, including diabetes, cancer, cerebrovascular, and cardiovascular disease. Inflammatory cytokines are associated with the formation of atherosclerotic plaques, a major contributor to the pathogenesis of CVD. Inflammatory markers also participate in the pathophysiology of CAD by direct effects on myocardial contractility and apoptosis. C-reactive protein (CRP), interleukin-6 (IL-6), tumor necrosis factor (TNF)-alpha, and interleukin-1 (IL-1) together are independent risk factors for cardiovascular disease.[3,32] Depression is associated with increased levels of inflammation, as repeatedly demonstrated by increased levels of inflammatory markers such as CRP and IL-6, a finding in both CVD patients and depressed patients without CVD, as demonstrated in a meta-analysis by Horwen.[33]

Depression and inflammatory processes are bidirectional—depression increases the inflammatory response, and inflammation promotes depression. Three meta-analyses have demonstrated increases in pro-inflammatory cytokines in patients with MDD compared to controls. There may be a causal pathway in that higher IL-6 and CRP concentrations predicted subsequent development of depressive symptoms.[34] Pro-inflammatory cytokines have been positively correlated to individual depressive symptoms such as fatigue, cognitive dysfunction, and impaired sleep.[34] Cytokines alter the production, metabolism, and transport of neurotransmitters that affect mood, including dopamine, glutamate, and serotonin.[34] Data from the National Health and Nutrition Examination Survey provide a rough estimate of the prevalence of increased inflammation in the depressed population: 47% of those who scored above threshold for depression had a CRP level that was ≥3 mg/L and 29% had a CRP level that was ≥5 mg/L.[34] This suggests that inflammatory markers are considerably higher in depressed patients; Raison and Miller reported a 35% rate compared to the non-depressed comparison subjects. Raison and Miller coined the phrase "immune response element amplification," suggesting that lower levels of inflammation could cause depression in vulnerable individuals.[35]

It is also well established that inflammation plays a major pathogenic role in the progression of atherosclerosis in CAD. There is also widespread evidence of coronary artery inflammation during unstable angina.[36] Arterial inflammation is triggered by noxious stimuli that damage the arterial wall, including low-density lipoprotein (LDL) cholesterol, tobacco smoke, and hypertension. Local endothelial dysfunction promotes LDL accumulation, which is then oxidized. The oxidized LDL triggers an inflammatory reaction, which then activates immune cells, including monocytes, macrophages, neutrophils, T lymphocytes, and mast cells.[37] There is an intrinsic repair process involving these cells that attempts to maintain arterial wall integrity. If the arterial repair is not possible or is incomplete, the inflammatory reaction persists, which can then lead to further destruction of the arterial wall.[5] One of the most widely used markers of systemic inflammation is CRP. CRP has been implicated as an independent predictor of MI, stroke, and cardiovascular death in primary prevention as well as in patients already suffering from CAD.[37] CRP has also not only been suggested to be a marker of inflammation, but it also seems to exert complex modulatory effects that participate in inflammatory processes associated with plaque vulnerability and progression of coronary stenosis.[37]

There have been several studies that demonstrated elevated levels of CRP in patients with depression. In a study in the Czech Republic of 6,126 middle-aged individuals (45–69 years), the patients with more severe depressive symptoms had higher CRP levels than the healthy controls.[38] A similar study in Finland also demonstrated that there was a statistically significant positive correlation between severe depression as assessed by the Beck Depression Index and CRP concentrations in men and women.[39] In both of these studies, the relationship between CRP and depression persisted after controlling for other major risk factors (age, obesity, smoking, high triglycerides, low high-density lipoprotein [HDL] levels).

There have only been a few studies that have examined whether the effects of depression on cardiac prognosis may be mediated by inflammation. Vaccarino et al. (2007) found that depressed women with an acute coronary syndrome (ACS) had an increased chance of adverse cardiac events compared to their non-depressed controls. Although the increased risk was only partly associated with increased levels of CRP and IL-6, it was statistically significant.[32] The PRIME study (Prospective Epidemiologic Study of Myocardial Infarction) compared 355 future cases of CVD with 670 control cases for five years and found a statistically significant correlation between depression severity and levels of IL-6 and CRP. The men with depression also had a 50% increase in the odds ratio for CVD.[5,40] In the Canadian Nova Scotia Health Survey of 1,794 participants, both depression and increases in inflammatory markers predicted an increased risk of CAD. Increased severity of depression has also been reported to be associated with increased concentrations of TNF-alpha.[41,42]

Mostowik and colleagues recently showed that percutaneous stent implantation can cause an early increase in CRP in stable CAD patients, even when on optimal cardiac pharmacological treatment (i.e., statin therapy, antiplatelet drugs, and beta blockers). A prolonged post-angioplasty increase in CRP was associated with higher thrombin generation and lower platelet response to clopidogrel. The association between high CRP and thrombin generation in CAD has been previously reported for CAD patients and those with unstable angina, but no other studies showed a correlation between post-angioplasty CRP increase and higher thrombin generation in patients with CAD.[37] Thrombin impacts plaque formation in the advanced stages of plaque progression and destabilization.

Wium-Andersen demonstrated in a cross-sectional analysis that an increase in fibrinogen was associated with an increase in psychological distress, use of antidepressants, and hospitalization for depression (p ≤ 0.005). The association between depression and fibrinogen was attenuated in patients with CVD, discrepant from what others have reported. Fibrinogen can stimulate the synthesis of IL-6 and TNF-alpha.[43] In the Heart and Soul Study, Duivis and colleagues found that CVD patients' higher levels of inflammatory markers (specifically IL-6 and CRP) were correlated with increased depression severity, mainly mediated by physical inactivity, smoking, and obesity.[3,5,43–45] Similar findings in the Meta Health Study of elevated CRP levels and more severe depressive symptoms in 512 patients continued to show this strong correlation between depression and inflammation. In the Whitehall II Cohort Study, the patients who were more physically active had lower baseline levels of IL-6 and CRP over a 10-year follow-up period.[46]

The Carlscrona Heart Attack Prognosis Study (CHAPS) comprised 5,292 patients admitted to the intensive care unit with acute chest pain. A diagnosis of acute coronary syndrome was confirmed in 908 patients aged 30–74, who were divided into two groups, those experiencing at least one acute MI ($n = 527$), and those not experiencing an acute MI but having at least one episode of unstable angina ($n = 381$). When they evaluated the inflammatory markers, elevation of CRP was significantly associated with MI versus unstable angina (odds ratio [OR] 1.75). MI was also significantly associated with higher fibrinogen levels compared to the angina group (p = 0.01). They demonstrated that the magnitude of inflammation at the time of admission was associated with a more severe outcome in the case of ACS. Preexisting inflammation predisposed to a more severe outcome in ACS as well.[36] Elevation of inflammatory biomarkers in patients with ACS may reflect myocardial injury instead of underlying inflammation. However, fibrinogen and CRP are induced by IL-1, IL-6, and TNF-alpha signaling, and there is a time lag between the secretion of the proteins and when the rise in plasma concentration becomes detectable during the acute phase of inflammation. The authors also observed a correlation between CRP and time in patients with an MI, where the duration between symptom onset and blood sampling was longer than four hours. Another interesting conclusion from the CHAPS study was that there was also an increase in both neutrophils and monocytes following the ACS. The results were similar to what was found with CRP and fibrinogen levels, that a preexisting inflammation before the ACS led to higher neutrophil and monocyte levels in the patients with an MI compared to those with only unstable angina.[36] This was also found in a population cohort study by Adamsson Eryd et al., who demonstrated an association between increased neutrophil count and the incident of coronary events and increased fatality rate during follow-up.[47]

In a rat model of depression, Wang et al. evaluated vulnerability markers of myocardial apoptosis (Bax:Bcl-2 ratio and caspase-3 levels) in the heart post-MI depression. A high Bax:Bcl-2 ratio is associated with greater vulnerability to apoptotic activation, while a high caspase-3 level is associated with apoptosis. They concluded that there was an increased myocardial Bax:Bcl-2 ratio in the depression, MI, and post-MI depression groups of the rats, particularly in the post-MI depression group. It was suggested that there might be greater vulnerability to apoptosis of myocardial cells after an acute MI in the presence of comorbid major depression. It also suggested that depression after MI may increase the Bax:Bcl-2 ratio and induce further cardiomyocyte apoptosis. There was no difference between any of the groups in the caspase-3 in the myocardium, which may suggest that it is not an active pathway to apoptosis in the myocardium in MI patients with depression.[48]

Gianaros et al. studied community volunteers (n = 157) without depression or CVD and tested whether prefrontal engagement by reappraisal as assessed with functional magnetic resonance imaging (fMRI) would be associated with atherosclerotic CVD risk and if the association would be mediated by inflammatory activity.[49] The participants were part of the Adult Health and Behavioral Project, Phase II. They showed that greater reappraisal-related engagement of the dorsal anterior cingulate cortex was associated with greater preclinical atherosclerosis and higher levels of IL-6. IL-6 also mediated the association of the dorsal anterior cingulate cortex engagement with preclinical atherosclerosis. They concluded that the regulation of emotion might relate to CVD risk through a pathway involving functional interplay between the anterior cingulate region of the prefrontal cortex and inflammatory activity, although further research is needed.[49]

Lafitte et al. investigated the role of atherosclerosis-induced inflammation and how that can mediate/affect major depression. They sought to determine if there was any prognostic value in CRP or fibrinogen as potential markers of inflammation in identifying new depressive symptoms in patients following an acute coronary event. Eighty-seven patients were studied and monitored over a nine-month period and depression and inflammatory markers measured. Although the incidence of depression was high in this study, no associations were found between CRP, fibrinogen, and MDD following an ACS. Because this study excluded patients with a history of depression, the relationship with inflammation may have been different.[50]

The Copenhagen General Population Study and the Copenhagen City Heart Study, comprising over 73,000 participants, were prospective studies in which fibrinogen, depression, use of antidepressants, and hospitalization were measured for all participants. In cross-sectional analyses, an increase in fibrinogen was associated with an increased risk of psychological distress, use of antidepressant medications, and hospitalization for depression (p trend 2×10^{-11} to 5×10^{-95}). In prospective analyses, increasing fibrinogen was also associated with increasing risk of hospitalization with depression (p trend 7×10^{-6}). These results indicate that increased fibrinogen is associated with psychological distress, use of antidepressants, and hospitalization with depression.[43,51]

Heart Rate Variability

Heart rate variability (HRV) is a direct measure of the ability of the heart to respond to physiological demands and reflects sympathetic–vagal balance.[5,26,31] It is a noninvasive measurement of autonomic nervous system activation of the heart.[5,26,31,32,52] Increases in HRV are associated with positive emotions, social connectedness, and longevity; whereas decreases are associated with depression, anxiety, CVD, and cardiac mortality. Decreased HRV may precede inflammation-mediated atherosclerosis and ventricular fibrillation.[52,53] HRV may, in part, be a marker for one's capacity for self-regulation, social engagement, and psychological flexibility. Geisler et al. reported that young adults with higher resting HRV have more adaptive self-regulation and more social engagement than those with lower HRVs. They were more inclined to seek social support than those with lower HRV.[9,54]

In a study, 19 CAD patients with depression were compared to 19 CAD patients without depression; Carney et al. reported that HRV was significantly reduced in depressed patients compared to the non-depressed group. This can help explain the increased risk of cardiac morbidity and mortality in patients with CAD and depression.[55,56,57] The Heart and Soul Study demonstrated that somatic depressive symptoms in CVD patients were associated with reduced HRV.[5] Gehi and colleagues showed that the somatic symptoms of depression (fatigue, psychomotor changes) were associated with lower HRV, while the cognitive symptoms (negative self-image) were not.[32,57,60]

In the Twins Heart Study, a component of the Vietnam-era twin registry, both depressive symptoms and HRV were highly heritable. The association between depression and reduced HRV was posited to be due to a shared genetic pathway, suggesting a common neurobiological substrate between depression and autonomic dysfunction. Of the total genetic variation of depression and HRV, about 80–90% was found to be due to the same genetic factors.[11,53,58–60] The findings were similar to previous studies'—that lower HRV is associated with depression in both patients with CAD and control subjects. Common genes that may be involved in the pathogenesis of both depression and autonomic function were suggested by Su and colleagues to include those in the hypothalamic-pituitary-adrenal (HPA) axis or in the sympathetic, parasympathetic, and serotonin pathways.[58,59] These have all previously been related to depression and may be relevant to autonomic regulation as well.

Measures of HRV and particularly the high-frequency component are a more accurate index of vagal activity than heart rate. Vagal activity plays an important role in mental and physical health. Increases are associated with positive emotions, social connectedness, and longevity. Decreases in the vagal activity are associated with depression, anxiety, CVD, and mortality. Kemp and colleagues suggested that vagal activity might provide the link between day-to-day emotional experiences and the morbidity and mortality associated with chronic medical conditions.[61] In one of their earlier studies, Kemp et al. also examined the impact of depression and anxiety on HRV in a search for psychiatric indicators of CVD risk reduction. They found that HRV is most reduced in comorbid generalized anxiety disorder (GAD), and that the reductions were not due to depression severity, as all of the depressive groups were fairly similar.[52]

The Brazilian Longitudinal Study of Adult Health (ELSA-Brasil) is a multicenter cohort study of adult health in Brazil, which is studying the relationship between CVD and diabetes, as well as risk factors. Kemp et al. used this population to determine if individuals diagnosed with mood and anxiety disorders exhibit decreased vagal activity and if antidepressant treatment would further reduce HRV. HRV was reduced in the GAD group compared to the control group. All of the antidepressants (tricyclic antidepressants [TCAs], selective serotonin reuptake inhibitors [SSRIs], serotonin-norepinephrine reuptake inhibitors [SNRIs]) were associated with lower HRV. Specifically, those on TCAs were lowest, but those on both SSRIs and SNRIs were also lower compared to the control group. Although only GAD was associated with a reduction in vagal activity, depression and GAD are linked such that each disorder increases the likelihood of developing the other over time. HRV was lowest in the un-medicated, depressed patient group compared to the healthy control subjects.[61]

Kemp and colleagues also performed a meta-analysis of the impact of depression and its treatment on HRV. After looking at 46 studies, they found that there was a negative correlation between depression severity and HRV ($p < 0.001$). HRV was also found to be significantly reduced after treatment with a TCA compared to the other antidepressants ($p = 0.1$). They also found a significant reduction in HRV after TCA treatment compared with HRV before treatment (Hedges' $g = -1.236$, $p = 0.008$). Although this analysis did not include patients with both depression and CVD, it is noteworthy because those with severe depression are likely to have lower HRV than those with less severe depression, which can affect both patients with CVD and those without. In addition, the study highlights that HRV is reduced in un-medicated patients with depression (relative to control subjects) and that antidepressant treatment (other than TCAs) in contrast to the study just cited neither increases nor decreases HRV. Therefore, depression without CVD reduces HRV, and antidepressants do not necessarily reverse the reduction. This is important for health care providers, especially cardiologists, who should be mindful of the impact that depression can have on the cardiovascular system.[62,63]

HPA Axis and Hypothalamic-Pituitary-Thyroid (HPT) Axis Alterations

The HPA axis plays an important role in the human stress response, and cortisol plays manifold roles in normal physiology. HPA-axis hyperactivity can be associated with many CAD risk factors, such as abdominal obesity, hypercholesterolemia, hypertriglyceridemia, hypertension, and glucose intolerance. In CAD patients, dysregulated cortisol secretion has been observed and there is a suggestion by many researchers that HPA dysfunction is implicated in the pathogenesis of CAD.[9,32,64] The HPA axis is also dysregulated in major depression and/or after continued exposure to stress, which can result in a chronically excessive secretion of cortisol or in a chronically hypoactive HPA axis. These can be due to decreased corticosteroid receptor sensitivity and a continuously increased hypothalamic secretion of CRH (corticotrophin-releasing hormone).[34] Conditions that cause sympatho-adrenal activation include coronary artery ischemia, heart failure, and mental stress. Sudden emotional stress can cause transient left ventricular dysfunction, even in patients without CAD, an effect that is possibly mediated by increased plasma cortisol/catecholamine levels.[21,53]

Many patients with depression have increases in plasma, urinary, and cerebrospinal fluid (CSF) levels of cortisol, increased plasma adrenocorticotropic hormone (ACTH) and β-endorphin levels, and increased CSF concentrations of CRF. In addition, a blunted ACTH response to exogenous CRF and suppression of cortisol after administration of the glucocorticoid dexamethasone can also be seen.[5] The contribution of the HPA-axis dysfunction to the pathogenesis of depression and comorbid CVD may be partly mediated by the loss of the glucocorticoid receptor–mediated negative feedback on inflammatory signaling. In addition, disruptions of the HPA axis can also be regulated by altered expression of pro-inflammatory cytokines, suggesting a complex bidirectional crosstalk between these systems. Dysregulation of the HPA axis can also lead to sympatho-adrenal hyperactivity which can lead to an increase in vasoconstrictive tone, heart rate, and platelet activation, which have all been implicated in CVD. The increased sympathetic drive can result in decreased HRV, which can increase vulnerability to arrhythmia and morbidity and mortality in CVD.[65]

A study of 508 men and women between ages of 53 and 76 years, using the Whitehall II epidemiological cohort, found that there was a significant association between cortisol response and a detectable cardiac troponin, which is a measure of cardiac cellular damage (OR 3.83, p < 0.001). Even after controlling for coronary calcification, a marker for preclinical coronary atherosclerosis, the findings remained significant.[66]

HPA-axis dysregulation, common in depression, has been implicated in the pathogenesis of coronary artery disease and predicted CAD death in depressed male cardiovascular patients.[67] Cortisol might also be a shared risk factor for depression and CAD.[34] In the Invecchiare in Chianti, aging in the Chianti area (CHIANTI) prospective cohort study, there were 861 patients over 65 years. Urinary cortisol levels predicted cardiovascular mortality risk. Those with the highest level of urinary cortisol had a five times higher risk of cardiovascular death (hazard ratio [HR] 5.00, CI 2.02–12.37).[68] Jokinen et al. studied 382 patients with MDD hospitalized at the Karolinska University Hospital over a 20-year span (1980–2000). The patients who exhibited hyperactivity of the HPA axis, demonstrated by non-suppression of cortisol on the dexamethasone-suppression test, and increased baseline levels of cortisol in serum, had a higher risk of mortality from cardiac death.[67]

Conrad et al. scrutinized circadian mood variation and HPA and autonomic function in elderly (>55 y.o.a.) depressed and non-depressed volunteers who were at risk of CVD. They measured diurnal positive and negative affect, cortisol levels, and cardiopulmonary variables. Cortisol levels did not differ between the depressed and non-depressed groups, but, positive affect was lower and negative affect higher in the depressed subgroup. The diurnal positive and negative affect helped distinguish depressed from non-depressed patients at risk of CVD.[69]

PLATELET CLOTTING ABNORMALITIES

Platelets serve multiple functions, including a role in the attachment of endothelial stem cells and bone marrow cells to arterial walls, as well as their repair activity. When there is a depletion of repair cells (secondary to, for example, age), platelets may be involved in the recruitment of inflammatory cells that contribute to the development of atherosclerosis. Platelets are responsible for thrombus formation, which is the ultimate cause of an MI and stroke, and intimately involved in atherosclerosis formation.[5,21,53] Activated platelets stimulate atherosclerotic plaque progression, which is why anticoagulation therapy with platelet antagonists can help prevent further or a new MI. Activated platelets are very adhesive, and they provide a unique boundary between the injured arterial wall and the circulating inflammatory cells.[5] Markovitz and Matthews first suggested that enhanced platelet response to physiological stress can trigger adverse coronary artery ischemic events.[8] Platelets might contribute to the remodeling of arteries and atheroma formation by recruiting inflammatory cells that induce apoptosis of the arterial cells. They also may produce platelet-derived growth factor, which promotes the proliferation of smooth muscle cells in the atheroma. Platelet microparticles help initiate coagulation and thrombosis as well as smooth muscle proliferation, which can then lead to rupture of the arterial plaque, resulting in thrombus formation with partial or total occlusion of the vessel lumen and adverse cardiac outcomes.[70–73]

Over the past 15–20 years, a number of researchers have demonstrated that alterations during platelet activation, platelet aggregation, and the clotting cascade are associated with depression. These alterations have been hypothesized to contribute to depression and added increased risk of thrombus formation. Musselman and Nemeroff showed that in drug-free patients with depression, there was an increased activation of platelet fibrinogen receptor integrin αIIb-β3 complex, which is the critical final common pathway for platelet activation.[74,75] Plasma concentrations of platelet factor IV (PF4) and β-thromboglobulin (βTG), which are markers of the intermediate steps of the platelet clotting cascade, are elevated in depressed patients with ischemic heart disease compared to non-depressed patients with heart disease, and the controls.[21,76,77] These increases in the markers of platelet activation in patients with depression were impressive because most of the patients were treated prophylactically with aspirin in this study.[77] In contrast, in the Heart and Soul Study, there was no evidence of increased platelet activation in patients with CAD—regardless of the presence of depression.[78] However, many of these patients were already receiving antidepressants and/or antiplatelet medications, and depression severity was not assessed. Although these findings have been confirmed in some (but not all) subsequent research studies, these differences in the findings can be due to differences in methods for detecting platelet activation and in the depression severity and age of the patients.[5]

In a study of 26 depressed CAD patients, there was a significant association between depressive symptom severity, as based on the Hamilton Depression Rating Scale, and an increase in platelet activating factor (PAF) lipids. This suggested that there are PAFs associated with depression in CAD patients, which is an area of future potential research for biomarkers of depressive symptoms in CAD.[79] In a community-based study, mean platelet volume was used as an indicator of platelet activity. This was found to be significantly elevated in patients with depression compared to those without depression. Piletz et al. also found that PF4, βTG, and P-selectin were increased in depressed patients compared to non-depressed controls.[80,81] P-selectin helps facilitate platelet–monocyte interactions that contribute to thrombosis and endothelial dysfunction. PAF-mediated platelet activation is higher in hypertensive patients compared to controls, which suggests that PAFs may interact with CVD risk factors that contribute to the development and progression of CAD.[80]

Delle Chiaie et al. studied 19 hospitalized MDD patients treated with electroconvulsive therapy (ECT), and measured PF4 and β-thromboglobulin (βTG). Their depression was quite severe at the start of the study, but upon completion, the patients no longer met criteria for MDD. As expected, the platelet aggregation factors, PF4 and βTG, were elevated at baseline, but were not reduced when the patients were euthymic. The observed reduction in measures of platelet activation and aggregation observed after sertraline treatment may be due to direct effects of the SSRI and not a "state" effect of recovery.

These platelet alterations may therefore represent a "trait," rather than a state, marker of depression.[82]

Lopez-Vilchez et al. sought to determine if a prothrombotic condition existed in depressed patients and whether treatment with an SSRI altered this state. To that end, 19 patients with MDD were compared to 20 healthy matched controls. The depressed patients were subsequently treated with escitalopram following the initial intake. At baseline, the platelets from the depressed patients showed higher levels of enhanced aggregating responses to arachidonic acid ($p < 0.01$) and higher levels of glycoprotein Ib (GPIb), fibrinogen, Factor V, and anionic phospholipids ($p < 0.05$). Clot firmness and procoagulant activity of PAFs were also significantly elevated in the depressed patients ($p < 0.05$), in addition to increased fibrin formation in the early-diagnosed depressed patients. After 24 months of SSRI treatment, the majority of these alterations normalized, except for a residual increased expression of preglycoprotein IIb/IIIa (PGIIbIIIa) ($p < 0.05$) and persistent alterations in certain thrombotic parameters. This data revealed the existence of a platelet related prothrombotic phenotype at the time of depression diagnosis. Treatment with an SSRI offers a potential approach for down-regulation of the platelet-related contribution to thrombogenesis.[83]

ENDOTHELIAL DYSFUNCTION AND IMPAIRED ARTERIAL REPAIR

Endothelial dysfunction is thought to contribute to the increased risk of developing CAD in patients with depression. Functions of endothelial cells include regulation of the coagulation cascade, platelet adhesion, immune function, and control of the volume and electrolyte content of the intravascular and extravascular spaces.[84,85] Tomfohr et al. studied 102 adolescent girls who had had no prior health issue to determine endothelial function by measuring finger arterial plethysmography. Endothelial function was inversely related to severity of depressive symptoms.[85] A meta-analysis of 12 studies of healthy adults and those with CVD supported the inverse relationship between depression and endothelial function.[86]

Both endothelial dysfunction and oxidative damage to lipids are thought to contribute to the development of atherosclerosis, important factors for those with increased risk of CAD. In a study of 73 depressed patients and 72 controls, biomarkers of oxidative damage were significantly higher in the depressed group compared to the healthy controls.[87] In another, smaller, study, 54 depressed patients had significantly higher levels of plasma peroxides and titers of antibodies to oxidized LDL when compared to the 37 patients in the control group.[88]

Atherosclerosis risk increases significantly with age, which could in part be due to the progressive breakdown of the body's ability to repair arteries. This process requires lineage-negative bone marrow cells (Lin-BMC), which circulate in the body with other endothelial progenitor cells (EPC). Whether it is due to age or to CVD, the loss of these cells has been associated with an increased risk of thromboembolic events and death.[70,71,89] A reduction of the progenitor cells might represent a risk of CAD. Dome et al. studied 33 depressed patients compared to 16 healthy controls, and found that EPC levels were lower in depressed patients. They also found that TNFα, an inflammatory cytokine, was increased in the depressed group and inversely related to the EPCs.[90] This demonstrates the possible link between depression and CVD; with the negative effect of depression on the body's ability to maintain EPCs for arterial repair.

Apoptosis or programmed cell death is a process of ordered, active, non-inflammatory cell death. There is a family of genes that mediates apoptosis: *Bcl-2*. One group promotes apoptosis—*Bax, Bak, Bad*, and *Bcl-xS*—whereas the other group inhibits cell death, including *Bcl-2* and *Bcl-xl*. In the presence of stress, the *Bcl-2* plays an active role in the regulation of cell death.[91] Wang et al. studied the apoptosis pathways in the heart, using a rat model, and sought to determine the role for *Bcl-2* genes in the interaction of CVD and depression. An upregulated *Bax:Bcl-2* ratio in the depressed, MI, and post-MI depression groups was observed, with the greatest ratio being in the post-MI depression group. This suggests that an active pro-apoptotic pathway may be involved in the connection between MI and depression.[91]

BIOLOGICAL AND PSYCHOSOCIAL MECHANISMS OF DEPRESSION

Lifestyle and Psychosocial Factors

In the 1980s, the "type A" personality was defined as an individual who is ambitious, aggressive, hostile, and competitive, with a chronic sense of urgency. This was linked to an increased risk of heart disease approximately 30 years ago. More recent studies have differed in their findings as to whether or not all of the symptoms that compose a type A personality are risk factors for heart disease, but hostility remains one of the few validated factors. "Type D" personality is another, more recently posited psychosocial risk factor for CAD, in which patients experience negative emotions paired with social inhibition. This might be a greater risk factor for CAD than hostility and the type A personality.

The increased risk that patients with depression exhibit for serious medical conditions, including CAD, is probably at least partly attributable to lifestyle factors. Depressed patients have higher rates of tobacco and alcohol use/abuse, use more illicit substances, engage in less physical activity, and typically exhibit poorer adherence rates to medical regimens.[5] The Heart and Soul Study, a landmark prospective trial of 1,017 patients with CAD, examined how depression contributed to the incidence of subsequent cardiac events.[45,92,93] They demonstrated that there was an association between depression and CVD, and that it was mainly secondary to physical inactivity and noncompliance with medication. However, behavioral factors alone probably do not solely account for the increased risk of CVD in patients with depression. Nevertheless, controversy remains as to whether depression worsens outcome in CVD patients, largely as an indirect consequence of depression-associated changes in one's lifestyle and behavior.[5,94]

In the Effect of Potentially Modifiable Risk Factors Associated with Myocardial Infarction (INTERHEART) case control study, attributable risk of MI in 52 countries was studied. Stress, low generalized locus of control, and depression accounted for 32.5% of the attributable risk of an MI, which is only slightly less than that of lifetime smoking, but greater than for hypertension and obesity, known risk factors for MI.[5,21,53] In the

Look AHEAD (Action for Health in Diabetes) trial of weight loss in type 2 diabetics, Rubin et al. studied the association of depression or antidepressant use in patients with cardiac risk factors. They hypothesized that an increase in depressive symptoms or use of an antidepressant would be associated with an increased risk of CVD over a four-year period. They reported that elevated symptom-severity scores of depression on the Beck Depression Index (BDI) or being treated with an antidepressant were positively associated with increased CVD risk factors, even when controlling for prior risk factor status. At least one indicator out of glycemia, lipids, blood pressure, smoking, and body mass index (BMI) was increased with the presence of depression and medication use. There were more significant associations with antidepressant use compared to just having increased depressive symptoms. The results suggest that both depression and perhaps certain antidepressants may place patients, especially those with type 2 diabetes, at a higher risk of CVD.[95]

Women are well known to have a significantly higher prevalence rate of major depression compared to men; heart disease remains the leading cause of death for both men and women (25.4% and 24.5%). Windle and Windle investigated a link between depression (MDD specifically), CVD, and diabetes in women. They found that recurrent MDD in middle-aged women predicted a significant increase in CVD risk factors, including hypertension and hypercholesterolemia, and an increase in diabetes over a five-year period. However, a single episode of MDD did not, even when controlling for age, BMI, and education-level increased risk.[96]

Gehi et al. examined the link between depression and adverse outcomes in patients with CAD, with a focus on medication nonadherence. They studied 204 participants with depression; 28 (14%) were not compliant with their medication. This was compared with 40 (5%) of the non-depressed patients.[11] Twice as many depressed patients reported forgetting to take their medications (OR 2.4, 95% CI 1.6–3.8, p < 0.001) and 9% of depressed patients reported deciding to skip their medications (OR 2.2, 95% CI 1.2–4.2, p = 0.01). Gehi and colleagues took these findings to conclude that depression was associated with medication nonadherence in patients with CVD and that medication nonadherence could contribute to adverse cardiovascular outcomes in depressed patients.[11,97]

TRAUMA, ABUSE, LIFE STRESSORS

Chronic exposure to stressors often leads to worsening cognitive and behavioral coping strategies. Cognitive appraisals are important to how one copes with stress, how one manages the balance between one's stressors and one's individual resources for coping.[98] Frequent chronic stress leads to learned helplessness and eventually MDD. Patients who experience early life trauma, including childhood physical or sexual abuse, neglect, bullying, or the death of a parent, may contribute to a feeling of helplessness and depression.[99,100] Cognitive schemas are developed early on in one's life, as ways to transform memories and data into long-term memories. Negative schemas can be inactive for long periods of time, but they can be reactivated when adults are faced with stressful situations. Many times the dysfunctional schemas formed during childhood can lead to negative cognitive appraisals and feelings of helplessness and depression.[100] Although not directly studied in patients with CVD or CVD risk factors, the connection between depression and cardiac disease makes these issues important and relevant.

Adverse events early in life, especially traumatic events such as abuse, neglect, and loss, are associated with later-life development of mood and anxiety disorders, specifically after additional stressful events in adulthood.[101] Abuse and/or neglect can lead to long-term alterations in the HPA axis. This has clinical implications for both depressed patients and those with significant CVD, because of the potential influence that the HPA axis has on both cardiac disease as well as depression. Adverse early-life events have been repeatedly shown to induce long-lasting changes in the neural and neuroendocrine systems involved in adaptive responses to stress, particularly in CRF neural transmission.[100,102] Increased availability of CRF can lead to hyperactivity of the HPA axis and increased levels of cortisol, which cause many changes in the central nervous system, including reduced hippocampal volume. Based on the results of many studies, the effects of child abuse and/or neglect on the HPA axis are impacted by the nature of the early-life stress, number of episodes, time length of the period of abuse, age when first abused/neglected, and the chronicity. Also affecting the HPA axis is the presence or absence of psychosocial support, presence of traumatic events in adulthood, having a family history of psychiatric disorders, and various genetic/epigenetic factors.[100,103]

Some of the first evidence that child abuse and neglect can be associated with an increased risk of depression and medical disorders, including cardiovascular disease (as well as many others), is derived from the Adverse Childhood Experiences (ACE) studies. The risk of CVD and depression was directly proportional to the number and degree of early life stress.[103,104] In a meta-analysis of 24 studies of 48,801 children, child abuse was significantly associated with gastrointestinal, respiratory, and most significant to the current subject, cardiovascular disorders.[105] There is also a correlation between high levels of inflammatory markers in adults and a history of early life stress. Markedly increased levels of IL-6 were observed in depressed men with a history of child abuse and neglect when presented with a standard laboratory stressor.[106] In the Dunedin Multidisciplinary Health and Development Study, Danese et al. reported that patients who were mistreated as children showed a significant and graded increase in CRP concentrations more than 20 years later. Interestingly, this effect was independent of any stressful life events in adulthood.[107,108] As discussed earlier in the chapter, increased inflammation has been observed in depressed individuals and is a significant risk factor for CVD and morbidity and mortality. Other studies have shown that not only childhood abuse, but also prenatal adversity is associated with increased CRP levels in adulthood.[103] When young people have experienced early adverse events as children, such as social isolation, low socioeconomic status, or parental maltreatment, they exhibit higher risk markers for cardiovascular disease. This includes higher blood pressure, abnormal lipid profiles, increased CRP, and an elevated glycosylated hemoglobin.[107,109] More recent research on childhood abuse has revealed higher levels of IL-6 in depressed breast cancer survivors. This suggests that inflammation may contribute to the poor outcomes in depressed breast cancer patients and opens the door for further research in the depressed cardiovascular disease patients.[110]

Both major depression and cardiovascular disease are complex diseases in which the risk of developing these illnesses is clearly related to both genetic and environmental contributions. There have been major advances in our understanding of the genetic contributions to the major cardiovascular risk factors (hypertension, dyslipidemia, and atherosclerosis), but little research has been done on any of the common genetic mechanisms that might mediate the depression-associated increase in the risk of CAD.[5]

Child abuse and neglect has been shown in many studies to be a major environmental risk factor for depression later on in life. There are literally hundreds of reports on the many possible genetic polymorphisms that are potential modifiers for the development of major depression in victims of early adversity.[103] "Epigenetics" refers to the heritable characteristics that are not determined by structural changes in the underlying genetic sequence.[100] This is accomplished by changes in the methylation of histone proteins or chromatin that increase or decrease gene expression without changing the original DNA sequence.[100,111] There is a major effect of early-life abuse/neglect on the epigenetic regulation of the glucocorticoid receptor NR3C1, which has been documented in postmortem brain tissue of suicide victims as well as in blood samples of patients with MDD.[112,113]

Genetic risk factors for depression and cardiac disease have been a focus of researchers over the past several years. Mannie et al. studied young men and women who had a parent with depression but no depression themselves, and healthy controls. They evaluated their cardiovascular risk profile by measuring fasting insulin, glucose, lipids, and CRP, as well as blood pressure, arterial stiffness, and cortisol levels. The group with the family history of depression showed an increase in peripheral and central blood pressure, increased arterial stiffness, and decreased insulin sensitivity. They did not differ from the control group in their lipids, CRP, or cortisol levels.[76] The data from this study suggest that, for individuals with an increased risk of depression due to family history, there is evidence of greater cardiovascular risk as well, even in the absence of depressive symptoms. The authors suggested that genetic factors are likely to explain both the increased risk of familial depression and the increase in cardiovascular risk factors, though no specific gene has been identified.[76,114]

In the Twins Heart Study, a common genetic pathway involved in the relationship between depression/depressive symptoms and inflammation was sought. Because depression was associated with increased levels of IL-6 and CRP, there was likely to be a causal relationship between the two. By utilizing the Vietnam Twins Registry, an association was observed between the severity of current depressive symptoms and increased levels of the inflammatory markers, including IL-6 ($p = 0.002$). The heritability of IL-6, CRP, and depressive symptoms were estimated to be 0.37, 0.65, and 0.48, respectively.[58,59] By using genetic modeling, a significant genetic correlation between IL-6 and depressive symptoms was demonstrated, indicating that 66% of the covariance between them can be explained by shared genetic influences ($p = 0.046$). These data suggest that depression and inflammation may be the expression of a common biological pathway that is genetically driven.[115,116]

CONCLUSION

Depression is a major public health concern, with significant and severe morbidity (a leading cause of disability) and mortality that affect many, and it continues to be insufficiently addressed. World Health Organization in March 2017 stated that Depression is the illness causing the greatest burden of health in the world, is the leading cause of death, disability, and disease burden in the developed world today. Depression adversely affects the cardiovascular system and can increase the risk of CVD—including CAD, acute coronary symptoms, and MI. Depression is also associated with a two-fold increase in mortality following an MI. Prevention and optimal treatment of depression would probably improve quality of life and longevity in those with CVD. It is also imperative that patients with significant cardiac risk factors—that is, recent history of MI, CAD, and heart failure—be evaluated and treated for depression.[3,117,118]

Increased inflammation is likely to contribute to both CVD and depression. Inflammation has a direct effect on arterial walls and the development of atherosclerosis and its complications. Unfortunately, our mechanistic understanding continues to be limited, and we do not yet know how depression increases inflammation. As also noted in this chapter, disruptions in the HPA axis are frequently observed in patients with depression and increased cardiovascular risk. It appears that perhaps the hormonal dysregulation seen in depressed individuals can reduce HRV, which then might affect cardiovascular risk factors. Genetic and epigenetic factors that affect both depression and CVD risk factors need more thorough investigation, especially as regards a shared genetic pathway. Pathophysiological mechanisms for depression and cardiovascular disease have a bidirectional influence on each other, and more research is needed to further clarify the exact impact that they have on each other.

REFERENCES

1. Shapiro P. Heart disease. In: *The textbook of psychosomatic medicine: psychiatric care of the medically ill*. New York: American Psychiatric Publishing; 2011:Chapter 18.
2. Dowlati Y, Herrmann N, Swardfager WL, Reim EK, Lanctot KL. Efficacy and tolerability of antidepressants for treatment of depression in coronary artery disease: A meta-analysis. *Can J Psychiatry*. 2010;55(2):91–99.
3. Celano CM, Huffman JC. Depression and cardiac disease. A review. *Cardiol Rev*. 2011;19(3):130–142.
4. Maltzberg B. Mortality among patients with involution melancholia. *Am J Psychiatry*. 1937;93:1231–1238.
5. Nemeroff CB, Goldschmidt-Clermont PJ. Heartache and heartbreak—the link between depression and cardiovascular disease. *Nat Rev Cardiol*. Jun 2012;26:1–14.
6. Garfield LD, Scherrer JF, Hauptman PJ, et al. Association of anxiety disorders and depression with incident heart failure. *Psychosom Med*. 2014;76:128–136.
7. Bucknall C, Brooks D, Curry PV, Bridges PK, Bouras N, Ankier SI. Mianserin and trazodone for cardiac patients with depression. *Eur J Clin Pharmacol*. 1988;33(6):565–569.
8. Scherrer JF, Chrusciel T, Garfield LD, et al. Treatment-resistant and insufficiently treated depression and all-cause mortality following myocardial infarction. *Br J Psychiatry*. 2012;200:137–142.
9. Kemp A, Quintana D. The relationship between mental and physical health: Insights from the study of heart rate variability. *Int J Psychophysiol*. 2013;89:288–296.

10. Lesperance F, Frasure-Smith N, Koszycki D, et al. Effects of citalopram and inter-personal psychotherapy on depression in patients with coronary artery disease. The Canadian Cardiac Randomized Evaluation of Antidepressant and Psychotherapy Efficacy (CREATE) trial. *JAMA*. 2007;297:367–379.

11. Gehi A, Haas D, Pipkin S, Whooley MA. Depression and medication adherence in out-patients with coronary heart disease: findings from the Heart and Soul Study. *Arch Intern Med*. Nov 28 2005;165(21):2508–2513.

12. Berry JD, Dyer A, Cai X, et al. Lifetime risks of cardiovascular disease. *NEJM*. 2012;366:321–329.

13. Glassman AH, Bigger JT. Depression and cardiovascular disease: the safety of antidepres-sant drugs and their ability to improve mood and reduce medical morbidity. In: *Depression and Heart Disease*. New York: Wiley and Sons; 2011:Chapter 5.

14. Holahan CJ, Pahl SA, Cronkite RC, et al. Depression and vulnerability to incident physical illness across 10 years. *J Affect Disord*. 2010;123:222–229.

15. McIntyre RS, Schaffer A, Beaulieu S. The Canadian Network for Mood and Anxiety Treatments (CANMAT) task force recommendations for the management of patients with mood disorders and comorbid conditions. *Ann Clin Psychiatry*. 2012;24(1):1–3.

16. Frasure-Smith N, Lesperance F, Talajic M. Depression following myocardial infarction. Impact on 6 month survival. *JAMA*. 1993;270:1819–1825.

17. Orth-Gomer K, Wamala SP, Horsten M, et al. Marital stress worsens prognosis in women with coronary heart disease. The Stockholm Female Coronary Risk Study. *JAMA*. 2000;284(23):3008–3014.

18. Van Melle JP, de Jonge P, Spijkerman TA, et al. Prognostic association of depression fol-lowing myocardial infarction with mortality and cardiovascular events: a meta-analysis. *Psychosom Med*. 2004;66(6):814–822.

19. Ford DD, Mead LA, Chang PF, et al. Depression is a risk factor for coronary artery disease in men: the Precursors Study. *Arch Intern Med*. 1998;158:1422–1426.

20. Janszky I, Ahlbom A, Hallqvist J, et al. Hospitalization for depression is associated with an increased risk for myocardial infarction not explained by lifestyle, lipids, coagulation, and inflammation: the SHEEP Study. *Biol Psychiatry*. 2007;62(1):25–32.

21. Mavrides N, Nemeroff C. Treatment of depression in cardiovascular disease. *Depress Anxiety*. April 30 2013;4:328–341.

22. Blumenthal JA, Sherwood A, Babyak MA, et al. Exercise and pharmacological treatment of depressive symptoms in patients with coronary heart disease: results from the UPBEAT (Understanding the Prognostic Benefits of Exercise and Antidepressant Therapy) study. *J Am Coll Cardiol*. 2012;60:1053–1063.

23. Rutledge T, Linke SE, Krantz DS, et al. Comorbid depression and anxiety symptoms as predictors of cardiovascular events: results from the NHLBI-sponsored Women's Ischemia Syndrome Evaluation (WISE) study. *Psychosom Med*. Nov 2009;71(9):958–964.

24. Frasure-Smith N, Lesperance F, Talajic M. Depression following myocardial infarc-tion: impact on 6-month survival. *JAMA*. 1993;270:1819–1825.

25. Frasure-Smith N, Lesperance F, Talajic M. Depression and 18-month prognosis after myocardial infarction. *Circulation*. 1995;91:999–1005.

26. Egede LE, Netert PJ, Zheng D. Depression and all-cause and coronary heart disease mor-tality among adults with and without diabetes. *Diabetes Care*. 2005;28:1339–1345.

27. Ramsey CM, Leoutsakos JM, Mayer LS, et al. History of manic and hypomanic episodes and risk of incident cardiovascular disease: 11.5-year follow up from the Baltimore Epidemiologic Catchment Area Study. *J Affect Disord*. 2010;125:35–41.

28. May H, Horne BD, Carlquist JF, et al. Depression after coronary artery disease is associated with heart failure. *J Am Coll Cardiol.* 2009;53:1440–1447.

29. Lesman-Leegte I, van Veldhuisen DJ, Hillege HL, et al. Depressive symptoms and outcomes in patients with heart failure: data from the COACH study. *Eur J Heart Fail.* 2009;15:912–919.

30. Frasure-Smith N, Lesperance F, Habra M, et al. Elevated depression symptoms predict long-term cardiovascular mortality in patients with atrial fibrillation and heart failure. *Circulation.* 2009;120:134–140.

31. Iosifescu DV, Clementi-Craven N, Fraguas R, et al. Cardiovascular risk factors may moderate pharmacological treatment effects in major depressive disorder. *Psychosom Med.* 2005;67:703–706.

32. De Jonge P, Rosmalen JGM, Kema IP. Psychophysiological biomarkers explaining the association between depression and prognosis in coronary artery patients: a critical review of the literature. *Neurosci Biobehav Rev.* Sep 2010;35(1):84–90.

33. Howren MB, Lamkin DM, Suls J. Associations of depression with C-reactive protein, IL-1, and IL-6: a meta-analysis. *Psychosom Med.* Feb 2009;71(2):171–186.

34. Kiecolt-Glaser JK, Derry HM, Fagundes CP. Inflammation: depression fans the flames and feasts on the heat. *Am J Psychiatry.* Nov 2015;172(11):1075–1091.

35. Raison CL, Miller AH. Is depression an inflammatory disorder? *Curr Psychiatry Rep.* Dec 2011;13(6):467–475.

36. Odeberg J, Freitag M, Forssell H, et al. Open influence of pre-existing inflammation on the outcome of acute coronary syndrome: a cross-sectional study. *BMJ Open.* Jan 12 2016;6(1):e009968.

37. Mostowik M, Siniarski A, Golebiowska-Wiatrak R, et al. Prolonged CRP increase after percutaneous coronary intervention is associated with high thrombin concentrations and low platelet response to clopidogrel in patients with stable angina. *Adv Clin Exp Med.* 2015:24(6):979–985.

38. Pikhart H, Hubacek JA, Kubinova R, et al. Depressive symptoms and levels of C-reactive protein: a population-based study. *Soc Psychiatry Psychiatr Epidemiol.* 2009;44:217–222.

39. Elovainio M, Aalto AM, Kivimaki M, et al. Depression and C-reactive protein: population-based Health 2000 study. *Psychosom Med.* 2009;71:423–430.

40. Cowles MK, Musselman DL, McDonald W, Nemeroff CB. Effects of mood and anxiety disorders on the cardiovascular system. In: *Hurt's The Heart,* 13th ed. New York: McGraw-Hill; 2010:2128–2145.

41. Davidson LW, Schwartz JE, Kirkland SA, et al. Relation of inflammation to depression and incident coronary heart disease (from the Canadian Nova Scotia Health Survey [NSHS95] Prospective Population Study). *Am J Cardiol.* 2006;103:755–761.

42. Ferketich AK, Ferguson JP, Binkley PE. Depressive symptoms and inflammation among heart failure patients. *Am Heart J.* 2005;150:132–136.

43. Wium-Andersen MK, Orsted DD, Nordestgaard BG. Elevated plasma fibrinogen, psychological distress, antidepressant use, and hospitalization with depression: two large population-based studies. *Psychoneuroendocrinology.* 2013;38:638–647.

44. Blumenthal JA, Sherwood A, Babyak MA, et al. Exercise and pharmacological treatment of depressive symptoms in patients with coronary heart disease: results from the UPBEAT (Understanding the Prognostic Benefits of Exercise and Antidepressant Therapy) study. *J Am Coll Cardiol.* 2012;60:1053–1063.

45. Ruo B, Rumsfeld JS, Hlatky MA, et al. Depressive symptoms and health related quality of life: the Heart and Soul Study. *JAMA.* 2003;290:215–221.

46. Hamer M, Batty GD, Seldenrijk A, Kivimaki M. Antidepressant medication use and future risk of cardiovascular disease: the Scottish Health Study. *Eur Heart J.* 2010;32(4):737–442.
47. Adamsson ES, Smoth JG, Melander O, et al. Incidence of coronary events and case fatality rate in relation to blood lymphocyte and neutrophil counts. *Arterioscler Thromb Vasc Bio.* 2012;32:533–539.
48. Wang Y, Xingde L, Zhang D, et al. The effects of apoptosis vulnerability markers on the myocardium in depression after myocardial infarction. *BMC Medicine.* 2013;11:32–40.
49. Gianaros PJ, Marsland AL, Kuan DCH, et al. An inflammatory pathway links atheroscle-rotic cardiovascular disease risk to neural activity evoked by the cognitive regulation of emotion. *Biol Psychiatry.* 2014;75:738–745.
50. Lafitte M, Tastet S, Perez P, et al. High sensitivity C-reactive protein, fibrinogen levels and the onset of major depressive disorder in post-acute coronary syndrome. *BMC Cardiovascular Disorders.* 2015;15:23–31.
51. Wium-Andersen MK, Orsted DD, Nordestgaard BG, et al. Association between elevated plasma fibrinogen and psychological distress and depression in 73,367 individuals from the general population. *Mol Psychiatry.* Aug 2013;18(8):854–855.
52. Kemp AH, Quintana DS, Felmingham KL, et al. Depression, comorbid anxiety disorders, and heart rate variability in physically healthy, unmedicated patients: implications for car-diovascular risk. *PloS One.* 2012;7(2):e30777.
53. Mavrides N, Nemeroff C. Treatment of depression in cardiovascular disease. *Depress Anxiety.* April 30 2013;(4):328–341.
54. Geisler FC, Vennewald N, Kubiak T, et al. The impact of heart rate variability on subjec-tive well-being is mediated by emotion regulation. *Pers Individ Dif.* 2010;49:723–728.
55. Seligman F, Nemeroff CB. The interface of depression and cardiovascular disease: thera-peutic implications. *Ann NY Acad Sci.* 2015;1345:25–35.
56. Carney RM, Steinmeyer B, Freedland KE, et al. Nocturnal patterns of heart rate and the risk of mortality after acute myocardial infarction. *Am Heart J.* Jul 2014;168(1):117–125.
57. Carney RM, Freedland KE. Depression and heart rate variability in patients with coronary heart disease. *Cleve Clin J Med.* Apr 2009;76(Suppl 2):S13–S17.
58. Su S, Lampert R, Lee F, et al. Common genes contribute to depressive symptoms and heart rate variability: the Twins Heart Study. *Twin Res Hum Genet.* 2010;13(1):1–9.
59. Su S, Miller AH, Sneider H, et al. Common genetic contributions to depressive symptoms and inflammatory markers in middle-aged men: the Twins Heart Study. *Psychosom Med.* 2009;71:152–158.
60. Gehi A, Rumsfeld JS, Stein PK, et al. Relation of self-reported angina pectoris to inducible myocardial ischemia in patients with known coronary disease: the Heart and Soul Study. *Am J Cardiol.* 2003;92:705–707.
61. Kemp AH, Brunoni AR, Santos IS, et al. Effects of depression, anxiety, comorbidity, and antidepressants on resting-state heart rate and its variability: an ELSA-Brasil Cohort base-line study. *Am J Psychiatry.* Dec 2014;171(12):1328–1334.
62. Kemp AH, Quintana DS, Gray MA, et al. Impact of depression and antidepres-sant treatment on heart rate variability: a review and meta-analysis. *Biol Psychiatry.* 2010;67:1067–1074.
63. Quintana DS, McGregor IS, Guastella AJ, et al. A meta-analysis on the impact of alcohol dependence on short-term resting-state heart rate variability: implications for cardiovas-cular risk. *Alcohol Clin Exp Res.* 2013;37:E23–E29.
64. Nijm J, Jonasson L. Inflammation and cortisol response in coronary artery disease. *Ann Med.* 2009;4(3):224–233.

65. Baune BT, Stuart M, Gilmour A, et al. The relationship between subtypes of depression and cardiovascular disease: a systemic review of biological models. *Transl Psychiatry*. Mar 13 2012;2:e92.

66. Lazzarnio A, Hamer M, Gaze D, et al. The association between cortisol response to mental stress and high-sensitivity cardiac troponin T plasma concentration in healthy adults. *J Am Coll Cardiol*. Oct 29 2013;62(18):1694–1701.

67. Jokinen J, Nodstrom P. HPA axis hyperactivity and cardiovascular mortality in mood disorder inpatients. *J Affect Disord*. 2009;116:88–92.

68. Volgelzangs N, Beekman AT, Milaneschi Y, et al. Urinary cortisol and six-year risk of all-cause and cardiovascular mortality. *J Clin Endocrinol Metab*. 2010;95:4959–4964.

69. Conrad A, Wilhelm FH, Roth WT, et al. Circadian affective, cardiopulmonary, and cortisol variability in depressed and nondepressed individuals at risk for cardiovascular disease. *J Psychiatr Res*. July 2008;42(9):769–777.

70. Goldschmidt-Clermont PJ. Loss of bone marrow-derived vascular progenitor cells leads to inflammation and atherosclerosis. *Am Heart J*. 2003;146(Suppl. 4):S5–S12.

71. Asahara T, Murohara T, Sullivan A, et al. Isolation of putative progenitor endothelial cells for angiogenesis. *Science*. 1997;275:964–967.

72. Ross R. Atherosclerosis—an inflammatory disease. *N Engl J Med*. 1999;340:115–126.

73. Libby P. Inflammation in atherosclerosis. *Nature*. 2002;420:868–874.

74. Musselman DL, Tomer A, Manatunga AK, et al. Exaggerated platelet reactivity in major depression. *Am J Psychiatry*. 1996;153:1313–1317.

75. Musselman DL, Marzec UM, Mantunga AK, et al. Platelet reactivity in depressed patients treated with paroxetine: preliminary findings. *Arch Gen Psychiatry*. 2000;57:875–882.

76. Mannie ZN, Williams C, Diesch J, Steptoe A, Leeson P. Cardiovascular and metabolic risk profile in young people at familial risk of depression. *Br J Psychiatry*. July 2013;203(1):18–23.

77. Pozuelo L, Zhang J, Franco K, Tesar G, Penn M, Jiang W. Depression and heart disease: what do we know, and where are we headed? *Cleve Clin J Med*. 2009;76(1):59–70.

78. Gehi A, Musselman D, Otte C, et al. Depression and platelet activation in outpatients with stable coronary heart disease: findings from the Heart and Soul Study. *Psychiatry Res*. 2010;175:200–204.

79. Mazereeuw G, Herrmann N, Bennett SAL, et al. Platelet activating factors in depression and coronary artery disease: a potential biomarker related to inflammatory mechanisms and neurodegeneration. *Neurosci Biobehav Rev*. 2013;37:1611–1621.

80. Mazereeuw G, Herrmann N, Xu H, et al. Platelet activating factors are associated with depressive symptoms in coronary artery disease patients: a hypothesis-generating study. *Neuropsychiatr Dis Treat*. 2015;11:2309–2314.

81. Piletz JE, Zhu H, Madakasira S, et al. Elevated P-selectin on platelets in depression: response to bupropion. *J Psychiatr Res*. 2000;64:397–404.

82. Delle Chiaie R, Capra E, Salviati M, et al. Persistence of subsyndromal residual symptoms after remission of major depression in patients without cardiovascular disease may condition maintenance of elevated platelet factor 4 and β-thromboglobulin plasma levels. *J Affect Disord*. 2013;150:664–667.

83. Lopez-Vilchez I, Serra-Millas M, Navarro V, et al. Prothrombotic platelet phenotype in major depression: downregulation by antidepressant treatment. *J Affect Disord*. 2014;159:39–45.

84. Van Zyl LT, Lesperance F, Frasure-Smith N, et al. Platelet and endothelial activity in comorbid major depression and coronary artery disease patients treated with citalopram: the Canadian Cardiac Randomized Evaluation of Antidepressant and Psychotherapy Efficacy Trial (CREATE) biomarker sub-study. *J Thromb Thrombolysis*. 2009;27:48–56.

85. Tomfohr LM, Martin TM, Miller GE. Symptoms of depression and impaired endothelial function in healthy adolescents. *J Behav Med.* 2008;31:137–143.

86. Cooper DC, Tomfohr LM, Milic MS, et al. Depressed mood and flow-mediated dilation: a systematic review and meta-analysis. *Psychosom Med.* 2011;73:360–369.

87. Yager S, Forlenza MJ, Miller GE. Depression and oxidative damage to lipids. *Psychoneuroendocrinology.* 2010;35:1356–1362.

88. Maes M, Mihaylova I, Kubera M, et al. Increased plasma peroxides and serum oxidized low density lipoprotein antibodies in major depression: markers that further explain the higher incidence of neurodegeneration and coronary artery disease. *J Affect Disord.* 2010;125:287–294.

89. Shantsila E, Watson T, Lip GY. Endothelial progenitor cells in cardiovascular disorders. *J Am Coll Cardio.* 2007;49:741–752.

90. Dome P, Teleki Z, Rihmer Z, et al. Circulating endothelial progenitor cells and depression: a possible novel link between heart and soul. *Mol Psychiatry.* 2009;14:523–531.

91. Wang Y, Zhang H, Chai F, et al. The effects of escitalopram on myocardial apoptosis and the expression of *Bax* and *Bcl-2* during myocardial ischemia/reperfusion in a model of rats with depression. *BMC Psychiatry.* Dec 2014;14:349.

92. Whooley MA, de Jonge P, Vittinghoff E, et al. Depressive symptoms, health behaviors, and risk of cardiovascular events in patients with coronary heart disease. *JAMA.* 2008;300:2379–2388.

93. Chone BE, Panguluri P, Na B, et al. Psychological risk factors and the metabolic syndrome in patients with coronary heart disease: findings from the Heart and Soul Study. *Psychiatry Res.* 2010;175:133–137.

94. Hoen PW, Denollet J, de Jonge P, Whooley MA. Positive affect and survival in patients with stable coronary heart disease: findings from the Heart and Soul Study. *J Clin Psychiatry.* July 2013;74(7):716–722.

95. Rubin RR, Peyrot M, Gaussoin SA, et al. Four-year analysis of cardiovascular disease risk factors, depression symptoms, and antidepressant medicine use in the Look AHEAD (Action for Health in Diabetes) clinical trial of weight loss in diabetes. *Diabetes Care.* May 2013;36:1088–1094.

96. Windle M, Windle RC. Recurrent depression, cardiovascular disease, and diabetes among middle-aged and older adult women. *J Affect Disord.* 2013;150:895–902.

97. Ruo B, Rumsfeld JS, Hlatky MA, et al. Depressive symptoms and health-related quality of life: the Heart and Soul Study. *JAMA.* 2003;290:215–221.

98. Folkman S, Lazarus RS. The relationship between coping and emotion: implications for theory and research. *Soc Sci Med.* 1988;26:309–317.

99. Heim C, Binder EB. Current research trends in early life stress and depression: review of human studies on sensitive periods, gene-environment interactions, and epigenetics. *Exp Neurol.* 2012;233:102–111.

100. Tafet GE, Nemeroff CB. The links between stress and depression: psychoneuroendocrinological, genetic, and environmental interactions. *J Neuropsychiatry Clin Neurosci.* Spring 2016;28(2):77–88.

101. Heim C, Nemeroff CB. The role of childhood trauma in the neurobiology of mood and anxiety disorders: preclinical and clinical studies. *Biol Psychiatry.* 2001;49:1023–1039.

102. Arborelius L, Owens MJ, Plotsky PM, et al. The role of corticotrophin-releasing factor in depression and anxiety disorders. *J Endocrinol.* 1999;160:1–12.

103. Nemeroff CB. Paradise lost: The neurobiological and clinical consequences of child abuse and neglect. *Neuron.* March 2016;89:892–909.

104. Dube SR, Fairweather D, Pearson WS, et al. Cumulative childhood stress and autoimmune disease in adults. *Psychosom Med.* 2009;71:243–250.
105. Wegman HL, Stetler C. A meta-analytic review of the effects of childhood abuse on medical outcomes in adulthood. *Psychosom Med.* 2009;71:805–812.
106. Pace TW, Mletzko TC, Alagbe O, et al. Increased stress-induced inflammatory responses in male patients with major depression and increased early life stress. *Am J Psychiatry.* 2006;163:1630–1633.
107. Danese A, Pariante CM, Caspi A, et al. Childhood maltreatment predicts adult inflammation in a life-course study. *Proc Natl Acad Sci USA.* 2007;104:1319–1324.
108. Danese A, Moffitt TE, Pariante CM, et al. Elevated inflammation levels in depressed adults with a history of childhood maltreatment. *Arch Gen Psychiatry.* 2008;65:409–415.
109. Caspi A, Harrington H, Moffitt TE, et al. Socially isolated children 20 years later: risk of cardiovascular disease. *Arch Paediatr.* 2006;8:805–811.
110. Crosswell AD, Bower JE, Ganz PA. Childhood adversity and inflammation in breast cancer survivors. *Psychosom Med.* 2014;76:208–214.
111. Stankiewicz AM, Swiergiel AH, Lisowski P. Epigenetics of stress adaptations in the brain. *Brain Res Bull.* 2013;98:76–92.
112. McGowan PO, Sasaki A, D'Alessio AC, et al. Epigenetic regulation of the glucocorticoid receptor in human brain associates with childhood abuse. *Nat Neurosci.* 2009;12:342–348.
113. Perroud N, Paoloni-Giacobino A, Prada P, et al. Increased methylation of glucocorticoid receptor gene (*NR3C1*) in adults with a history of childhood maltreatment: a link with the severity and type of trauma. *Transl Psychiatry.* 2011;1;e59.
114. Mannie ZN, Hammer CJ, Cowen PJ. Increased waking salivary cortisol levels in young people at familial risk of depression. *Am J Psychiatry.* 2007;164:617–621.
115. Scherrer JF, Xian H, Bucholz KK, et al. A twin study of depression symptoms, hypertension, and heart disease in middle-aged men. *Psychosom Med.* 2003;65:548–557.
116. Pankow JS, Folsom AR, Cushman M, et al. Familial and genetic determinants of systemic markers of inflammation: the NHLBI family heart study. *Atherosclerosis.* 2001;154:681–690.
117. Holt RIG, Phillips DIW, Jameson KA, Cooper C, Dennison E, Peveler RC. The relationship between depression, anxiety, and cardiovascular disease: Findings from the Hertfordshire Cohort Study. *J Affect Disord.* 2013;150:84–90.
118. Scherrer JF, Garfield LD, Lustman PJ, et al. Antidepressant drug compliance: reduced risk of MI and mortality in depressed patients. *Am J Med.* 2011;124:318–324.
119. Alvarez W, Pickworth KK. Safety of antidepressant drugs in the patient with cardiac disease: a review of the literature. *Pharmacotherapy.* 2003;23(6):754–771.

5

Biological Effects of Depression
Risk for and Occurrence of Stroke

Bradleigh Hayhow and Sergio Starkstein

INTRODUCTION

This chapter examines the bidirectional relationship between depression and stroke. It is now clearly established that depression is a significant risk factor for stroke, and vice-versa. We review the main biological and demographic factors underlying the association between stroke and depression, the predicted mortality, the mechanism of post-stroke depression, and recent findings on its pharmacological prevention. We conclude by stressing the need for developing effective strategies to manage the burden of illness associated with these interacting conditions.

OVERVIEW

Stroke and depression are both highly prevalent disorders that are also entangled in a complex, bidirectional risk relationship. It has long been known that stroke acts as a significant risk factor for depression, but it has more recently become apparent that depression also acts as a risk factor for stroke. Such is the complexity of the relationship that it is not yet clear whether either risk can be effectively modified by primary or secondary prevention; in fact, there is some evidence that in some circumstances, pharmacological treatment could increase risk. There is nevertheless an urgent need to develop an effective management approach to modify the considerable burden of illness associate with these interacting diseases.

This chapter will review relevant biological factors linking depression with cerebrovascular disease in the light of recent advances in genetics and neuroinflammation, and it will also address additional medical factors underlying this association. The first section will address depression as a risk factor for cerebrovascular disease, while the second section will examine the mechanism, clinical correlates, and prevention of post-stroke depression (PSD).

DEPRESSION AS A RISK FACTOR FOR STROKE

Evidence that depression represents an independent risk factor for stroke arises from a number of large, prospective epidemiological studies and several associated meta-analyses. Ostir and co-workers reported that in a prospective cohort of 2,478 older adults, increasing depression scores on the modified version of the Centre for Epidemiological Studies Depression Scale (CES-D) were significantly associated with stroke incidence (risk ratio [RR] = 1.04 for each 1-point increase, 95% confidence interval [CI] 1.01–1.09), even after adjusting for sociodemographic characteristics, blood pressure, body mass index, smoking status, and selected chronic diseases (Ostir, Markides, Peek, Goodwin 2001). This finding was extended by a large French study of 9,294 older adults assessed prospectively over 10 years, in whom each additional study visit with high levels of depressive symptoms (defined as a score >/= 16 on the CES-D) conferred a combined risk of coronary heart disease and stroke events of 1.15 (95% CI 1.06–1.25) (Pequignot et al. 2016). In a different setting, 901 rural Japanese adults followed over 10 years were found to be at significantly increased risk of incident stroke (RR = 1.9, 95% CI 1.1–3.5) if reporting scores within the upper third tertile on the Zung Self-Rating Depression Scale. While total figures included cases of both ischemic and hemorrhagic stroke, sub-group analysis demonstrated a stronger relationship for the former (RR = 2.7, 95% CI = 1.2–6.0) (Ohira et al. 2001). In Denmark, a national retrospective linkage study of hospital discharges found that patients previously hospitalized for depression were at significantly increased risk of cerebrovascular disease (hazard ratio [HR] = 1.22, 95% CI = 1.06–1.41), while those hospitalized for mania or bipolar disorder were not (Nilsson & Kessing 2004).

In a nine-year follow-up population-based matched cohort study of 5,015 patients (1,003 with major depressive disorder and 4,012 controls), Li et al. found significantly higher rates of stroke amongst the depressed subjects (4.3% vs 2.8%, p < 0.05), with greater severity conferring greater risk. The authors also reported the effect to be mediated by the development of major metabolic comorbidities (Li et al. 2012). A 2012 meta-analysis of prospective studies only (involving 206,641 participants) yielded a pooled, risk-adjusted risk estimate for the effect of baseline depression on incident stroke of 1.34 (95% CI 1.17–1.54) (Dong, Zhang, Tong, Qin 2012). An earlier meta-analysis addressing the contribution of depression to stroke morbidity and mortality yielded a pooled estimated hazard ratio of 1.55 (95% CI 1.25–1.93) for fatal stroke, accounting for 22 cases per 100,000 individuals per year (Pan, Sun, Okereke, Rexrode, Hu 2011).

The strongest challenge to the status of depression as a risk factor for stroke comes from the prospective Whitehall II cohort study in which 10,036 participants underwent multiple repeat measures of depression to elicit dose-response and reverse-causation effects in relation to both coronary heart disease and stroke. Over a five-year observational cycle, depression ascertained on serial General Health Questionnaire (GHQ-30) or Centre for Epidemiologic Studies Depression Scale (CES-D) administration predicted coronary heart disease with some evidence of dose-response, but the association of depression with stroke was found to arise wholly or partly through reverse causation (that is, that stroke was causing depression, rather than the other way around) (Brunner et al. 2014).

In conclusion, with few exceptions, most epidemiological studies suggest a strong association between depression and both coronary and cerebrovascular disease. Nevertheless, future studies should investigate the important confounder of reverse causation. We shall now examine potential causes for the association between depression and stroke.

Demographic Considerations

Several studies have drawn attention to the impact of race and gender on the risk of stroke conferred by baseline depression. Hamano and colleagues presented evidence of a stronger association between depression and stroke in men in a large national sample of 137,305 men and 188,924 women attending primary health care centers in Sweden over a period of two years (Hamano et al. 2015). In addition to a combined adjusted odds ratio of 1.22 (95% CI = 1.08–1.38), the greater effect of depression on stroke in men was demonstrated by a difference in the between-gender odds ratio of 1.30 (95% CI 1.01–1.68). A large, cross-sectional prevalence study in China also demonstrated a stronger relationship between depression and stroke in men than in women (Yu et al. 2016).

In the National Health and Nutrition Examination Survey (NHANES) of 6,095 North American adults aged 25–74 over an average follow-up period of 16 years, self-reported depressive symptomatology emerged as significant risk-adjusted predictor of stroke (RR = 1.73, 95% CI = 1.30–2.31). The risk was highest among Afro-American men and women (RR = 2.60, 95% CI = 1.40–4.80), but it was of borderline significance in white women (p = 0.7) (Jonas, Mussolino 2000). Pan and colleagues also found depression to be a significant risk factor for stroke in a prospective six-year cohort study of 80,574 women aged 54–79 years enrolled in the Nurses' Health Study. Current depression was associated with a significantly *increased* risk of stroke of 1.41 (95% CI 1.18–1.67), but historical depression was not. An interesting additional finding was that antidepressant use conferred an increased risk of stroke even in the absence of diagnosed depression or a significant Mental Health Index score (HR 1.31, 95% CI 1.18–1.67). Finally, the Australian Longitudinal Study on Women's Health followed 10,547 women aged 47–52 over a 12-year period. Women with depression demonstrated an odds ratio for stroke of 1.94 (95% CI = 1.37–2.74), with depression having been ascertained via CES-D or recent antidepressant use, and stroke by self-report and mortality data (Jackson, Mishra 2013). These findings challenge the notion that the association between depression and stroke is significant for men only.

Post-Stroke morbidity and mortality: the relevance of depression

In addition to being a risk factor for incident stroke, premorbid depression is associated with increased morbidity and mortality in stroke, and poorer post-stroke recovery. In the large, naturalistic Chichester/Salisbury Catchment Area study, boasting a follow-up period of 40 years, clinically diagnosed depression was found to be a significant risk factor for fatal stroke in men (Thomson 2014). The Multiple Risk Factor Intervention Trail followed 11,216 middle-aged men at high risk of heart disease over a period of 18 years to establish a hazard ratio of 2.03 for stroke mortality (95% CI 1.20–3.44) between subjects scoring in the highest and lowest quintiles of the CES-D, respectively (Gump, Matthews, Eberly, Chang, Group 2005).

Depressive symptoms have also been linked to increased stroke morbidity. In their follow-up study of 240 older adults who reported stroke, heart attack, or hip fracture over the course of six years, Ostir et al. showed that baseline depressive symptoms were associated with poorer recovery in activities of daily living (ADLs) (odds ratio [OR] 0.38, 95% CI = 0.16–0.94 versus non-depressed patients), even after adjustment for socio-demographic characteristics, smoking status, ADLs at time of event, cognitive status, and prior history of disease (Ostir et al. 2002).

In conclusion, there is a significant association between depression and post-stroke increased mortality and morbidity. We shall now review potential mechanisms underlying this association.

Mechanisms Underlying the Association between Depression and Stroke

There are two main hypotheses for the increased risk of stroke in patients with depression. On one hand, there are molecular mechanisms involving proinflammatory and pro-thrombotic effects, and on the other hand, there are increasing data emphasizing the consequences of increased medical comorbidity and poor chronic-disease self-management.

In a small proof-of-concept study, Cassidy and colleagues used flow cytometry to examine platelet glycoproteins involved in early adhesion and aggregation and found a significant increase in glycoprotein 1b (GP1b) amongst both depressed patients and stroke patients versus healthy controls. The increase in GP1b expression between depressed patients and stroke patients was of roughly the same magnitude, and no additive effect was observed in patients with both stroke and depression. The authors hypothesized that platelet dysfunction may therefore contribute to the association between depression and stroke, presumably via a pro-thrombotic pathway (Cassidy et al. 2003).

Rasmussen et al. used a ligand-binding technique and found that platelet serotonin transporter numbers were significantly reduced in acute stroke patients compared to sub-acute stroke patients and healthy controls, but no differences were observed between stroke patients with or without depression (Rasmussen, Christensen, et al. 2003), making the interpretation of the result uncertain.

Depressive symptoms may also influence stroke risk indirectly, for instance through the promotion or exacerbation of medical comorbidity. In a longitudinal study of 2,830 older Mexican American subjects with type 2 diabetes mellitus, Black et al. found that depression was associated with worse diabetes control and increased micro- and macro-vascular complications (Fireman et al. 2003). In general, patients with depression are at an increased risk of wide-range adverse health behaviors and chronic diseases that may in turn lead to cerebrovascular disease. Depressed individuals are more likely to be smokers than their non-depressed peers (Grant, Hasin, Chou, Stinson, Dawson 2004; Lawrence, Mitrou, Zubrick 2009) and have a higher risk of type II diabetes mellitus (Vancampfort et al. 2014), obesity (Stunkard, Faith, Allison 2003) and hypertension (Meng, Chen, Yang, Zheng, Hui 2012). Depressed patients may also suffer from poorer disease self-management and, as a consequence, poorer health outcomes (Ciechanowski, Katon, Russo 2000; Evans et al. 2005). Ultimately, the relationship between psychiatric and medical illness is a complex one, and it remains a daunting task to determine the underlying mechanisms of the interaction.

Treatment and Prevention

There is no specific evidence to support the view that the medical treatment of baseline depression prevents stroke; in fact, the majority of studies examining antidepressant use have demonstrated an increased risk of stroke in patients exposed to antidepressants. The mechanism for this is unclear, but a sub-analysis demonstrated that this association is unrelated to the risk imposed by having an affective disorder. In fact, the association was stronger for individuals without a history of pre-stroke antidepressant use.

Juang et al. followed 16,770 adults enrolled in the National Health Insurance Research Database in Taiwan who suffered incident stroke between 2000 and 2009. Antidepressant use was associated with an increased risk of stroke recurrence for ischemic stroke (HR 1.48, 95% CI 1.28–1.70) only (Juang, Chen, Chien 2015). Interestingly, Wang et al. reported an increase in stroke risk and recurrence associated with tricyclic antidepressant (TCA) use but, more particularly, with its abrupt cessation. The use of any TCA was associated with a risk of stroke recurrence of 1.41 (95% CI 1.19–1.67), and cessation within the past 30 days posed an even greater risk (OR 1.87, 95% CI 1.22–2.86). The mechanism behind this association is unclear, but it is not related to the presence of atrial fibrillation (a potential reason for discontinuation), or depression relapse. No risks were identified in relation to the use of other classes of antidepressants (Wang et al. 2015). In a longitudinal magnetic resonance imaging (MRI) study of 2,559 participants enrolled in the population-based Rotterdam Study, Akoudad and colleagues demonstrated increased cerebral microbleed incidence in patients without imaging-based evidence of microbleeds at baseline who were subsequently exposed to antidepressant medications (OR 2.22, 95% CI 1.31–3.76) (Akoudad et al. 2016). A meta-analysis of 13 studies of selective serotonin reuptake inhibitor (SSRI) use and stroke, incorporating both case-control and cohort designs, demonstrated an increased risk of all stroke types in SSRI users (OR 1.40, 95% CI 1.09–1.80) (Shin, Oh, Eom, Park 2014). Future studies are needed to clarify the mechanism of this association, which is independent of the severity of depression.

On the other hand, a recent study was unable to replicate these findings. Coupland et al. studied of 238,963 patients aged 20–64 years to explore associations between antidepressant exposure and stroke, myocardial infarction, and cardiac arrhythmia. Over a five-year follow-up period, no significant associations were found between antidepressant use and risk of incident stroke or transient ischemic attack (TIA), but neither was a specific protective effect demonstrated (Coupland et al. 2016).

While more studies are needed, there are thus some concerns about the safety of antidepressant exposure in relation to stroke risk and recurrence, and non-pharmacological interventions may be a preferred mode of stroke prevention. On the other hand, the treatment of depression may be an important consideration in its own right, not just in relation to stroke and stroke recovery, but in relation to a wide range of more general health outcomes.

STROKE AS A RISK FACTOR FOR DEPRESSION

Depression is a common neuropsychiatric consequence of stroke, though its frequency is quite variably reported, due to the wide range of diagnostic strategies, care settings, and time points framing its study. In a meta-analysis of 43 studies including 20,293 stroke patients, 11 different methods were used to diagnose depression, with only 13 studies evaluating patients at more than one time point, and only eight studies following patients beyond their first year post-stroke. The pooled prevalence of depression on this analysis was 29% (95% CI = 25–32%), with a cumulative incidence of 39–52% over five years. At 12-month follow-up, the rate of recovery from depression ranged from 15–57% (Ayerbe, Ayis, Wolfe, Rudd 2013). A more recent meta-analysis, conducted by Hackett et al., obtained similar results from a total of 61 studies involving 25,488 stroke patients. While ascertainment remained heterogeneous, the pooled incidence of depression among stroke survivors was 31% (95% CI 28 to 35%), with a prevalence at five years of 23% (95% CI 14 to 31%) (Hackett, Pickles 2014). Notwithstanding the methodological issues, it therefore seems that about one third of stroke patients experience incident depression during the early phases of stroke, and about one quarter still have prevalent disease at five years post-stroke. Because of the considerable morbidity and mortality this confers, it is important to understand the factors contributing both to the risk of post-stroke depression, and to subsequent recovery from it.

Demographic Considerations

A range of risk factors has been proposed for the development of depression after stroke, and several groups have conducted systematic reviews considering factors such as age, gender, past history of depression, stroke severity, degree of functional impairment, and level of family and social support (De Ryck et al. 2014; Hackett, Anderson 2005; Johnson, Minarik, Nystrom, Bautista, Gorman 2006; Kutlubaev, Hackett 2014). In the most recent systematic review, Kutlubaev and Hackett included data from 23 studies involving 18,374 patients to examine predictors of depression after stroke (Kutlubaev, Hackett 2014). Once again, there was considerable methodological heterogeneity. While 8/18 studies reported female gender and 3/16 reported older age to be associated with post-stroke depression, no consistent relationship was demonstrated on review. Stroke hemisphere, lesion location, and pathological subtype were also dismissed as risk factors. A personal history of depression was associated with later post-stroke depression in 4/7 studies, and cognitive impairment was associated with depression in 2/4 studies. The strongest predictors of post-stroke depression were found to be stroke severity (4/6 studies), early physical disability (4/5 studies), and later functional disability (mild–moderate 5/5, major 7/8). These findings were consistent with previous systematic reviews, although a near-contemporaneous review of 24 studies by De Ryck and colleagues described additional associations with family history of depression, comorbid diabetes mellitus, high levels of alcohol consumption in men, and living situations both before and after stroke onset (De Ryck et al. 2014). Somewhat surprisingly, no relationship between cardiovascular disease and post-stroke depression was demonstrated in any of the investigated studies. The authors also draw attention to the fact that while aphasia has often been an exclusion criterion in post-stroke depression research, it has also been proposed as an important risk factor that may warrant further investigation (Johnson et al. 2006).

Morbidity and Mortality of Post-Stroke Depression (PSD)

Post-stroke depression is associated with increase in both short- and long-term stroke mortality. Morris and coworkers were the first to examine mortality rates among a consecutive series of 103 patients assessed 10 years after their stroke. After controlling for confounding variables such as age, stroke severity, and coexistent medical conditions, the authors found that patients meeting *Diagnostic and Statistical Manual of Mental Disorders III* (DSM-III) criteria for depression within the first two weeks of their stroke were approximately three times more likely to have died during the follow-up period than patients who were not depressed (Morris, Robinson, Andrezejewski, Samuels, Price, 1993). The association between post-stroke depression and increased mortality was supported by the results of a retrospective analysis of 51,119 U.S. veterans hospitalized for ischemic stroke between 1990 and 1998 (Williams, Ghose, Swindle 2004). House and colleagues conducted a more robust study of mortality in a prospective cohort of 448 stroke patients enrolled in a randomized controlled trial of psychological therapy for post-stroke depression. They reported significant associations between depressive symptoms at one month post-stroke and subsequent mortality at both 12 and 24 months, with an odds ratio of 2.4 (95% CI = 1.3–4.5 and 1.4–4.1 respectively) at both time points. More recently, Ayerbe et al. reviewed epidemiological data obtained from 271,817 patients included in the South London Register from 1997–2010 (Ayerbe, Ayis, Crichton, Wolfe, Rudd 2014). They found that at three months post-stroke, depression was significantly associated with mortality (HR = 1.27, 95% CI = 1.04–1.55), disability (RR = 4.71, 95% CI = 2.96–7.48), anxiety (OR = 3.49, 95% CI = 1.71.7.12), and poorer quality of life (OR = 11.36, 95% CI = 14.86–7.85) up to Year 5 follow-up.

Potential Mechanisms of Post-Stroke Depression

Little is known about the specific mechanism of post-stroke depression, but several neuro-anatomical, neurophysiological, and genetic hypotheses have been advanced. In sympathy with hypotheses relating to idiopathic depression, a common hypothesis for post-stroke depression proposes the impingement of stroke lesions on ascending monoaminergic pathways as a possible mechanism (Robinson 2006). Mayberg and co-workers used the serotonergic PET ligand N-methyl-spiperone to demonstrate that stroke lesions arising in the right hemisphere produce a significantly higher ratio of ipsilateral-to-contralateral spiperone binding in uninjured temporal and parietal cortex than stroke lesions arising in the left hemisphere (Mayberg et al. 1988). Because they observed a significant inverse correlation between depression scores and spiperone binding in the left temporal cortex, the authors hypothesized that greater monoamine depletion in patients with right hemisphere lesions may result in compensatory upregulation of serotonin receptors, whereas a loss of upregulation with left hemisphere lesions could lead to left temporal dysfunction, resulting in depression. Evidence for more general serotonergic dysfunction in patients with post-stroke depression also includes the attenuated prolactin response observed in stroke patients treated with d-fenfluramine (a marker of serotonergic function) (Ramasubbu et al. 1998) and the finding that patients with polymorphisms of the serotonin transporter gene (specifically the *5-HTTLPR* and the *STin2 VNTR*) are three to four times more likely to have depression after stroke than patients with a different genotype (Kohen et al. 2008).

There is also preliminary evidence from magnetic resonance spectroscopy that glutamate levels in the anterior cingulate cortex are altered in depressed stroke patients (Glodzik-Sobanska et al. 2006). On the other hand, meta-analyses and systematic reviews have generally failed to demonstrate a reliable association between stroke lesion location and depression risk (De Ryck et al. 2014; Johnson et al. 2006; Kutlubaev, Hackett 2014), with the most recent review of 43 studies involving 5,507 stroke patients reporting an odds ratio of 0.99 (95% CI 0.88–1.11) (Wei et al. 2015).

Alexopolous and colleagues have proposed the more general hypothesis that chronic cerebrovascular disease may lead to depression via the progressive disruption of the cortico-subcortical circuits regulating mood via connections between the prefrontal cortex, basal ganglia, and limbic areas (Alexopoulos et al. 1997). Supporting evidence comes from Tang and colleagues, who found severe white matter hyper intensities to be associated with post-stroke depression in a case control study of 992 patients admitted to a hospital in Hong Kong with acute ischemic stroke (Tang et al. 2010). Autonomic dysfunction may also play a role in the mechanism of post-stroke depression, as Robinson and colleagues found that patients with post-stroke depression had decreased heart rate variability compared to non-depressed stroke patients (Robinson et al. 2010).

Because cerebral ischemia is associated with an increased production of proinflammatory cytokines, the inflammatory changes elicited by stroke and their downstream effects of neurogenesis have also been proposed as potential mediators of post-stroke depression. Patients with severe post-stroke depression have been found to exhibit significantly increased levels of the inflammatory cytokine interleukin-18 (IL-18) (Bossu et al. 2009) and the inflammatory marker leptin (Jimenez et al. 2009), and both human and animal studies suggest that proinflammatory cytokines alter hypothalamus-pituitary-adrenal (HPA) axis reactivity, decrease neurogenesis and plasticity in hippocampal circuits, and reduce serotonergic transmission (Feng, Fang, Liu 2014). In support of the crucial role of post-stroke neurogenesis and neuroplasticity, Yang and colleagues observes a significant reduction in brain-derived neurotrophic factor (BDNF) in patients with post-stroke depression (Yang et al. 2011), while Kim and colleagues have associated post-stroke depression with increased BDNF gene methylation status (Kim et al. 2013). The elucidation of additional epigenetic factors in the mechanism of post-stroke depression represents a promising avenue for future research.

PREVENTION OF POST-STROKE DEPRESSION

Recently, increased attention has been provided to the possibility of preventing PSD using psychoactive medication. Palomaki and colleagues (Palomaki et al., 1999) carried out a randomized controlled trial (RCT) using mianserin (60 mg/day) as the active treatment in a series of 100 consecutive acute-stroke patients recruited and treated during one year. The main result was a lack of difference in the frequency of major depression between patients on mianserin and placebo-treated patients at any time point. Narushima et al. compared the effect of nortriptyline vs. fluoxetine to prevent PSD in a series of 48 non-depressed patients with acute stroke. Patients were treated for three months and had an additional 21 months follow-up. The authors' main finding was that both nortriptyline and fluoxetine were effective in preventing depression after stroke among patients who completed the treatment trial. However, after stopping the antidepressants, there was an increase in both the frequency and the severity of depressive symptoms, particularly among nortriptyline-treated patients (Narushima, Kosier, Robinson 2002). Rasmussen and colleagues have also examined the effect of sertraline in the prevention of PSD among 137 non-depressed patients with an ischemic stroke who were randomly assigned to 12 months of double-blind treatment with either active drug (n = 70) or placebo (n = 67). The main finding was that sertraline had superior prophylactic efficacy compared to placebo, with approximately 10% of the sertraline-treated group developing depression, compared to 30% in the placebo group. Treatment was well tolerated, and patients experienced few adverse events (Rasmussen, Lunde, et al. 2003). A contrasting finding was reported by Almeida and colleagues, who randomly assigned 111 acute stroke patients to treatment with placebo (n = 56) or sertraline (n = 55, 50 mg once daily). There was no significant difference in the frequency of depressive symptoms during 24 weeks of treatment (17% sertraline vs. 22% placebo) (Almeida, Waterreus, Hankey 2006). A major limitation of this study, however, was the relatively short follow-up period.

In a multi-site RCT, Robinson and colleagues recruited 176 non-depressed patients within three months following acute stroke who were followed up over 12 months. Patients were randomized to receive escitalopram (n = 59), placebo (n = 58), or a non-blinded problem-solving therapy group (n = 59). Patients on placebo were significantly more likely to develop depression than individuals on either escitalopram (adjusted hazard ratio [HR], 4.5; P < .001) or problem-solving therapy (adjusted HR, 2.2; P < .001). These results remained significant after adjusting for history of mood disorders, age, gender, treatment site, and severity of impairment (Robinson et al. 2008). A meta-analysis including eight randomized-controlled trials for the prevention of PSD using SSRIs found a reduced likelihood of developing PSD after a one-year treatment (Salter, Foley, Zhu, Jutai, Teasell 2013).

Hackett and co-workers carried out a systematic review of the efficacy of psychotherapy in preventing PSD (Hackett, Anderson, House, Halteh 2008). Outcome data were analyzed from four trials including 902 participants with interventions including supportive psychotherapy, cognitive behavior therapy, problem-solving therapy, and motivational interviewing. Treatment duration varied from four weeks to one year. All of the studies used "standard care" as a comparator, and one study also included an "attention-control group," in which subjects spent time in focused conversation with a trained therapist, but did not receive structured psychotherapy. Pooled results demonstrated a small effect for the prevention of depression as well as an improvement in psychological distress scores. There was no evidence for improved functional outcome, although fewer subjects reported adverse events in the intervention groups compared to controls. One major limitation with these reviews and meta-analyses is that they compare studies with important methodological differences, such as treatment agent, time since stroke, duration of treatment, assessment methods, and outcome measures.

EFFECTS OF ANTIDEPRESSANTS ON STROKE RECOVERY

Common antidepressants are pleiotropic substances that have other effects than the ones related to mood regulation. They may certainly influence neuroplasticity and inflammatory responses elicited by stroke and, consequently, affect recovery. A systematic review and meta-analysis of 52 RCTs including 4,059 patients suggest that antidepressants improve rehabilitation outcomes (Hackett, Anderson, House, Xia 2008). More recently, it has been shown that fluoxetine enhances motor recovery following cerebral ischemia, an effect that is considered to be unrelated to depression (Chollet et al. 2011), and several studies reported beneficial effects of antidepressants on memory function (Jorge, Acion, Moser, Adams, Robinson 2010), disability (Mikami et al. 2011), and mortality following stroke (Jorge, Robinson, Arndt, Starkstein 2003).

CONCLUSION

Important aspects of the association between depression and cerebrovascular disease were reviewed. First, the evidence for depression as a risk factor for stroke was reviewed. Most studies to date have found that depression is a significant predictor of stroke, and several mechanisms have been proposed, such as pro-thrombotic and proinflammatory effects, as well as increased clinical morbidity. The epidemiology, underlying mechanisms, and prevention of PSD were examined. There is strong consensus that stroke is associated with depression, which has a highly negative impact on the morbidity of stroke and is also related to increased mortality. Recent studies have examined a variety of potential mechanisms for PSD, and the main findings include autonomic dysfunction and abnormalities in noradrenergic and glutamatergic neurotransmission, inflammatory systems, and neuroplasticity.

The prevention of PSD remains an open question, although there is evidence in favor of using SSRIs. Future studies will hopefully unravel the mechanism of PSD and guide the prophylactic treatment on solid physiopathological bases.

REFERENCES

Akoudad S, Aarts N, Noordam R, et al. Antidepressant use is associated with an increased risk of developing microbleeds. *Stroke.* 2016;47(1):251–254. doi:10.1161/STROKEAHA.115.011574

Alexopoulos GS, Meyers BS, Young RC, Campbell S, Silbersweig D, Charlson M. "Vascular depression" hypothesis. *Arch Gen Psychiatry.* 1997;54(10):915–922.

Almeida OP, Waterreus A, Hankey GJ. Preventing depression after stroke: results from a randomized placebo-controlled trial. *J Clin Psychiatry.* 2006;67(7):1104–1109.

Ayerbe L, Ayis S, Crichton S, Wolfe CD, Rudd AG. The long-term outcomes of depression up to 10 years after stroke; the South London Stroke Register. *J Neurol Neurosurg Psychiatry.* 2014;85(5):514–521. doi:10.1136/jnnp-2013-306448

Ayerbe L, Ayis S, Wolfe CD, Rudd AG. Natural history, predictors and outcomes of depression after stroke: systematic review and meta-analysis. *Br J Psychiatry.* 2013;202(1):14–21. doi:10.1192/bjp.bp.111.107664

Bossu P, Salani, F, Cacciari C, et al. Disease outcome, alexithymia and depression are differently associated with serum IL-18 levels in acute stroke. *Curr Neurovasc Res.* 2009;6(3):163–170.

Brunner EJ, Shipley MJ, Britton AR, et al. Depressive disorder, coronary heart disease, and stroke: dose-response and reverse causation effects in the Whitehall II cohort study. *Eur J Prev Cardiol.* 2014;21(3):340–346. doi:10.1177/2047487314520785

Cassidy EM, Walsh MT, O'Connor R, et al. Platelet surface glycoprotein expression in post-stroke depression: a preliminary study. *Psychiatry Res*. 2003;118(2):175–181.

Chollet F, Tardy J, Albucher JF, et al. Fluoxetine for motor recovery after acute ischaemic stroke (FLAME): a randomised placebo-controlled trial. *Lancet Neurol*. 2011;10(2):123–130. doi:10.1016/S1474-4422(10)70314-8

Ciechanowski PS, Katon WJ, Russo JE. Depression and diabetes: impact of depressive symptoms on adherence, function, and costs. *Arch Intern Med*. 2000;160(21):3278–3285.

Coupland C, Hill T, Morriss R, Moore M, Arthur A, Hippisley-Cox J. Antidepressant use and risk of cardiovascular outcomes in people aged 20 to 64: cohort study using primary care database. *BMJ*. 2016;352:i1350. doi:10.1136/bmj.i1350

De Ryck A, Brouns R, Geurden M, Elseviers M, De Deyn PP, Engelborghs S. Risk factors for poststroke depression: identification of inconsistencies based on a systematic review. *J Geriatr Psychiatry Neurol*. 2014;27(3):147–158. doi:10.1177/0891988714527514

Dong JY, Zhang YH, Tong J, Qin LQ. Depression and risk of stroke: a meta-analysis of prospective studies. *Stroke*. 2012;43(1):32–37. doi:10.1161/STROKEAHA.111.630871

Evans DL, Charney DS, Lewis L, et al. Mood disorders in the medically ill: scientific review and recommendations. *Biol Psychiatry*. 2005;58(3):175–189. doi:10.1016/j.biopsych.2005.05.001

Feng C, Fang M, Liu XY. The neurobiological pathogenesis of poststroke depression. *Sci World J*. 2014; 521349. doi:10.1155/2014/521349

Fireman B, Black SB, Shinefield HR, Lee J, Lewis E, Ray P. Impact of the pneumococcal conjugate vaccine on otitis media. *Pediatr Infect Dis J*. 2003;22(1):10–16. doi:10.1097/01.inf.0000045221.96634.7c

Glodzik-Sobanska L, Slowik A, McHugh P, et al. Single voxel proton magnetic resonance spectroscopy in post-stroke depression. *Psychiatry Res*. 2006;148(2–3):111–120. doi:10.1016/j.pscychresns.2006.08.004

Grant BF, Hasin DS, Chou SP, Stinson FS, Dawson DA. Nicotine dependence and psychiatric disorders in the United States: results from the National Epidemiologic Survey on Alcohol and Related Conditions. *Arch Gen Psychiatry*. 2004;61(11):1107–1115. doi:10.1001/archpsyc.61.11.1107

Gump BB, Matthews KA, Eberly LE, Chang YF, Group MR. Depressive symptoms and mortality in men: results from the Multiple Risk Factor Intervention Trial. *Stroke*. 2005;36(1):98–102. doi:10.1161/01.STR.0000149626.50127.d0

Hackett ML, Anderson CS. Predictors of depression after stroke: a systematic review of observational studies. *Stroke*. 2005;36(10):2296–2301.

Hackett ML, Anderson CS, House A, Halteh C. Interventions for preventing depression after stroke. *Cochrane Database Syst Rev*. 2008(3):CD003689. doi:10.1002/14651858.CD003689.pub3

Hackett ML, Anderson CS, House A, Xia J. Interventions for treating depression after stroke. *Cochrane Database Syst Rev*. 2008(4):CD003437. doi:10.1002/14651858.CD003437.pub3

Hackett ML, Pickles K. Part I: frequency of depression after stroke: an updated systematic review and meta-analysis of observational studies. *Int J Stroke*. 2014;9(8):1017–1025. doi:10.1111/ijs.12357

Hamano T, Li X, Lonn SL, et al. Depression, stroke and gender: evidence of a stronger association in men. *J Neurol Neurosurg Psychiatry*. 2015;86(3):319–323. doi:10.1136/jnnp-2014-307616

Jackson CA, Mishra GD. Depression and risk of stroke in middle-aged women: a prospective longitudinal study. *Stroke*. 2013;44(6):1555–1560. doi:10.1161/STROKEAHA.113.001147

Jimenez I, Sobrino T, Rodriguez-Yanez M, et al. High serum levels of leptin are associated with post-stroke depression. *Psychol Med*. 2009;39(7):1201–1209. doi:10.1017/S0033291709005637

Johnson JL, Minarik PA, Nystrom KV, Bautista C, Gorman MJ. Poststroke depression incidence and risk factors: an integrative literature review. *J Neurosci Nurs*. 2006;38(4 Suppl):316–327.

Jonas BS, Mussolino ME. Symptoms of depression as a prospective risk factor for stroke. *Psychosom Med.* 2000;62(4):463–471.

Jorge RE, Acion L, Moser D, Adams HP Jr., Robinson RG. Escitalopram and enhancement of cognitive recovery following stroke. *Arch Gen Psychiatry.* 2010;67(2):187–196. doi:10.1001/archgenpsychiatry.2009.185

Jorge RE, Robinson RG, Arndt S, Starkstein S. Mortality and poststroke depression: a placebo-controlled trial of antidepressants. *Am J Psychiatry.* 2003;160(10):1823–1829.

Juang HT, Chen PC, Chien KL. Using antidepressants and the risk of stroke recurrence: report from a national representative cohort study. *BMC Neurol.* 2015;15:86. doi:10.1186/s12883-015-0345-x

Kim JM, Stewart R, Kang HJ, et al. A longitudinal study of BDNF promoter methylation and genotype with poststroke depression. *J Affect Disord.* 2013;149(1–3):93–99. doi:10.1016/j.jad.2013.01.008

Kohen R, Cain KC, Mitchell PH, et al. Association of serotonin transporter gene polymorphisms with poststroke depression. *Arch Gen Psychiatry.* 2008;65(11):1296–1302. doi:10.1001/archpsyc.65.11.1296

Kutlubaev MA, Hackett ML. Part II: predictors of depression after stroke and impact of depression on stroke outcome: an updated systematic review of observational studies. *Int J Stroke.* 2014;9(8):1026–1036. doi:10.1111/ijs.12356

Lawrence D, Mitrou F, Zubrick SR. Smoking and mental illness: results from population surveys in Australia and the United States. *BMC Public Health.* 2009;9:285. doi:10.1186/1471-2458-9-285

Li CT, Bai YM, Tu PC, et al. Major depressive disorder and stroke risks: a 9-year follow-up population-based, matched cohort study. *PLoS One.* 2012;7(10):e46818. doi:10.1371/journal.pone.0046818

Mayberg HS, Robinson RG, Wong DF, et al. PET imaging of cortical S2 serotonin receptors after stroke: lateralized changes and relationship to depression. *Am J Psychiatry.* 1988;145(8):937–943.

Meng L, Chen D, Yang Y, Zheng Y, Hui R. Depression increases the risk of hypertension incidence: a meta-analysis of prospective cohort studies. *J Hypertens.* 2012;30(5):842–851. doi:10.1097/HJH.0b013e32835080b7

Mikami K, Jorge RE, Adams HP Jr., et al. Effect of antidepressants on the course of disability following stroke. *Am J Geriatr Psychiatry.* 2011;19(12):1007–1015. doi:10.1097/JGP.0b013e31821181b0

Morris PL, Robinson RG, Andrezejewski P, Samuels J, Price TR. Association of depression with 10-year post-stroke mortality. *Stroke.* 1993;150:124–129.

Narushima K, Kosier JT, Robinson RG. Preventing poststroke depression: a 12-week double-blind randomized treatment trial and 21-month follow-up. *J Nerv Ment Dis.* 2002;190(5):296–303.

Nilsson FM, Kessing LV. Increased risk of developing stroke for patients with major affective disorder—a registry study. *Eur Arch Psychiatry Clin Neurosci.* 2004;254(6):387–391. doi:10.1007/s00406-004-0519-9

Ohira T, Iso H, Satoh S, et al. Prospective study of depressive symptoms and risk of stroke among Japanese. *Stroke.* 2001;32(4):903–908.

Ostir GV, Goodwin JS, Markides KS, Ottenbacher KJ, Balfour J, Guralnik JM. Differential effects of premorbid physical and emotional health on recovery from acute events. *J Am Geriatr Soc.* 2002;50(4):713–718.

Ostir GV, Markides KS, Peek MK, Goodwin JS. The association between emotional well-being and the incidence of stroke in older adults. *Psychosom Med.* 2001;63(2):210–215.

Palomaki H, Kaste M, Berg A, et al. Prevention of poststroke depression: 1 year randomised placebo controlled double blind trial of mianserin with 6 month follow up after therapy. *J Neurol Neurosurg Psychiatry.* 1999;66(4):490–494.

Pan A, Sun Q, Okereke OI, Rexrode KM, Hu FB. Depression and risk of stroke morbidity and mortality: a meta-analysis and systematic review. *JAMA.* 2011;306(11):1241–1249. doi:10.1001/jama.2011.1282

Pequignot R, Dufouil C, Prugger C, et al. High level of depressive symptoms at repeated study visits and risk of coronary heart disease and stroke over 10 years in older adults: the Three-City Study. *J Am Geriatr Soc.* 2016;64(1):118–125. doi:10.1111/jgs.13872

Ramasubbu R, Flint A, Brown G, et al. Diminished serotonin-mediated prolactin responses in non-depressed stroke patients compared with healthy normal subjects. *Stroke.* 1998;29(7):1293–1298.

Rasmussen A, Christensen J, Clemmensen PM, et al. Platelet serotonin transporter in stroke patients. *Acta Neurol Scand.* 2003;107(2):150–153.

Rasmussen A, Lunde M, Poulsen DL, Sorensen K, Qvitzau S, Bech P. A double-blind, placebo-controlled study of sertraline in the prevention of depression in stroke patients. *Psychosomatics.* 2003;44(3):216–221.

Robinson RG. *The clinical neuropsychiatry of stroke* (2nd ed.). Cambridge; New York: Cambridge University Press; 2006.

Robinson RG, Jorge RE, Moser DJ, et al. Escitalopram and problem-solving therapy for prevention of poststroke depression: a randomized controlled trial. *JAMA.* 2008;299(20):2391–2400.

Robinson RG, Spaletta G, Jorge RE, et al. Decreased heart rate variability is associated with poststroke depression. *Am J Geriatr Psychiatry.* 2008;16(11):867–873. doi:10.1097/JGP.0b013e318180057d

Salter KL, Foley NC, Zhu L, Jutai JW, Teasell RW. Prevention of poststroke depression: does prophylactic pharmacotherapy work? *J Stroke Cerebrovasc Dis.* 2013;22(8):1243–1251. doi:10.1016/j.jstrokecerebrovasdis.2012.03.013

Shin D, Oh YH, Eom CS, Park SM. Use of selective serotonin reuptake inhibitors and risk of stroke: a systematic review and meta-analysis. *J Neurol.* 2014;261(4):686–695. doi:10.1007/s00415-014-7251-9

Stunkard AJ, Faith MS, Allison KC. Depression and obesity. *Biol Psychiatry.* 2003;54(3):330–337.

Tang WK, Chen YK, Lu JY, et al. White matter hyperintensities in post-stroke depression: a case control study. *J Neurol Neurosurg Psychiatry.* 2010;81(12):1312–1315. doi:10.1136/jnnp.2009.203141

Thomson W. Rate of stroke death after depression: a 40-year longitudinal study extension of Chichester/Salisbury Catchment Area study. *J Stroke Cerebrovasc Dis.* 2014;23(7):1837–1842. doi:10.1016/j.jstrokecerebrovasdis.2014.03.013

Vancampfort D, Correll CU, Wampers M, et al. Metabolic syndrome and metabolic abnormalities in patients with major depressive disorder: a meta-analysis of prevalences and moderating variables. *Psychol Med.* 2014;44(10):2017–2028. doi:10.1017/S0033291713002778

Wang MT, Chu CL, Yeh CB, Chang LC, Malone DC, Liou JT. Antidepressant use and risk of recurrent stroke: a population-based nested case-control study. *J Clin Psychiatry.* 2015;76(7):e877–e885. doi:10.4088/JCP.14m09134

Wei N, Yong W, Li X, et al. Post-stroke depression and lesion location: a systematic review. *J Neurol.* 2015;262(1):81–90. doi:10.1007/s00415-014-7534-1

Williams LS, Ghose SS, Swindle RW. Depression and other mental health diagnoses increase mortality risk after ischemic stroke. *Am J Psychiatry.* 2004;161(6):1090–1095.

Yang L, Zhang Z, Sun D, et al. Low serum BDNF may indicate the development of PSD in patients with acute ischemic stroke. *Int J Geriatr Psychiatry.* 2011;26(5):495–502. doi:10.1002/gps.2552

Yu CQ, Chen YP, Lv J, et al. [Major depressive disorder in relation with coronary heart disease and stroke in Chinese adults aged 30–79 years]. *Beijing Da Xue Xue Bao.* 2016;48(3):465–471.

6

Depression and Cancer

Daniel C. McFarland and Jimmie Holland

INTRODUCTION

This chapter coalesces broad, sweeping epidemiological data with the potential underlying biological constructs of depression as a systemic disease in the context of cancer. It attempts to look at depression from this broader view, informing how depression as a systemic disease may impact and interact with cancer. It is clear, in the converse, that having cancer leads to sadness, depressed mood, and existential concerns about life, and if depression worsens, then the physical symptoms of fatigue, asthenia, slow cognition, and apathy develop, which constitute a major depressive episode. It is this more severe form of depression, composed of both mental and physical symptoms, that is the focus of this chapter. The less severe forms of adjustment disorders and sub-syndromal depression are responses to illness and are common experiences for patients who are adapting to the cancer diagnosis and its treatments.

At present, data do not support a malignant transformation potential resulting from depression or other emotional states, including grief.[1] However, current research suggests that depression, along with many other factors, may play a role in the metastatic progression of cancer mediated by the nervous system and the cancer environment (i.e., tumor stroma).[2] At an epidemiological level, there are tantalizing data to suggest that the manifestations of depression such as social isolation and poor social support are associated with worse survival in the cancer setting.[3]

Specifically, the chapter reviews several putative mechanisms of biologically based depression in the cancer setting: (1) the cytokine hypothesis, (2) hypothalamic-pituitary-adrenal (HPA) dysregulation, (3) abnormal diurnal cortisol rhythms, (4) glucocorticoid dysregulation, (5) enhanced sympathetic nervous system adrenergic activity, and (6) alterations in DNA protein products through transcription/epigenetics.

Depression in the cancer setting has provided substantial insights into the biological basis of cancer through the small but growing field of psychoneuroimmunology. Technological advances in cancer (e.g., those that harness the immune system) and continued work in discovering the epigenetic imprint of social factors associated with depression promise to further elucidate this overlapping relationship.

HISTORICAL OVERVIEW

The association between depression and cancer runs deep. Although both were elegantly described early on, their enigmatic roots have conjured up many fantasies in the public imagination. The Greeks astutely identified the mysteriously hardened crab-like shell that forms just beneath the skin of those with advanced cancers.[4] Once present, it meant death. But what was its cause? Similarly, depression was beautifully described in Robert Burton's *Anatomy of Melancholy* in 1621, and its origins were attributed to one of the four "humors," black bile.[5] It was equally without a known cause or treatment. It is easy to imagine how both have inspired fear and stigma.

For centuries, societies around the globe have stigmatized both diseases. In fact, in some countries where education is still limited, these fears linger on and often lead to a delay in or absence of treatment. There has been a long-held assumption that depression causes cancer. Theories have continued to inspire popular ideas that stress or depression cause cancer, leading to alternative anti-cancer approaches, such as (1) relinquishing bad emotions that caused the malignant transformation of cancer cells, or (2) enhancing the immune system to fight against cancer by imagining it shooting bullets at cancer cells. In fact, the absence of adequate tools to quantifiably measure mental states made it difficult to study the psychological aspects of cancer. This area of research, psychoneuroimmunology, has been slow to develop, but it is presently growing in stature with high-quality research studies that have laid to rest many of these initial theories, which initially led to enhanced societal fears of cancer and depression.

OVERVIEW OF DEPRESSION IN CANCER

Depression in the Context of Psycho-Oncology

Patients and their families experience recurrent emotional turmoil in the setting of cancer. The majority of depression in cancer comes on insidiously and is normalized by healthcare professionals. Therefore, it is frequently not recognized, nor treated in a timely fashion. Perhaps this is surprising, given that depression is universally common, accounting for the majority of worldwide health morbidity, and even more common in patients with cancer. The prevalence of psychiatric disorders is now recognized in approximately 30–60% of patients newly diagnosed with various types of cancer.[6–8] The consequences of untreated depression in cancer have been shown to lead to multiple adverse outcomes. Apart from the mental suffering that it imposes, depression has major implications for both morbidity and possibly mortality in cancer.[9]

Comorbid depression with cancer leads to worsened quality of life, increased sensitivity to pain, difficulties with treatment, communication difficulties, caregiver burnout, increased risk of suicide, longer periods of hospitalization, and a reduced expectation of survival.[9–13] Psychological disturbances may present at any time during the cancer trajectory, but they tend to occur with increased frequency at certain points: at diagnosis; with cancer recurrence or progression; and during advanced cancer states or even survivorship.[14,15] Some barriers for oncology clinicians to making an initial psychological or psychiatric diagnosis include inadequate training or interview skills, a low index of suspicion or awareness of common mental health complications of cancer, and a perceived lack of time.[6] At the same time, it is important to understand other potential reasons for not addressing these issues in the cancer setting: underestimating the prevalence of depressive symptoms; expectations that all patients will be depressed and therefore depressive symptoms are normalized; and having difficulty exploring emotional symptoms.[16,17] Psychological reactions to cancer should be recognized and assessed for underlying psychiatric morbidity and treated according to existing guidelines and patients' preferences. This effort often requires working collaboratively with patients' primary oncologists and other providers. The need for integrating psychosocial care within oncology settings is increasingly recognized.

Depressive disorders result in a spectrum of symptoms, severity, and dysfunction. In the cancer setting, the diagnosis is more difficult because adapting to losses related to illness is difficult to distinguish from depressive symptoms. Understanding the prevalence of depression in cancer is limited by our understanding of depression in general. In the layperson's parlance, "depression" can mean anything from a transient depressed mood to severe psychotic depression leading to suicide. As an illness, it can be conceptualized as either a dimension (e.g., a symptom spectrum) or a category (e.g., a disorder). Both conceptualizations are helpful in understanding depression. Specific depression criteria in medically ill patients, such as the Cavanaugh or Endicott criteria, have been examined and may be helpful for identifying depression in the cancer setting, although they are not frequently used.[18] In addition, several other barriers exist for diagnosing depression in the cancer context, including the following: the myth that all cancer patients are depressed; difficulty distinguishing between depression and normal sadness; misconception that depression is a normal part of the disease process; and the clinician's fear of fully exploring psychological symptoms at a vulnerable time.[19]

In recognition of this diagnostic problem, "distress screening" is now used early in the course of treatment to capture patients who are at greater risk of psychological complications and poorer coping. Screening is now mandated by the American College of Surgeon's Commission on Cancer as an accreditation requirement of cancer centers across the United States. The seamless management of psychological issues in the context of routine cancer care is the goal of collaborative or integrated care in psycho-oncology.

The psychosocial science of oncology has advanced in the past 20–30 years so that it now positively influences the routine practice of oncology. In 1996, the National Comprehensive Cancer Network (NCCN) assembled a multidisciplinary panel to explore ways to integrate psychosocial care into routine treatment. The panel recognized that discourse between patients and an oncologist about "psychiatric problems" was awkward and often avoided by both parties to reduce stigma. It was recognized that "distress" is present in all patients with cancer and is acceptable to patients as a non-psychiatric term. Thus, "distress" serves as an umbrella term for the range of emotional problems that arise during a patient's illness and his or her existential fears related to death. Distress covers the range of responses from the "normal" fear, worry, and anxiety in adapting to cancer, to formally defined psychiatric disorders, including depression. In 2008, the Institute of Medicine's report *Cancer Care for the Whole Patient: Meeting Psychosocial Health Needs* noted a sufficient evidence base for both psychosocial and psychopharmacological interventions to issue a policy statement that quality cancer care must integrate psychosocial treatments into routine cancer treatment.[20] The International Psycho-Oncology Society

(IPOS) and the International Union Against Cancer (UICC) have endorsed *distress* as the sixth vital sign, after pain. In fact, distress screening has been an important step forward in assuring the integration of psychological care in the oncology setting.

In the setting of cancer, the line between psychological reactions that are normal and abnormal is often difficult to draw and is not sufficiently studied. Sadness and worry are normal distressed responses to cancer and can even be helpful for some people who take steps to reduce their anxiety (e.g., information seeking, seeking out social supports) or deal with their sadness (e.g., take stock of what is important to them). An emotional reaction to a stressor out of proportion to the expected is an *adjustment disorder*. It is by far the most commonly diagnosed psychiatric disorder in patients with cancer and often occurs with anxiety.[6]

The recognition and treatment of comorbid distress and depression in accordance with clinical practice guidelines is required for oncology practice of the highest measure.[21] Collaboration with the primary oncology team and a deep clinical understanding of the interplay between cancer biology and the influence of anti-cancer treatments and depressive symptoms inclusive of a major depressive episode are central to delivering quality psychosocial cancer care.

EXPLORING THE ASSOCIATION OF DEPRESSION WITH CANCER

Prevalence of Depression

Depression is the most frequent psychological problem found throughout the cancer trajectory, though there are differences associated with sex, age, cancer type, and even the economic aspects of treatment.[22,23] Depression is more common in patients with pancreatic (33–50%), oropharyngeal (22–57%), breast (4.5–46%) and lung (11–44%) cancers.[24] The reason is not clear as to whether these tumors cause more distress or whether they are tumor-related responses, which include depressive symptoms. The "sickness behavior" model in animals is comparable.[25] This issue has been raised most often with pancreatic cancer.[26] Also, varying criteria used to define and measure depression, along with disparate cancer populations of study (e.g., diagnosis and stage, hospitalization status, time since diagnosis) account for tremendous variability in prevalence.[27,28]

A recent meta-analysis of 70 studies (*n* = 10,071) reported a 16.3% prevalence of all types of depression (minor, major [*Diagnostic and Statistical Manual* {DSM} and *International Classification of Diseases* {ICD}] criteria) and a 6% prevalence of major depressive episode (MDE) in cancer settings.[6] However, the prevalence of depressive symptoms rises for patients receiving palliative care to 25–29%, and the prevalence of MDE increases to 14–17%.[6] The average prevalence of MDE in cancer populations is 5–10%, which is two to three times higher than that of the general population.[29]

Despite diagnostic ambiguity, depression can be recognized in the cancer setting through clinical interpretation and with the aid of a screening instrument. Even relatively short instruments that screen for distress and depression have proven validity against gold standard measures of depression, such as the trained clinician.[30–32] However, no measure offers 100% sensitivity or specificity, and they always require a skilled clinical assessment and interpretation of findings in order to rule out confounding variables and provide adequate depression care.[33] After utilizing recognized measures, depression is certainly even more highly prevalent in people living with cancer than in the general population.[28] Although an increased prevalence is similarly seen in other chronic medical illness, the cancer setting offers several advantages for studying the biology of depression as a systemic illness. For instance, the cancer diagnosis offers variability in terms of severity of physical or biological illness that can also be compared at several time points within the same individual. Also, the cancer diagnosis is not uniform and provides several specific scenarios in which to study the relationship between physical illness biology and depression. We propose that studying depression in cancer will inform exploratory hypotheses about the biology of depression as a systemic illness and may lead to explanations that inform us about the links, the overlap in symptoms, and what might suggest possible therapeutic approaches to both.

Before exploring the underlying biology of depression and its associations with cancer, we will review the historical data regarding depression and cancer initiation and progression.

Reviewing the Data: Depression and Cancer Initiation

Stressful life events, chronic stress, personality, and a whole host of other risk factors have all been explored as possible etiological or contributing agents to the development of cancer. The International Agency for Research in Cancer has been tracking a multitude of possible cancer-causing factors since 1969. Multiple methodological problems need to be considered in exploring this research in order to avoid the temptation to attribute causation. For instance, although some studies reported an association,[34] others revealed no association between cancer initiation and severe life stressors or personality factors.[35,36] In several large-scale epidemiological Scandinavian studies over several decades, a significant association between major life events and stress has not been discovered.[1,37,38] Similarly, large epidemiological studies of cancer incidence and depression or depressed mood have been performed and have not found a significant association when controlling for socioeconomic factors, family history of cancer, parity, and health behavior.[39–41]

One study found that depression, anxiety, cynical distrust, or poor coping did not increase the risk for cancer.[40] One study from the United Kingdom of patients admitted to hospitals for either depression or anxiety found an increased incidence of cancer when the first year of follow-up was excluded.[42] However, this study could not distinguish between the causative factors of depression versus the lifestyle association with depression—a common confounder in many positive studies. Personality factors such as neuroticism, life satisfaction, type A personality, and hostility have not been significantly associated with the development of cancer and do not point to an association between personality traits and cancer.[36,43–45] A notable exception is a Japanese study that found that women who expressed *Ikigai*, a Japanese concept of "something to live for, the joy and goal of living, or the happiness and benefit of being alive"—something similar to a mix between purpose and gratefulness—had lower rates of breast cancer.[46] Other factors— ease of anger arousal and self-perceived stress of daily life—were not associated with breast cancer risk.[46]

Purely speculative data implicating stress and viral infections with cancer initiation are interesting to consider. Essentially, all major human tumor-associated viruses have been found to be responsive to beta-adrenergic receptor or glucocorticoid-dependent signaling cascades. The Epstein-Barr virus (e.g., lymphomas and nasopharyngeal carcinoma), high-risk variants of the human papilloma virus (e.g., cervical, anal, and oropharyngeal carcinoma), and human herpes virus 8 (e.g., Kaposi's sarcoma) are all subjected to the activation of glucocorticoids.[47-49] However, these data are speculative, and knowledge in this area remains limited and needs further investigation. For the most part, it should not be concluded that depression, stress, or personality are associated with cancer initiation.

Reviewing the Data: Depression and Cancer Progression

Overall, studies have been equivocal on the effect of depression on survival. However, stronger data exist for the effect of depression on cancer progression, but not necessarily survival. Recent studies continue to provide evidence that depression leads to inferior survival in the cancer setting.[9] A non-definitive argument for this conclusion is made by a series of reviews and meta-analyses. Other psychological or psychiatric variables (e.g., anxiety, distress) may influence cancer related outcomes but have not been as thoroughly studied as depression. Early studies even dating back to the 1970s have demonstrated worse survival outcomes in cancer when depression coexists, although not consistently.[9,50,51] Follow-up epidemiological and prospective studies showed mixed results and did not replicate this substantial effect.[52,53] A descriptive review that was not specific to depression (e.g., included descriptions of helplessness) found that the majority of studies showed a significant association between depression and worse survival outcomes.[54] But another review found mixed results with average sample sizes twice as large in the negative studies.[55] Subsequently, a recent in-depth meta-analysis of 25 independent studies found that mortality rates were 25% higher in patients experiencing depressive symptoms and up to 39% higher in patients who were diagnosed with either a major or minor depression.[9] Some studies have also shown that depression is also associated with cancer progression in addition to worsened survival.[9] In addition, the treatment of depression in the cancer setting has been found to mitigate the negative outcomes of depression such as poorer quality of life, adherence, and even the adverse survival findings.[56-58] Evidence exists that treatment of depression may prevent worsening mortality from cancer.[59]

Although there is mounting evidence for the association between depression and earlier mortality in cancer, the biological mechanism behind the association is still not entirely clear. Descriptive evidence is growing despite inherent challenges in this research and the shifting sands of the ever-changing cancer treatment landscape.[60,61] In the future, we may see a transition from research that indirectly measures peripheral blood to looking directly at tumor-relevant measurements, the tumor microenvironment, better understanding the central nervous system, biobehavioral risk factors, and the ecological perspective of cancer and survivorship.[60]

Exploring Biological Correlates of Depression and Cancer

The increased prevalence of depression in cancer is not solely explained by the psychosocial stress associated with the cancer diagnosis. Elevated rates of depression associated with some forms of cancer (e.g., pancreatic cancer) prior to diagnosis illustrate this association.[62] Despite the significant associations, prevalence rates, and adverse outcomes, the mechanism by which depression is increased in the cancer setting is not fully understood.[63] Essentially, several biological phenomena are associated with depression in the cancer setting, but a clear understanding of their interactions, causative or otherwise, remains only partially elucidated. Biology is affected by internal and external (social) influences/environments. Both cancer and depression represent chronic physiological stresses that the body and mind endure. Depression may be exacerbated by the physiological stresses in the cancer setting caused by inflammation, acute and chronic stress (e.g., glucocorticoid-related and adrenergic-related, respectively), sleep dysregulation (diurnal cortisol rhythms), and epigenetic phenomena.

The classical biological theories of depression include (1) the monoamine hypothesis, (2) neurotransmitter receptor hypothesis, (3) neurotrophic factor hypothesis, (4) hypothalamic-pituitary-adrenal (HPA) dysregulation, (5) cytokine hypothesis, (6) elevated hippocampal nitric oxide levels, (7) oxidative stress, and (8) neurodegeneration.[64]

Of these multiple biological explanations for the development of depression, a few in particular are putatively enhanced by cancer-related biology, and include (1) the cytokine hypothesis, (2) hypothalamic-pituitary-adrenal (HPA) dysregulation, and (3) abnormal diurnal cortisol rhythms (associated with HPA dysregulation). In addition, other physiological consequences of depression contribute to comorbidity, and perhaps tumor progression, in cancer and include (1) glucocorticoid dysregulation, (2) enhanced sympathetic nervous system and adrenergic activity, and (3) alterations in DNA protein transcription (e.g., epigenetic phenomena) (Table 6.1). The pathobiology of cancer interacts with several of these pathways simultaneously and may contribute to depressive mind states and worsened physical outcomes through nutrition deficiencies or elevated inflammation, for example.

Several classes of medications have been implicated in causing depression-like symptoms in patients with cancer (see Table 6.2).[65] Aside from the prototypical depression caused by interferon-α, other immunotherapies, including many new classes of immunotherapy (e.g., immune checkpoint blockade drugs) may be implicated in the development of depression. For instance, dopamine receptor antagonists used to manage emesis and nausea reduce dopamine transmission in the brain and have been linked with the development of depressive symptoms.[66]

"Sickness Behavior" of Advanced Cancer and Its Similarity to Depression

An immune system on overdrive may induce depressive states by causing a "sickness syndrome" of asthenia, malaise, and apathy that is similarly seen in both sickness and depression as a consequence of proinflammatory cytokines. For instance, roughly 50%

Table 6.1 Putative Mechanisms of Biologically Based Depression in the Cancer Setting

1. The cytokine hypothesis[67]	Proinflammatory cytokines have been found to induce depressive states	Many complex protein interactions makes causal relationship difficult to assess
2. Hypothalamic-pituitary-adrenal (HPA) dysregulation[138]	Hormonal dysregulation is common to both depression and advanced cancer	Found to normalize with anti-depressive treatments
3. Abnormal diurnal cortisol rhythms[55]	Sleep/wake dysregulation is common to both depression and advanced cancer	Tends to worsen in both advanced cancer states and depression
4. Glucocorticoid dysregulation[91]	A physiological manifestation of chronic stress states common to both depression and cancer	Has been associated with cancer progression
5. Enhanced sympathetic nervous system and adrenergic activity[2]	Increased sympathetic nervous system tone is common to both depression and cancer	Found to be associated with cancer progression
6. Alterations in DNA protein transcription/ epigenetics (social genomics)[133]	The social outcomes of depression (e.g., less stable relationships, isolation) mirror epigenetic phenomena	Associated with cancer progression

Table 6.2 Chemotherapeutic and Other Pharmacological Agents Linked to Depression (Borrowed from *Psychosomatic Medicine*, Blumenfield and Strain, 2006)[65]

Antineoplastic agents	Alkylating agents (e.g., Dacarbazine, Procarbazine)
	Corticosteroids
	Cyclosporine
	Interferon
	L-asparaginase
	Methotrexate
	Tamoxifen
	Vinblastine
	Vincristine
Analgesics	Codeine
	Indomethacin
	Oxycodone
Cardiovascular agents	Propranolol
	Reserpine
	α methyldopa
	Calcium channel blockers
Neurologic agents	Levodopa
	Phenobarbital
	Levetiracetam
Gastrointestinal agents	Cimetidine
Antibiotics	Amphotericin

of patients receiving therapeutic doses of interferon-α will meet criteria for a major depressive episode and many have to stop treatment.[67] The symptoms of "sickness syndrome" and consequent behavior overlap with clinical depression.[68] Similarly, chronic inflammation associated with stress underlies non–physically-ill-based depression and overlaps with the inflammation seen in many medical conditions, including cancer.[68] In vitro experiments reveal the underlying mechanistic activity of psychoneuroimmunological concepts, while proof of concept studies and in vivo experiments have met primary clinical outcomes, although not consistently. Early observations that depressed patients exhibit increases in inflammatory markers (e.g., acute phase reactant proteins, chemokines, adhesion molecules), innate immune cytokines (e.g., IL-1, IL-6, TNF-α), and their soluble receptors in the peripheral blood and cerebral spinal fluid (CSF) have been replicated, albeit not predictably.[25,67,69] Fueling this hypothesis, psychosocial stressors, which are associated strongly with depression, are also associated with immune signaling pathways (e.g., nuclear factor kappa B) and innate immune cytokines (e.g., IL-6).[70]

Also, depressed patients exhibit exaggerated stress-induced inflammatory responses.[71] In addition, early-life stress may be especially relevant since it leads to both higher rates of depressive symptomatology and exaggerated inflammatory responses in the cancer context.[72,73] Arguing further for this hypothesis is the fact that antagonism of innate immune cytokines (e.g., TNF-α inhibitor Etanercept) improves depressed mood in patients with excessive inflammation.[74] The association of inflammation with sickness syndrome and depression becomes even more interesting when one considers that several symptoms of advanced cancer and cachexia are similar to symptoms of aging. Cancer is a disease of aging and arguably accelerates the aging process, contributing to the physical, psychological, and cognitive changes associated with normal aging, which is associated with predictable immune system dysfunction.[75] The biology of depression and cytokine-mediated inflammation becomes even more complicated in the elderly populations when one considers that the prevalence of depression actually decreases in otherwise healthy elderly patients but increases for select groups of elderly individuals.[76]

Although exciting evidence exists for the role of inflammation in the development of depression in the setting of cancers, the majority of positive studies are correlational without substantive evidence for the underlying causative mechanisms. Over the last 20 years, cytokine research in depression has made several shifts that reflect enhanced technological expertise, greater oncological focus on the "tumor microenvironment," changing treatment paradigms, prolonged survivorship in certain oncological diseases, and awareness of how the immune system changes with aging. Now, cytokine research has taken on a more direct focus on the tumor microenvironment and the central nervous system specifically.[60] Early work in psychoneuroimmunology has led to a basic understanding that biobehavioral risk factors (e.g., obesity, chronic stress, depression, social isolation) interact physiologically with the central nervous system and peripherally through neuroendocrine signaling that is mediated bidirectionally from tumor biology itself.[77] These interactions are hypothesized to influence the clinical cancer course, which will again be mediated by changing clinical environments (e.g., new anti-cancer drugs and approaches to cancer care like enhanced supportive care, prolonged survivorship).[60]

Abnormal Diurnal Cortisol Rhythms in Depression and Cancer

Dysregulation of circadian physiology is readily apparent in patients with advancing cancer as well as in depressed patients.[78] Endocrine, immune, metabolic, and cellular systems may contribute to the disrupted circadian cycle.[78,79] Patients with advanced cancer display varied and idiosyncratic circadian rhythm abnormalities. The peaks and troughs that are seen add up to a disrupted curve that should be highest in the morning (e.g., around 8 a.m.) and lowest in the early morning (e.g., around 3 a.m.). Up to 70% of advanced cancer patients display a "flattened" profile without the normal cortisol peak 30–45 minutes after first awakening and nadir during sleep as measured by saliva samples.[80] Depressed patients, and patients with other psychiatric disorders, exhibit a similar flattened cortisol curve.[81,82] Although many common psychiatric disorders are associated with circadian disruptions, its causal influence is in question. Psychiatric disorders may lead to circadian disruption, but not vice versa. Similarly, circadian disruptions are found in cancer but may not be causative of cancer progression.

However, it is intriguing that both depression and diurnal cortisol rhythm disruption, also seen in depression, are both associated with decreased survival in the advanced cancer setting. For example, a study of metastatic breast cancer patients found that flattened slopes predicted early mortality independently of other associated biological factors (e.g., low natural killer activity and cytotoxicity, sleep disruption) or psychological factors (e.g., marital discord).[81] Another study found the a flattened diurnal rhythm in lung cancer patients followed for three years predicted early mortality independently of similarly biological and psychological factors.[83] The dysregulation of circadian HPA rhythms has also been associated specifically with accelerated tumor growth rates and biomarkers in advancing cancer.

PSYCHOSOCIAL STRESS AND NEUROENDOCRINE PROCESSES: INFLAMMATION, DEPRESSION, AND CANCER PROGRESSION

Depression and the Stress Response

Depression is a condition of human emotion that is associated with an underlying state of biological stress.[64] Many overlapping biological phenomena exist between depression and a chronically stressed state. For example, the somatic symptoms of depression such as decreased energy and appetite, and insomnia, are the direct result of altered physiology. In 1936, Hans Selye defined "physiological stress" as the state in which the autonomic nervous system and the hypothalamic-pituitary-adrenal (HPA) axis are co-activated.[84] Depressed states are associated with an overactive HPA similar to a physiological reaction to acute stress. However, HPA overactivity leads to a depleted HPA axis that is consistent with chronic stress. Elevated cortisol and over-secretion of corticotrophin-releasing hormone (CRP) from the hypothalamus are implicated in both the cognitive and arousal (e.g., agitated) symptoms of depression.[85]

Depression distorts a person's interpretation of experience (e.g., pessimism or catastrophic thinking), which may, in part, stem from the underlying physiology of the chronically stressed state. The translation of environmental or situational factors into physiological stress, as experienced by the patient, is a complex process that involves the interpretation, synthesis, and coordination of environmental and internal physiological stimuli by the peripheral, central, and autonomic nervous systems. Many of these feedback loops happen automatically, and a bidirectional influence exists with the patient's temperament and mental status.[86,87] Essentially, catecholamine (norepinephrine and/or epinephrine) is secreted from the sympathetic neurons and adrenal medulla, and cortisol is secreted from the adrenal cortex during the "fight or flight response," which is initiated by the autonomic nervous system or the defeat/withdrawal responses in the HPA. These adaptive processes are key for responding to environmental stressors and survival but have negative physiological effects in the long term due to excessive catecholamine exposure, as seen in depression.[88]

Essentially, the stress "fight or flight" response is largely mediated by the sympathetic nervous system and sustained by the HPA axis. Catecholamines and glucocorticoids are released either into the bloodstream or directly into various organs by neurons. During chronic stress, such as in a depressed state, catecholamines (e.g., norepinephrine and epinephrine) remain elevated, while dopamine levels are depleted following an initial elevation during the acute phase of stress. Also, this sustained inflammatory milieu of proinflammatory cytokines can lead to the "sickness syndrome" that is associated with depression and potentially cancer progression, as described earlier. For example, this shift in catecholamine levels has been shown to result in a cellular environment that is conducive to tumor growth in animal models (e.g., elevated catecholamines are associated with ovarian rat follicle growth and also appear to influence cancer progression in murine bone marrow).

Of all the possible theories of depression biology, the association of inflammation and both cancer and depression has garnered the most scientific attention through the variable parts of the inflammatory network (HPA axis, sympathomimetic system, cortisol regulation, cytokine release, leukocyte alteration). However, other relevant biological theories of depression such as (1) neurogenic and neurotrophic theories (e.g., BDNF, Glial-based synaptic dysfunction) and (2) epigenetic modifications (e.g., DNA methylation, histone alteration through methylation or acetylation) require adequate attention.

Effects of Stress on Cancer

Neuroendocrine stress responses can influence tumor biology and possibly contribute to cancer progression. The HPA axis is a major physiological pathway for homeostasis that becomes altered under chronic stress. Initially, following an acute stress exposure, an increased glucocorticoid response is observed; eventually chronic stress exposure leads to a blunting of the normal diurnal cortisol pattern. Notably, estrogen-independent breast cancer progression has been linked to high primary-tumor glucocorticoid receptor expression and increased glucocorticoid-mediated gene expression. Animal models of human breast cancer suggest that glucocorticoids inhibit tumor cell apoptosis, which could then lead to cancer progression.

These findings provide a conceptual basis for understanding the molecular mechanisms underlying the influence of an individual's stress response, and specifically glucocorticoid action, on solid tumors. How might increased glucocorticoid signaling affect cancerous states?

Well-defined physiological changes occur at the organismal and biochemical level when an individual encounters stressors in his or her social environment. A social network and its effect on an individual's physiology, to some extent, can buffer these changes. When life stressors are unrelenting and social support or other resources are insufficient, neuroendocrine pathways can become altered despite homeostatic forces. This deregulation of physiological pathways underlies the mechanisms whereby psychosocial stressors are hypothesized to influence the biology of chronic diseases, like cancer. Similar to the association between stress and heart disease, the stress response-disease relationship is seen in the biobehavioral influence on tumor progression in cancer research.[89,90]

The most important determinant of cortisol action is its cognate protein, the glucocorticoid receptor (GR). These receptors are ever-present in most tissues, and their primary action is as a ligand-dependent transcription factor regulating gene expression. Within the nucleus, the GR regulates the expression of target genes directly through interacting with glucocorticoid release elements (GRE) or indirectly through interacting with other transcription factors. GR regulates numerous biological processes, including metabolisms, behavior, growth and cellular apoptosis.[91] The specific glucocorticoid response is often dependent on the receptors present in the target cell or tissue type. However, what happens downstream is not currently known.

This approach is appealing to uncover the molecular underpinning linking psychosocial stress response to cancer. For example, the female Sprague-Dawley rats have an inherited genetic predisposition for spontaneous mammary tumor formation. An altered systemic glucocorticoid (GC) regulation following exposure to the chronic stress (i.e., similar in depression) of social isolation was associated with a significantly increased mammary tumor burden.[92] A related study found that an animal model of social isolation was associated with abnormal GC regulation in response to a superimposed acute stressor and also associated with increased mammary tumor growth.[93] The GR antagonist, mifepristone, when used to block GR signaling led to increased chemotherapy efficacy in a human breast cancer xenograft model.[91]

Biologically relevant concentrations of glucocorticoids were found to enhance the proliferation of mammary carcinoma cells in vitro by almost two-fold.[94] Similarly, cortisol and cortisone can stimulate the growth of prostate cancer cells in the absence of androgens and increase the secretion rate of prostate-specific antigen (PSAs) through mutated androgen receptors.[95] Also the growth of normal cells, such as keratinocytes, may be slowed by catecholamines and impair wound healing in the context of stress. However, in some cases, the effects of a stress hormone can inhibit cell proliferation depending on its receptor, its expression, and the pathway that is blocked.[96] Although the role of glucocorticoid hormones on cancer cell proliferation has been examined, there are limited data describing concomitant interactions with other neuroendocrine hormones, and this needs to be further examined in the future.

An important aside is that acute inflammation must be distinguished from chronic inflammation that tends to have more adverse physical and mental health implications. Acute inflammation, from an infection or foreign-body induced, has been known for over 100 years to be able to cause "spontaneous cancer remissions" in the form of "Coley's vaccine."[97] Modern cancer therapeutics now harness "Coley's vaccine," the body's innate ability to form anti-cancer antigens that can be used to treat many forms of cancer in the form of "checkpoint inhibitors" or "immunotherapy."[98] Moreover, the absence of an intact immune system via an innate immune deficiency, immunosuppressant drugs (e.g., for solid organ transplant or autoimmune diseases), bone marrow transplant, or AIDS can promote the development of many cancers. However, an overactive immune system (e.g., autoimmune disease), an example of chronic inflammation, is not effective at preventing cancers. Clearly, there is an intimate relationship between inflammation and cancer. Cancer increases systemic inflammation via an immune response. The bidirectional relationship between cancer and inflammation is complex. Malignant cells are created and destroyed by the body's immune system continuously.

Inflammatory Associations of Stress (and Possibly Depression) and Tumor Progression

Inflammation may contribute to tumor progression as mediated by glucocorticoid signaling and other inflammatory pathways described later. Psychosocial stressors contribute to increased metastatic progression through GR signaling through in vivo models that have observed that altering the social environment has observed effects on cancer growth.[99] GC-mediated mechanisms influencing solid tumor progression are not limited to the effects of GCs directly on tumor cells. Tumor progression involves the tumor microenvironment, which supports the cancer cell's proliferation, the host, and the individual's environment. Neuroendocrine pathways have diverse effects. Indeed, nearly every mammalian tissue is believed to express the GR. Therefore, attempting to integrate stress physiology with aspects of cancer progression also requires examining the tumor microenvironment and an individual's systemic physiology to fully understand the stress response influencing tumor progression.[91]

Tumor progression is only partially dependent on cell autonomous programming. Stromal signals from cells in the microenvironment are increasingly appreciated as significant factors influencing tumor progression. Bidirectional "cross-talk" forms a dialogue involving enzymes, metabolites, growth factors, and other cytokines on both compartments. Gene-expression profiling studies have compared tumor-associated stroma to normal stroma and suggest that cancerous cells can dramatically alter stromal mRNA expression.[100] However, the specific cells of the tumor microenvironment that display altered tumor-promoting signals in response to GCs have yet to be determined.

Tumorigenesis is the biological process of cancer initiation and progression. Genetic and epigenetic processes that cause the transition of a normal cell to a malignant clone influence tumorigenesis. Six essential acquired alterations in cell physiology, as described by Hanahan and Weinberg, can portend malignant growth, and each one of these processes could be influenced by the chronic inflammation that accompanies depression.[101,102] They are the following: (1) self-sufficiency in growth signals, (2) insensitivity to anti-growth signals, (3) evasion of apoptosis, (4) limitless replicative potential, (5) sustained angiogenesis, and (6) tissue invasion and metastasis.

Firstly, inflammation enhances tumor growth signals. Both breast and prostate cancer models show less restricted, unencumbered proliferation (i.e., *self-sufficiency*) in the presence of inflammation without normal hormonal regulation.[94,95]

Secondly, inflammation reduces anti-proliferation signals from the tumor stroma (i.e., *insensitivity to anti-growth signals*). Stress hormones modulate tumor–stroma interactions. Ultimately, the only way for a tumor cell to survive is to adhere to the extracellular matrix within tissues, which consists of collagens, laminins, fibronectin, and other noncollagenous glycoproteins. Adhesion via integrin function can be modulated by the beta-agonist isoproterenol and has been shown to promote ovarian cell spread.[103] For example, this may be particularly relevant in ovarian cancer since it spreads by direct adhesion throughout the pelvic and abdominal cavities.

Thirdly, inflammation and stress hormones help cancer cells *evade apoptosis*. For example, dopamine, substance P, and norepinephrine had a stimulating effect on the migration of breast cancer cells.[104] Specifically, norepinephrine has been found to have a chemotactic effect on the breast cancer cells and is a potent inducer of colon and prostate cancer cells, and this action can be inhibited by beta-blockers.[105,106]

Fourthly, dysregulated inflammation permits unregulated tumor cell reproductive potential and also permits dysregulated angiogenesis (i.e., *limitless replicative potential*).

Fifthly, tumors require new blood vessels for growth beyond 1–2 mm in diameter, and metastasis requires the recruitment of nearby blood vessels (e.g., angiogenesis), which is mediated by such factors as vascular endothelial growth factor (VEGF) and IL-6 (i.e., *sustained angiogenesis*). Both of these growth factors are increased under stressful conditions. Specifically, norepinephrine upregulates VEGF in ovarian cell lines, but this action can be blocked by beta-adrenergic modulation.[107,108] Similarly, IL-6 enhances ovarian tumor cell proliferation and migration in vitro and is clinically associated with a worse prognosis in ovarian cancer.[109] Social support has been shown to be associated with decreased levels of IL-6 in ovarian cancer patients blood and ascites samples.[110] Cortisol has also been shown to cause significant increases in VEGF, while exogenous glucocorticoid has been shown to decrease VEGF mRNA in a non-hypoxic rat glioma model, depending on the glucocorticoid receptor function.[108,111] However, the overall data pertaining to the effects of glucocorticoids on angiogenesis remain limited.

Lastly, stress hormones and inflammation may assist tumor cell survival by helping them *invade tissues and metastasize*. In prostate and breast cancer cell lines, epinephrine reduced the sensitivity of cancer cells to apoptosis through interactions with ADRB2 receptors followed by protein kinase A–dependent *BAD* phosphorylation.[112] Although large-scale prospective data are lacking, these effects may be translated epidemiologically. A reduction of prostate cancer incidence has been reported in patients taking beta blockers, thereby implying the importance of the activation of B-adrenergic receptors in the development of prostate cancer.[113]

In addition, other major stress mediators such as prolactin, oxytocin, dopamine, and substance P are affected by stress (i.e., inflammation) and may play a role in tumor cell proliferation. Dopamine, a precursor in the synthesis of catecholamines, has been shown to have direct effects on the inhibition of breast, head and neck, melanoma, and neuroblastoma cancer cell lines and may have anti-angiogenic properties.[114,115] Chronic psychosocial stress depletes dopamine and may limit its potential anti-cancer effects.[116] By extension, rates of cancer in patients with schizophrenia, a disease of dopamine excesses, are lower than what might be expected, given their rates of smoking and lifestyle factors.[117] An anti-cancer role of the phenothiazines—the primary drug class used to treat schizophrenia—has been proposed.

SOCIAL INFLUENCES ON INFLAMMATION PROCESSES

Social Implications: Depression and Cancer Progression Through Epigenetics

The science of inflammation connects human beings to their environments. In order to deal with our environment, human beings have adapted the autonomic, parasympathetic, and sympathetic nervous systems—three separate but interconnected systems. The original discoveries of Eric Kandel using the marine mollusks revealed the epigenetic protein production as a result of physical environment alterations and has led to further scientific insights into how our social/physical environments may influence our genetics.[118] Social environments reflect a person's mental status, which is typically damaged or conflicted after a person has been suffering with depression. The sympathetic nervous system responds immediately to external environmental threats and regulates the function of virtually all human organ systems through gene expression. The parasympathetic and autonomic nervous systems are equally responsive to environmental stimuli but are more passively situated. Modulated transcriptional dynamics stem from evolutionarily conserved molecular genetics that adapt a broad range of cellular functions to detect and respond more effectively to challenging, threatening, or novel environments.[2] These adaptations are conserved evolutionarily and may explain how certain social or human environment scenarios are interpreted physiologically. Not only are certain genes, but also the expression of these genes, conserved and the emerging field of "social genomics" is beginning to understand the influence of social environment on gene expression. This field promises to understand the long-observed relationship between social conditions and the distribution of health and disease, including cancer.

That is, although the environment may not change our DNA make-up during our lifetimes, its expression can be modulated by epigenetic factors (e.g., methylation, acetylation, histones). These epigenetic factors (i.e., proteins) influence gene expression and are partially responsible with the variability in genetic penetration that is witnessed clinically. It is plausible to imagine how one's DNA could be manipulated by pro- and anti-regulatory factors that are either up- or down-regulated due to environmental stimuli (e.g., stress, anxiety, and depression).

The sympathetic nervous system (SNS) not only works acutely through α and β adrenergic receptors and direct stimulation of organs but also influences the post-translational modification of proteins through chronic and circadian variations in activity, which regulates constitutive gene expression. Abnormal regulation of SNS seen in depression and chronically stressed states may influence cancer biology as mediated by β adrenergic signaling. Many of the in vitro animal models show that β adrenergic antagonists can block stress-mediated tumor progression. Also, β adrenergic signaling may inhibit DNA repair and p53-associated apoptosis, thus raising the possibility that SNS activity might potentially contribute to chromosomal instability; but this has not been seen in vivo.[119] β adrenergic signaling may influence several oncogenic pathways, including SRC and HER-2, that drive many solid tumors such as breast, gastric, lung, or pancreatic cancer.[120,121] Additionally, β adrenergic signaling stimulates the transcription of proinflammatory cytokines such as IL-6 and IL-8 by tumor cells mediated by myeloid lineage immune cells.[122,123] And studies have shown that SNS stimulation of inflammatory signaling can enhance tumor progression and metastasis, but no studies have shown any effect on tumor initiation in vivo.[124,125] β adrenergic signaling also stimulates macrophage expression of genes that promote tumor progression, including transforming growth factor-β, vascular endothelial growth factor, IL-6, matrix metalloproteinase 9, and PTGS1.[125] Thereby, the SNS also influences the tumor stroma where the cancer cells are embedded onto fibroblasts, adipocytes, and mesenchymal cells by sending activating signals.[126] It can also block the programmed cell death (i.e., apoptosis), one of the key mediators of tumor progression, and has been shown to influence leukemic cells in vivo.[127,128] Tumors become innervated by the SNS, which then directly and indirectly influence the tumor humoral microenvironment.[129]

Strong evidence for β adrenergic signaling leading to cancer progression has therapeutic implications in its blockade, which is easily achieved with β and non-selective adrenergic antagonist drugs. Observational epidemiological studies have documented associations between β adrenergic antagonists and reduced progression of primary solid malignancies such as prostate, breast, lung, melanoma, and ovarian cancers. However, these studies are not entirely consistent, and prospective trials have yet to be performed. And high expression of adrenergic receptors on tumor cells has not substantially predicted tumor responsiveness to β antagonists in vivo. Even so, there is a need for a randomized controlled, biomarker-enriched trials to assess this proof-of-concept.[2]

Most of the genetic transcription in these studies comes from peripheral blood leukocytes, which show distinct, proinflammatory or anti-antiviral patterns in settings of adverse life circumstances (e.g., bereavement, traumatic stress, social isolation, low socioeconomic status, and cancer diagnoses). Animal models of these stressors reveal similar gene expression, and it appears to be common to mammalian immune systems.[130] These patterns can be seen in HSV (*Herpes simplex* virus) or human immunodeficiency virus (HIV) containment under personal or social stressors (e.g., concealment of sexual identity).[131,132] This has been termed the "conserved transcriptional response to adversity" (CTRA) and it induces a proinflammatory/anti-antiviral skew in the circulating lymphocyte transcriptome when environments are interpreted as threatening for an extended period of time.[133] In the context of cancer, these transcriptional genomes have been studied and contribute the genetic basis to the idea that social adversity may not only predict worsening psychological function but also breast and ovarian cancer progression.[134,135]

Other mediators of CTRA include the tendency for social isolation and loneliness to worsen inflammatory parameters, apart from the influence of depression itself. However, a distinct purpose or identified goal in life tends to stabilize the disharmonious effects of stress.[3] That is, studies have shown that CTRA gene expression is upregulated with loneliness and downregulated in association with well-being characterized by *eudaimonia* (Greek) or *ikigai* (Japanese) for a sense of purpose in life.[136,137] However, the directionality of the leukocyte transcription has not been fully elucidated.

Chronic stress, negative affect, and social adversity are associated with biobehavioral alterations that increase the SNS signaling, HPA axis dysregulation, and inflammation, but decrease cellular immunity activity, which putatively interacts with the tumor microenvironment to promote factors favoring tumor growth, invasion, and metastatic signaling.[138] And cancer patients with less social support and greater anxiety have molecular evidence of impaired transcription of glucocorticoid response genes and increased activity of proinflammatory transcription control pathways.[139] Thus, behavioral interventions to decrease the psychological and biological consequences of stress in the cancer setting make therapeutic sense.

Antoni and colleagues have summarized some of the biological outcomes of drug and psychosocial interventions in patients with cancer.[140] In essence, some evidence suggests that psychosocial interventions can improve biological measures of psychological and physiological adaptation in cancer patients, but less is known about whether these interventions can influence tumor activity and tumor growth–promoting processes or whether these biological changes account for the psychosocial intervention effects on recurrence and survival documented to date. Interventions have been designed to cognitively modify outlook, stress appraisals, and coping via cognitive behavioral therapy (CBT); behaviorally reduce tension, anxiety, and distress through relaxation training, mindfulness, hypnosis, yoga, and other techniques; and efforts to interpersonally build skills to cope in a group format to improve perceived social support and communication. The vast majority of interventions have occurred in the breast cancer setting to influence health behaviors such as physical exercise, diet, sleep, and medication adherence. Reviews have concluded that psychosocial interventions that teach relaxation techniques and stress management among other interventions have been effective in increasing quality of life (QOL) indicators.[141,142] Many effects were still apparent at 12-month follow-up.[143]

Fewer studies have looked at biological correlates specifically. Of those that have, Andersen and colleagues found that the women with breast cancer in their intervention group had increases in cellular immune measures such as lymphocyte proliferative response to mitogens, in addition to improved clinical outcomes. In that study, women whose cancer ultimately recurred revealed greater serum cortisol and leukocytosis at an average of 17 months prior to their recurrence, which suggested that pre-intervention levels might have been relevant in explaining differences in outcome, despite the intervention.[144] Also, women who recurred at a distant metastatic site tended to have weaker immune responses (e.g., natural killer cell activity and lymphocyte proliferation rates to mitogens). Stress-reducing techniques and cognitive behavioral therapies have also produced decreases in late afternoon serum cortisol, and increases in IL-2 and IFN-Υ (anti-inflammatory cytokines) from anti-CD3 stimulated peripheral blood mononuclear cells (PMBCs).[145,146]

Negative affect associated with depression also influences gene expression with greater than 50% differential expression of 201 genes including upregulated expression of proinflammatory cytokines (IL-1A, IL1B, IL-6, TNF) and metastasis-promoting genes involved with tissue remodeling and epithelial–mesenchymal transition.[134] In addition, interventions such as CBT and interpersonal therapy have been shown to downregulate those same genes that were upregulated by negative affect. The immune cell types most likely mediating therapeutic interventions such as CBT or interpersonal therapy transcriptional alterations have previously been linked to distress states.[147]

CONCLUSION

Depression is of great interest in cancer *because* of its systemic nature, producing both psychological (e.g., anhedonia, depressed mood) and profound physical symptoms of fatigue, weakness, reduced stamina, insomnia, and apathy. These physical symptoms are also common in patients with many sites of cancer, and particularly in advanced cancer, in general. The overlap has made the diagnosis of depression difficult in cancer, in fact, leading to Endicott's substitutive diagnostic criteria for diagnosing depression, and is a reason for a deeper biological look at this relationship. We have attempted to summarize current knowledge about how depression impacts tumor biology and have highlighted some of the common links we need to understand to treat both more effectively. The field of psychoneuroimmunology remains in its infancy, and it has had to overcome negative stigma related to early misguided and simplistic assumptions by society about personality features, depression, and cancer. This field, while still in an early stage of development, is producing important studies that will continue to elucidate the underlying biological nature of depression as it relates to cancer.

At this point, the major hypotheses of depression and cancer interactions relate to four distinct areas in psychoneuroimmunology: (1) the cytokine hypothesis of depression; (2) dysregulation of the HPA, glucocorticoids, and diurnal circadian rhythms; (3) enhanced SNS adrenergic activity; and (4) alterations in DNA protein transcription/epigenetics. Of these, the latter two, the sympathetic nervous system and epigenetics, have garnered the most attention recently.

REFERENCES

1. Lillberg K, Verkasalo PK, Kaprio J, Teppo L, Helenius H, Koskenvuo M. Stressful life events and risk of breast cancer in 10,808 women: a cohort study. *Am J Epidemiol.* 2003;157(5):415–423.
2. Cole SW, Nagaraja AS, Lutgendorf SK, Green PA, Sood AK. Sympathetic nervous system regulation of the tumour microenvironment. *Nat Rev Cancer.* 2015;15(9):563–572.
3. Cole SW, Levine ME, Arevalo JM, Ma J, Weir DR, Crimmins EM. Loneliness, eudaimonia, and the human conserved transcriptional response to adversity. *Psychoneuroendocrinology.* 2015;62:11–17.

4. Gallucci BB. Selected concepts of cancer as a disease: from the Greeks to 1900. *Oncol Nurs Forum*. 1985;12(4):67–71.

5. Burton R. *The Anatomy of Melancholy*. Reprint ed. Originally published London, 1621.

6. Mitchell AJ, Chan M, Bhatti H, et al. Prevalence of depression, anxiety, and adjustment disorder in oncological, haematological, and palliative-care settings: a meta-analysis of 94 interview-based studies. *Lancet Oncol*. 2011;12(2):160–174.

7. Mitchell AJ. Pooled results from 38 analyses of the accuracy of distress thermometer and other ultra-short methods of detecting cancer-related mood disorders. *J Clin Oncol*. 2007;25(29):4670–4681.

8. Mehnert A, Brahler E, Faller H, et al. Four-week prevalence of mental disorders in patients with cancer across major tumor entities. *J Clin Oncol*. 2014;32(31):3540–3546.

9. Satin JR, Linden W, Phillips MJ. Depression as a predictor of disease progression and mortality in cancer patients: a meta-analysis. *Cancer*. 2009;115(22):5349–5361.

10. Skarstein J, Aass N, Fossa SD, Skovlund E, Dahl AA. Anxiety and depression in cancer patients: relation between the Hospital Anxiety and Depression Scale and the European Organization for Research and Treatment of Cancer Core Quality of Life Questionnaire. *J Psychosom Res*. 2000;49(1):27–34.

11. Prieto JM, Blanch J, Atala J, et al. Psychiatric morbidity and impact on hospital length of stay among hematologic cancer patients receiving stem-cell transplantation. *J Clin Oncol*. 2002;20(7):1907–1917.

12. Misono S, Weiss NS, Fann JR, Redman M, Yueh B. Incidence of suicide in persons with cancer. *J Clin Oncol*. 2008;26(29):4731–4738.

13. Colleoni M, Mandala M, Peruzzotti G, Robertson C, Bredart A, Goldhirsch A. Depression and degree of acceptance of adjuvant cytotoxic drugs. *Lancet*. 2000;356(9238):1326–1327.

14. Delgado-Guay M, Parsons HA, Li Z, Palmer JL, Bruera E. Symptom distress in advanced cancer patients with anxiety and depression in the palliative care setting. *Support Care Cancer*. 2009;17(5):573–579.

15. Kangas M, Henry JL, Bryant RA. The course of psychological disorders in the 1st year after cancer diagnosis. *J Consult Clin Psychol*. 2005;73(4):763–768.

16. Fann JR, Thomas-Rich AM, Katon WJ, et al. Major depression after breast cancer: a review of epidemiology and treatment. *Gen Hosp Psychiatry*. 2008;30(2):112–126.

17. Chochinov HM. Depression in cancer patients. *Lancet Oncol*. 2001;2(8):499–505.

18. Akechi T, Ietsugu T, Sukigara M, et al. Symptom indicator of severity of depression in cancer patients: a comparison of the DSM-IV criteria with alternative diagnostic criteria. *Gen Hosp Psychiatry*. 2009;31(3):225–232.

19. Snyderman D, Wynn D. Depression in cancer patients. *Prim Care*. 2009;36(4):703–719.

20. Cancer Care for the Whole Patient: Meeting Psychosocial Health Needs [press release]. Washington, DC: National Academies Press; 2008.

21. Wein S, Sulkes A, Stemmer S. The oncologist's role in managing depression, anxiety, and demoralization with advanced cancer. *Cancer J*. 2010;16(5):493–499.

22. van't Spijker A, Trijsburg RW, Duivenvoorden HJ. Psychological sequelae of cancer diagnosis: a meta-analytical review of 58 studies after 1980. *Psychosom Med*. 1997;59(3):280–293.

23. Carlson LE, Bultz BD. Efficacy and medical cost offset of psychosocial interventions in cancer care: making the case for economic analyses. *Psychooncology*. 2004;13(12):837–849; discussion 850–836.

24. Newport DJ, Nemeroff CB. Assessment and treatment of depression in the cancer patient. *J Psychosom Res*. 1998;45(3):215–237.

25. Maes M. Evidence for an immune response in major depression: a review and hypothesis. *Prog Neuropsychopharmacol Biol Psychiatry.* 1995;19(1):11–38.
26. Olson SH, Xu Y, Herzog K, et al. Weight loss, diabetes, fatigue, and depression preceding pancreatic cancer. *Pancreas.* 2016 Aug;45(7):986–991.
27. Walker J, Holm Hansen C, Martin P, et al. Prevalence of depression in adults with cancer: a systematic review. *Ann Oncol.* 2013;24(4):895–900.
28. Massie MJ. Prevalence of depression in patients with cancer. *J Natl Cancer Inst Monogr.* 2004(32):57–71.
29. Dauchy S, Dolbeault S, Reich M. Depression in cancer patients. *EJC Suppl.* 2013;11(2):205–215.
30. Vodermaier A, Linden W, Siu C. Screening for emotional distress in cancer patients: a systematic review of assessment instruments. *J Natl Cancer Inst.* 2009;101(21):1464–1488.
31. Grassi L, Caruso R, Sabato S, Massarenti S, Nanni MG, The UniFe Psychiatry Working Group C. Psychosocial screening and assessment in oncology and palliative care settings. *Front Psychol.* 2014;5:1485.
32. Wakefield CE, Butow PN, Aaronson NA, et al. Patient-reported depression measures in cancer: a meta-review. *Lancet Psychiatry.* 2015;2(7):635–647.
33. Mitchell AJ, Hussain N, Grainger L, Symonds P. Identification of patient-reported distress by clinical nurse specialists in routine oncology practice: a multicentre UK study. *Psychooncology.* 2011;20(10):1076–1083.
34. Price MA, Tennant CC, Smith RC, et al. The role of psychosocial factors in the development of breast carcinoma: Part I. The cancer prone personality. *Cancer.* 2001;91(4):679–685.
35. Duijts SF, Zeegers MP, Borne BV. The association between stressful life events and breast cancer risk: a meta-analysis. *Int J Cancer.* 2003;107(6):1023–1029.
36. Bleiker EM, Hendriks JH, Otten JD, Verbeek AL, van der Ploeg HM. Personality factors and breast cancer risk: a 13-year follow-up. *J Natl Cancer Inst.* 2008;100(3):213–218.
37. Kroenke CH, Hankinson SE, Schernhammer ES, Colditz GA, Kawachi I, Holmes MD. Caregiving stress, endogenous sex steroid hormone levels, and breast cancer incidence. *Am J Epidemiol.* 2004;159(11):1019–1027.
38. Surtees PG, Wainwright NW, Luben RN, Khaw KT, Bingham SA. No evidence that social stress is associated with breast cancer incidence. *Breast Cancer Res Treat.* 2010;120(1):169–174.
39. Nyklicek I, Louwman WJ, Van Nierop PW, Wijnands CJ, Coebergh JW, Pop VJ. Depression and the lower risk for breast cancer development in middle-aged women: a prospective study. *Psychol Med.* 2003;33(6):1111–1117.
40. Aro AR, De Koning HJ, Schreck M, Henriksson M, Anttila A, Pukkala E. Psychological risk factors of incidence of breast cancer: a prospective cohort study in Finland. *Psychol Med.* 2005;35(10):1515–1521.
41. Kroenke CH, Bennett GG, Fuchs C, et al. Depressive symptoms and prospective incidence of colorectal cancer in women. *Am J Epidemiol.* 2005;162(9):839–848.
42. Goldacre MJ, Wotton CJ, Yeates D, Seagroatt V, Flint J. Cancer in people with depression or anxiety: record-linkage study. *Soc Psychiatry Psychiatr Epidemiol.* 2007;42(9):683–689.
43. Lillberg K, Verkasalo PK, Kapr J, Teppo L, Helenius H, Koskenvuo M. A prospective study of life satisfaction, neuroticism and breast cancer risk (Finland). *Cancer Causes Control.* 2002;13(2):191–198.
44. Lillberg K, Verkasalo PK, Kaprio J, Helenius H, Koskenvuo M. Personality characteristics and the risk of breast cancer: a prospective cohort study. *Int J Cancer.* 2002;100(3):361–366.

45. Sturmer T, Hasselbach P, Amelang M. Personality, lifestyle, and risk of cardiovascular disease and cancer: follow-up of population based cohort. *BMJ.* 2006;332(7554):1359.

46. Wakai K, Kojima M, Nishio K, et al. Psychological attitudes and risk of breast cancer in Japan: a prospective study. *Cancer Causes Control.* 2007;18(3):259–267.

47. Cacioppo JT, Kiecolt-Glaser JK, Malarkey WB, et al. Autonomic and glucocorticoid associations with the steady-state expression of latent Epstein-Barr virus. *Horm Behav.* 2002;42(1):32–41.

48. Glaser R, Kutz LA, MacCallum RC, Malarkey WB. Hormonal modulation of Epstein-Barr virus replication. *Neuroendocrinology.* 1995;62(4):356–361.

49. Chang M, Brown HJ, Collado-Hidalgo A, et al. Beta-adrenoreceptors reactivate Kaposi's sarcoma-associated herpes virus lytic replication via PKA-dependent control of viral RTA. *J Virol.* 2005;79(21):13538–13547.

50. Pinquart M, Duberstein PR. Depression and cancer mortality: a meta-analysis. *Psychol Med.* 2010;40(11):1797–1810.

51. Shekelle RB, Raynor WJ, Jr., Ostfeld AM, et al. Psychological depression and 17-year risk of death from cancer. *Psychosom Med.* 1981;43(2):117–125.

52. Zonderman AB, Costa PT, Jr., McCrae RR. Depression as a risk for cancer morbidity and mortality in a nationally representative sample. *JAMA.* 1989;262(9):1191–1195.

53. Kaplan GA, Reynolds P. Depression and cancer mortality and morbidity: prospective evidence from the Alameda County study. *J Behav Med.* 1988;11(1):1–13.

54. Milo KM. The relationship between depression and cancer survival. *Med Health R I.* 2003;86(8):249–250.

55. Spiegel D, Giese-Davis J. Depression and cancer: mechanisms and disease progression. *Biol Psychiatry.* 2003;54(3):269–282.

56. Spiegel D, Bloom JR, Kraemer HC, Gottheil E. Effect of psychosocial treatment on survival of patients with metastatic breast cancer. *Lancet.* 1989;2(8668):888–891.

57. Fawzy FI, Fawzy NW, Hyun CS, et al. Malignant melanoma. Effects of an early structured psychiatric intervention, coping, and affective state on recurrence and survival 6 years later. *Arch Gen Psychiatry.* 1993;50(9):681–689.

58. Kissane DW. Letting go of the hope that psychotherapy prolongs cancer survival. *J Clin Oncol.* 2007;25(36):5689–5690.

59. Giese-Davis J, Collie K, Rancourt KM, Neri E, Kraemer HC, Spiegel D. Decrease in depression symptoms is associated with longer survival in patients with metastatic breast cancer: a secondary analysis. *J Clin Oncol.* 2011;29(4):413–420.

60. Green McDonald P, O'Connell M, Lutgendorf SK. Psychoneuroimmunology and cancer: a decade of discovery, paradigm shifts, and methodological innovations. *Brain Behav Immun.* 2013;30(Suppl):S1–S9.

61. Kling MA, Coleman VH, Schulkin J. Glucocorticoid inhibition in the treatment of depression: can we think outside the endocrine hypothalamus? *Depress Anxiety.* 2009;26(7):641–649.

62. Boyd AD, Riba M. Depression and pancreatic cancer. *J Natl Compr Canc Netw.* 2007;5(1):113–116.

63. Kissane DW, Maj M, & Sartorius N (ed.). *Depression and Cancer.* Oxford: Wiley-Blackwell; 2011:244.

64. Chopra K, Kumar B, Kuhad A. Pathobiological targets of depression. *Expert Opin Ther Targets.* 2011;15(4):379–400.

65. Blumenfield M, Strain JJ. Depression as a systemic illness. *Psychosomatic Medicine*, Vol 2. Philadelphia, PA: Lippincott Williams & Williams; 2006:50.

66. Patten SB, Barbui C. Drug-induced depression: a systematic review to inform clinical practice. *Psychother Psychosom*. 2004;73(4):207–215.
67. Raison CL, Capuron L, Miller AH. Cytokines sing the blues: inflammation and the pathogenesis of depression. *Trends Immunol*. 2006;27(1):24–31.
68. Sotelo JL, Musselman D, Nemeroff C. The biology of depression in cancer and the relationship between depression and cancer progression. *Int Rev Psychiatry*. 2014;26(1):16–30.
69. Irwin MR, Miller AH. Depressive disorders and immunity: 20 years of progress and discovery. *Brain Behav Immun*. 2007;21(4):374–383.
70. Bierhaus A, Wolf J, Andrassy M, et al. A mechanism converting psychosocial stress into mononuclear cell activation. *Proc Natl Acad Sci U S A*. 2003;100(4):1920–1925.
71. Pace TW, Mletzko TC, Alagbe O, et al. Increased stress-induced inflammatory responses in male patients with major depression and increased early life stress. *Am J Psychiatry*. 2006;163(9):1630–1633.
72. McFarland DC, Andreotti C, Harris K, Mandeli J, Tiersten A, Holland J. Early childhood adversity and its associations with anxiety, depression, and distress in women with breast cancer. *Psychosomatics*. 2016;57(2):174–184.
73. Danese A, Moffitt TE, Pariante CM, Ambler A, Poulton R, Caspi A. Elevated inflammation levels in depressed adults with a history of childhood maltreatment. *Arch Gen Psychiatry*. 2008;65(4):409–415.
74. Tyring S, Gottlieb A, Papp K, et al. Etanercept and clinical outcomes, fatigue, and depression in psoriasis: double-blind placebo-controlled randomised phase III trial. *Lancet*. 2006;367(9504):29–35.
75. Danese A, McEwen BS. Adverse childhood experiences, allostasis, allostatic load, and age-related disease. *Physiol Behav*. 2012;106(1):29–39.
76. Fiske A, Wetherell JL, Gatz M. Depression in older adults. *Annu Rev Clin Psychol*. 2009;5:363–389.
77. Dantzer R. Depression and inflammation: an intricate relationship. *Biol Psychiatry*. 2012;71(1):4–5.
78. Mormont MC, Levi F. Circadian-system alterations during cancer processes: a review. *Int J Cancer*. 1997;70(2):241–247.
79. Mazzoccoli G, Vendemiale G, De Cata A, Carughi S, Tarquini R. Altered time structure of neuro-endocrine-immune system function in lung cancer patients. *BMC Cancer*. 2010;10:314.
80. Sephton S, Spiegel D. Circadian disruption in cancer: a neuroendocrine-immune pathway from stress to disease? *Brain Behav Immun*. 2003;17(5):321–328.
81. Sephton SE, Sapolsky RM, Kraemer HC, Spiegel D. Diurnal cortisol rhythm as a predictor of breast cancer survival. *J Natl Cancer Inst*. 2000;92(12):994–1000.
82. Jones SG, Benca RM. Circadian disruption in psychiatric disorders. *Sleep Med Clin*. 2015;10(4):481–493.
83. Sephton SE, Lush E, Dedert EA, et al. Diurnal cortisol rhythm as a predictor of lung cancer survival. *Brain Behav Immun*. 2013;30(Suppl):S163–S170.
84. Chrousos GP. The hypothalamic-pituitary-adrenal axis and immune-mediated inflammation. *N Engl J Med*. 1995;332(20):1351–1362.
85. Masand PS, Culpepper L, Henderson D, et al. Metabolic and endocrine disturbances in psychiatric disorders: a multidisciplinary approach to appropriate atypical antipsychotic utilization. *CNS Spectr*. 2005;10(Suppl 14):11–15.
86. Sapolsky RM. *Why zebras don't get ulcers: a guide to stress, stress-related diseases, and coping*. New York: Macmillan; 1994.

87. Weiner H. *Perturbing the organism: the biology of stressful experience.* Chicago, IL: University of Chicago Press; 1992.

88. McEwen BS. Sex, stress and the hippocampus: allostasis, allostatic load and the aging process. *Neurobiol Aging.* 2002;23(5):921–939.

89. Costanzo ES, Sood AK, Lutgendorf SK. Biobehavioral influences on cancer progression. *Immunol Allergy Clin North Am.* 2011;31(1):109–132.

90. Armaiz-Pena GN, Lutgendorf SK, Cole SW, Sood AK. Neuroendocrine modulation of cancer progression. *Brain Behav Immun.* 2009;23(1):10–15.

91. Volden PA, Conzen SD. The influence of glucocorticoid signaling on tumor progression. *Brain Behav Immun.* 2013;30(Suppl):S26–S31.

92. Hermes GL, Delgado B, Tretiakova M, et al. Social isolation dysregulates endocrine and behavioral stress while increasing malignant burden of spontaneous mammary tumors. *Proc Natl Acad Sci U S A.* 2009;106(52):22393–22398.

93. Williams JB, Pang D, Delgado B, et al. A model of gene-environment interaction reveals altered mammary gland gene expression and increased tumor growth following social isolation. *Cancer Prev Res (Phila).* 2009;2(10):850–861.

94. Simon WE, Albrecht M, Trams G, Dietel M, Holzel F. In vitro growth promotion of human mammary carcinoma cells by steroid hormones, tamoxifen, and prolactin. *J Natl Cancer Inst.* 1984;73(2):313–321.

95. Zhao XY, Malloy PJ, Krishnan AV, et al. Glucocorticoids can promote androgen-independent growth of prostate cancer cells through a mutated androgen receptor. *Nat Med.* 2000;6(6):703–706.

96. Carie AE, Sebti SM. A chemical biology approach identifies a beta-2 adrenergic receptor agonist that causes human tumor regression by blocking the Raf-1/Mek-1/Erk1/2 pathway. *Oncogene.* 2007;26(26):3777–3788.

97. Jessy T. Immunity over inability: the spontaneous regression of cancer. *J Nat Sci Biol Med.* 2011;2(1):43–49.

98. Pardoll DM. The blockade of immune checkpoints in cancer immunotherapy. *Nat Rev Cancer.* 2012;12(4):252–264.

99. Cao L, Liu X, Lin EJ, et al. Environmental and genetic activation of a brain-adipocyte BDNF/leptin axis causes cancer remission and inhibition. *Cell.* 2010;142(1):52–64.

100. Finak G, Bertos N, Pepin F, et al. Stromal gene expression predicts clinical outcome in breast cancer. *Nat Med.* 2008;14(5):518–527.

101. Thaker PH, Sood AK. Neuroendocrine influences on cancer biology. *Semin Cancer Biol.* 2008;18(3):164–170.

102. Hanahan D, Weinberg RA. The hallmarks of cancer. *Cell.* 2000;100(1):57–70.

103. Enserink JM, Price LS, Methi T, et al. The cAMP-Epac-Rap1 pathway regulates cell spreading and cell adhesion to laminin-5 through the alpha3beta1 integrin but not the alpha6beta4 integrin. *J Biol Chem.* 2004;279(43):44889–44896.

104. Sood AK, Bhatty R, Kamat AA, et al. Stress hormone-mediated invasion of ovarian cancer cells. *Clin Cancer Res.* 2006;12(2):369–375.

105. Drell TLT, Joseph J, Lang K, Niggemann B, Zaenker KS, Entschladen F. Effects of neurotransmitters on the chemokinesis and chemotaxis of MDA-MB-468 human breast carcinoma cells. *Breast Cancer Res Treat.* 2003;80(1):63–70.

106. Masur K, Niggemann B, Zanker KS, Entschladen F. Norepinephrine-induced migration of SW 480 colon carcinoma cells is inhibited by beta-blockers. *Cancer Res.* 2001;61(7):2866–2869.

107. Fredriksson JM, Lindquist JM, Bronnikov GE, Nedergaard J. Norepinephrine induces vascular endothelial growth factor gene expression in brown adipocytes through a beta-adrenoreceptor/cAMP/protein kinase A pathway involving Src but independently of Erk1/2. *J Biol Chem.* 2000;275(18):13802–13811.

108. Lutgendorf SK, Cole S, Costanzo E, et al. Stress-related mediators stimulate vascular endothelial growth factor secretion by two ovarian cancer cell lines. *Clin Cancer Res.* 2003;9(12):4514–4521.

109. Lutgendorf SK, Johnsen EL, Cooper B, et al. Vascular endothelial growth factor and social support in patients with ovarian carcinoma. *Cancer.* 2002;95(4):808–815.

110. Costanzo ES, Lutgendorf SK, Sood AK, Anderson B, Sorosky J, Lubaroff DM. Psychosocial factors and interleukin-6 among women with advanced ovarian cancer. *Cancer.* 2005;104(2):305–313.

111. Machein MR, Kullmer J, Ronicke V, et al. Differential downregulation of vascular endothelial growth factor by dexamethasone in normoxic and hypoxic rat glioma cells. *Neuropathol Appl Neurobiol.* 1999;25(2):104–112.

112. Sastry KS, Karpova Y, Prokopovich S, et al. Epinephrine protects cancer cells from apoptosis via activation of cAMP-dependent protein kinase and BAD phosphorylation. *J Biol Chem.* 2007;282(19):14094–14100.

113. Perron L, Bairati I, Harel F, Meyer F. Antihypertensive drug use and the risk of prostate cancer (Canada). *Cancer Causes Control.* 2004;15(6):535–541.

114. Wick MM. Levodopa and dopamine analogs as DNA polymerase inhibitors and antitumor agents in human melanoma. *Cancer Res.* 1980;40(5):1414–1418.

115. Chakroborty D, Sarkar C, Mitra RB, Banerjee S, Dasgupta PS, Basu S. Depleted dopamine in gastric cancer tissues: dopamine treatment retards growth of gastric cancer by inhibiting angiogenesis. *Clin Cancer Res.* 2004;10(13):4349–4356.

116. Isovich E, Mijnster MJ, Flugge G, Fuchs E. Chronic psychosocial stress reduces the density of dopamine transporters. *Eur J Neurosci.* 2000;12(3):1071–1078.

117. Grinshpoon A, Barchana M, Ponizovsky A, et al. Cancer in schizophrenia: is the risk higher or lower? *Schizophr Res.* 2005;73(2–3):333–341.

118. Kandel E. *In search of memory: the emergence of a new science of mind.* New York: W.W. Norton & Company; 2007.

119. Wolter JK, Wolter NE, Blanch A, et al. Anti-tumor activity of the beta-adrenergic receptor antagonist propranolol in neuroblastoma. *Oncotarget.* 2014;5(1):161–172.

120. Armaiz-Pena GN, Allen JK, Cruz A, et al. Src activation by beta-adrenoreceptors is a key switch for tumour metastasis. *Nat Commun.* 2013;4:1403.

121. Shi M, Liu D, Duan H, et al. The beta2-adrenergic receptor and Her2 comprise a positive feedback loop in human breast cancer cells. *Breast Cancer Res Treat.* 2011;125(2):351–362.

122. Cole SW, Arevalo JM, Takahashi R, et al. Computational identification of gene-social environment interaction at the human IL6 locus. *Proc Natl Acad Sci U S A.* 2010;107(12):5681–5686.

123. Shahzad MM, Arevalo JM, Armaiz-Pena GN, et al. Stress effects on FosB- and interleukin-8 (IL8)-driven ovarian cancer growth and metastasis. *J Biol Chem.* 2010;285(46):35462–35470.

124. Sloan EK, Priceman SJ, Cox BF, et al. The sympathetic nervous system induces a metastatic switch in primary breast cancer. *Cancer Res.* 2010;70(18):7042–7052.

125. Armaiz-Pena GN, Gonzalez-Villasana V, Nagaraja AS, et al. Adrenergic regulation of monocyte chemotactic protein 1 leads to enhanced macrophage recruitment and ovarian carcinoma growth. *Oncotarget.* 2015;6(6):4266–4273.

126. Hori Y, Ishii K, Kanda H, et al. Naftopidil, a selective {alpha}1-adrenoceptor antagonist, suppresses human prostate tumor growth by altering interactions between tumor cells and stroma. *Cancer Prev Res (Phila)*. 2011;4(1):87–96.

127. Sood AK, Armaiz-Pena GN, Halder J, et al. Adrenergic modulation of focal adhesion kinase protects human ovarian cancer cells from anoikis. *J Clin Invest*. 2010;120(5):1515–1523.

128. Inbar S, Neeman E, Avraham R, Benish M, Rosenne E, Ben-Eliyahu S. Do stress responses promote leukemia progression? An animal study suggesting a role for epinephrine and prostaglandin-E2 through reduced NK activity. *PLoS One*. 2011;6(4):e19246.

129. Ayala GE, Dai H, Powell M, et al. Cancer-related axonogenesis and neurogenesis in prostate cancer. *Clin Cancer Res*. 2008;14(23):7593–7603.

130. Irwin MR, Cole SW. Reciprocal regulation of the neural and innate immune systems. *Nat Rev Immunol*. 2011;11(9):625–632.

131. Padgett DA, Sheridan JF, Dorne J, Berntson GG, Candelora J, Glaser R. Social stress and the reactivation of latent herpes simplex virus type 1. *Proc Natl Acad Sci U S A*. 1998;95(12):7231–7235.

132. Cole SW, Kemeny ME, Taylor SE, Visscher BR, Fahey JL. Accelerated course of human immunodeficiency virus infection in gay men who conceal their homosexual identity. *Psychosom Med*. 1996;58(3):219–231.

133. Cole SW. Social regulation of human gene expression: mechanisms and implications for public health. *Am J Public Health*. 2013;103(Suppl 1):S84–S92.

134. Antoni MH, Lutgendorf SK, Blomberg B, et al. Cognitive-behavioral stress management reverses anxiety-related leukocyte transcriptional dynamics. *Biol Psychiatry*. 2012;71(4):366–372.

135. Lutgendorf SK, DeGeest K, Sung CY, et al. Depression, social support, and beta-adrenergic transcription control in human ovarian cancer. *Brain Behav Immun*. 2009;23(2):176–183.

136. Ryff CD. Psychological well-being revisited: advances in the science and practice of eudaimonia. *Psychother Psychosom*. 2014;83(1):10–28.

137. Cacioppo JT, Hawkley LC. Perceived social isolation and cognition. *Trends Cogn Sci*. 2009;13(10):447–454.

138. Lutgendorf SK, Sood AK. Biobehavioral factors and cancer progression: physiological pathways and mechanisms. *Psychosom Med*. 2011;73(9):724–730.

139. Lutgendorf SK, Mullen-Houser E, Russell D, et al. Preservation of immune function in cervical cancer patients during chemoradiation using a novel integrative approach. *Brain Behav Immun*. 2010;24(8):1231–1240.

140. Antoni MH. Psychosocial intervention effects on adaptation, disease course and biobehavioral processes in cancer. *Brain Behav Immun*. 2013;30(Suppl):S88–S98.

141. Newell SA, Sanson-Fisher RW, Savolainen NJ. Systematic review of psychological therapies for cancer patients: overview and recommendations for future research. *J Natl Cancer Inst*. 2002;94(8):558–584.

142. McGregor BA, Antoni MH. Psychological intervention and health outcomes among women treated for breast cancer: a review of stress pathways and biological mediators. *Brain Behav Immun*. 2009;23(2):159–166.

143. Andersen BL, Farrar WB, Golden-Kreutz DM, et al. Psychological, behavioral, and immune changes after a psychological intervention: a clinical trial. *J Clin Oncol*. 2004;22(17):3570–3580.

144. Thornton LM, Andersen BL, Carson WE 3rd. Immune, endocrine, and behavioral precursors to breast cancer recurrence: a case-control analysis. *Cancer Immunol Immunother*. 2008;57(10):1471–1481.

145. Phillips KM, Antoni MH, Lechner SC, et al. Stress management intervention reduces serum cortisol and increases relaxation during treatment for nonmetastatic breast cancer. *Psychosom Med*. 2008;70(9):1044–1049.

146. Antoni MH, Lechner S, Diaz A, et al. Cognitive behavioral stress management effects on psychosocial and physiological adaptation in women undergoing treatment for breast cancer. *Brain Behav Immun*. 2009;23(5):580–591.

147. Cole SW, Hawkley LC, Arevalo JM, Cacioppo JT. Transcript origin analysis identifies antigen-presenting cells as primary targets of socially regulated gene expression in leukocytes. *Proc Natl Acad Sci U S A*. 2011;108(7):3080–3085.

7

Depression in Neurological Disorders
Comorbidity or Another Clinical Manifestation?

Andres M. Kanner

INTRODUCTION

Depressive disorders are more common in patients with neurological disease than in the general population. Thus, in the general population, their lifetime prevalence has been estimated to be 26% for women and 12% for men, while in neurological patients, it has been found to range between 30% and 50%.[1,2] Depressive disorders in neurological patients may be clinically identical to primary mood disorders, but they can also have atypical clinical manifestations, as seen in epilepsy, stroke, Alzheimer's dementia (AD), and Parkinson's disease (PD), creating an obstacle to their identification during individual evaluations and in epidemiological studies.

Typically, depressive disorders are considered to be one of the "complications" of the underlying neurological disorder, despite the fact that they often precede the latter by months to years and, in fact, a bidirectional relationship between depression and several neurological disorders (e.g., stroke, migraine, epilepsy, PD, and AD) has been suggested by several population-based studies.[3–10] Furthermore, depressive disorders have a negative impact on the course and recovery of the neurological disorder.

Yet, despite their relatively high prevalence and complex relationship with neurological disorders, depressive disorders remain under-recognized and under-treated. For example, in a study of 100 consecutive patients with epilepsy, 69 patients were found to experience symptoms of depression severe enough to warrant referral for treatment[11]; 63% of patients with spontaneous depression and 54% of patients with an iatrogenic depression had been symptomatic for more than one year before treatment was initiated.

The aim of this chapter is to briefly review some of the epidemiological data and atypical clinical manifestations of depression in neurological disorders, to highlight the possible bidirectional relationship between depressive and neurological disorders, to analyze potential pathogenic mechanisms that may explain this phenomenon, and to review the negative impact that depressive disorders have on the course and management of the neurological disorder. Given the complex problems associated with the treatment of depression in neurological disorders, it will not be addressed in this chapter.

EPIDEMIOLOGICAL DATA

As stated, depressive disorders are more frequent in neurological patients than in the general population and represent, with anxiety disorders, the most frequent psychiatric comorbidity. Yet the epidemiological data of psychiatric comorbidities in neurological disorders have several limitations; first, the reported prevalence rates vary widely among studies, based on the methodology used to identify psychiatric phenomena, with some studies using screening instruments designed to identify "psychiatric symptoms," while others rely on structured and semi-structured interviews aimed at identifying categorical psychiatric diagnoses based on the *Diagnostic and Statistical Manual of Mental Disorders* (DSM) classifications.[12] Secondly, the atypical clinical manifestations of depressive disorders may fail to meet the diagnostic criteria suggested in the DSM editions.

Epilepsy

A lifetime prevalence of 34.2% (25.0–43.3%) of mood /anxiety disorders (vs. 19% in people without epilepsy) was identified in a Canadian population-based study in patients with epilepsy[13]; a major depressive disorder and a history of suicidal ideation was found in 17.2% and 25%, respectively (vs. 19% and 13.3%). Three population-based studies have also reported higher prevalence rates among patients with treatment-resistant epilepsy.[14-16] While depressive disorders had been typically associated with focal epilepsy of temporal lobe origin, high prevalence rates have also been identified in generalized epilepsy and in pediatric populations.

Multiple Sclerosis

Prevalence rates of depression in multiple sclerosis have ranged between 27% and 65% among the various studies.[17] For example, in a population-based study that included 115,071 subjects aged 18 and older, a 12-month prevalence-rate of 25.7% of major depression was found in a population-based study among people with multiple sclerosis (MS), compared to 8.9% of those without it.[18] In a Canadian study where psychiatric interviews were used, a current or lifetime diagnosis of depression was found in 34.4% of 221 MS patients, and 50.3% of patients were estimated to have a cumulative risk for depression by age 59,[19] while a 42% lifetime prevalence rate of major depression was found in a separate Canadian study conducted in 100 patients, using a combination of self-report measures and psychiatric interviews.[20] In a study that relied on screening instruments, symptoms of depression were identified in 65% of outpatients.[21]

Stroke

The prevalence rates of post-stroke depression (PSD) have ranged from 30–50% in several cross-sectional studies,[22] with one study estimating a pooled prevalence rate of all types of depression at 31.8% (range: 30–44%) in population-based studies and prevalence rates of major depressive disorder (MDD) ranging from 11–15%, and minor depression from

8–12%.[23-25] In hospital-based studies, the overall prevalence rates ranged from 25–47%, with those of MDD ranging from 10–27% and minor depression between 11 and 20%.[26-28] In studies done in rehabilitation institutions, overall rates ranged from 35–72%, with rates of major depressive episodes (MDE) ranging from 10–40% and of minor depression from 21–44%.[29-31] The occurrence of PSD peaks between three and six months after a stroke.[32] In a population-based study conducted in Denmark, which included 135,417 stroke patients and a matched control group of 145,499, PSD was diagnosed in the first two years in 25.4% of stroke patients compared to 7.8% of controls, yielding a hazard ratio of 8.99 (range: 8.61–9.39).[33] Of note, in more than half of the stroke patients, depression was identified within the first three months, while this was the case in fewer than one quarter of the controls.

Parkinson's Disease

A systematic review of the prevalence of depression in patients with Parkinson's Disease (PD) revealed a 17% prevalence of MDD, 22% of minor depression, and 13% of dysthymia, according to DSM-IV criteria,[34] while clinically significant depressive symptoms were reported by an average of 35% of patients. In contrast, a separate study found high prevalence rates of "symptoms" of depression with estimates ranging from 40–50%,[35] with some studies suggesting prevalence rates as high as 90%. However, the similarity of symptoms of depression and Parkinsonian symptoms, such as apathy and psychomotor retardation, may falsely increase the prevalence rate of depressive symptoms. Severe depressive episodes are more often identified in patients with an akinetic, rigid form of PD, while less severe depressive symptomatology has been reported in PD with akinetic rigid and tremor form.[36]

Alzheimer's Dementia

As in the case of PD, the identification of depression in patients with AD can be difficult, particularly in patients with moderate to severe dementia, as the symptoms of depression in these patients can often be masked by the underlying dementing process and result in erroneous data. Nonetheless, the prevalence of depression in AD patients has been estimated to range from 30–50%, presenting as major or minor depression, with the lowest rates in community samples.[37]

Migraine

Several epidemiological studies have found that migraine is associated with a relatively high prevalence of mood disorders. In a Canadian population study of 36,984 subjects, the prevalence of MDD, bipolar disorder, panic disorder, and social phobia was more than two times higher in patients with migraine than in those without.[38] Furthermore, patients with MDD have higher prevalence of comorbid migraine. Other types of headache have been linked to depressive disorders, but migraine seems to be the one with the closest relationship. The type of headache more commonly associated with depression was investigated in a case-control study of 1,259 patients with recurrent MDE in which their headache type was compared with that of 859 healthy controls.[39] Patients with recurrent MDE had more than a five-fold higher prevalence of migraine with aura, more than a three-fold higher prevalence of migraine without aura, and a two-fold higher prevalence of other non-migraine chronic headaches than controls; all of these differences were statistically significant.

Several studies have shown that suicide attempts seem to be more frequent in young patients suffering from migraine with aura. For example, Breslau and colleagues conducted a study of 1,007 young adults and found that persons with migraine had higher rates of suicide attempts than persons without migraine, with patients with migraine with aura being at significantly higher risk of suicide (odds ratio [OR] for suicide attempts in migraine with aura: 3.0 [95% confidence interval {CI}, 1.4–6.6], after adjusting for coexisting MDD and other psychiatric disorders).[40] Migraine without aura was not associated with an increase in suicide risk. These findings were reproduced in a study of 121 adolescents with chronic daily headache, in which patients with migraine were found to have significantly higher suicidal risk.[41] In this study, migraine with aura was the only type of headache that was found to be a significant and independent predictor of a high suicidal risk, after controlling for gender, depression, and anxiety disorders.

ARE DEPRESSIVE DISORDERS A RISK FOR THE DEVELOPMENT OF NEUROLOGICAL DISORDERS?

Depressive disorders are often considered to be a complication of the underlying neurological disorder. However, depressive and neurological disorders appear to have a very complex relationship, whereby not only are patients with neurological disorders at greater risk of developing a depressive disorder, but patients with primary depressive disorders appear to be at greater risk of developing several neurological disorders. As stated before, this bidirectional relationship has been suggested by several population-based studies of patients with migraines, epilepsy, stroke, PD, and AD.[3–10] This observation is not recent; indeed, Hippocrates was the first clinician to identify a bidirectional relationship between depression and epilepsy when he wrote, 26 centuries ago: "Epileptics become melancholics and melancholics epileptics."[42]

Of note, symptoms of depression may be the initial clinical manifestations of certain neurological disorders such as PD and AD, which in these two disorders raise the question of the existence of an actual bidirectional relationship with depression. (This complex relationship is examined later in the chapter).

Epilepsy

Data from four population-based studies have suggested that patients with a primary depressive disorder have a two- to seven-fold higher risk of developing epilepsy.[3–6] Likewise, patients with a prior history of suicidality have a four to five times higher risk of developing epilepsy.[3]

Stroke

Several studies have suggested that a history of a primary depressive disorder and/or of symptoms of depression is associated with an increased risk of stroke. For example, a meta-analysis of 28 prospective cohort studies that encompassed a total of 317,540 subjects and 8,478 stroke cases followed for a period ranging from 2–29 years identified an increased risk for total stroke (hazards ratio [HR] = 1.45; 95% CI, 1.29–1.63), fatal stroke (HR = 1.55, 95% CI, 1.25–1.93), and ischemic stroke (HR = 1.25, 95% CI, 1.11–1.40).[7]

Parkinson's Disease

Data from two population-based studies appear to suggest that depressive disorders may increase the risk of developing PD.[8,9] In one study from the Netherlands, subjects diagnosed with depression between 1975 and 1990 had a three-fold higher risk of developing PD than subjects matched by birth year who were never diagnosed with depression (HR of 3.13; 95% CI: 1.95–5.01).[8] In the second study, which included 105,416 subjects, investigators compared the lifetime incidence of depressive disorders in patients later diagnosed with PD with that of a matched control population.[9] At the time of their diagnosis of PD, these patients had a greater than two-fold higher risk of a past history of depression (9.2% of the patients had a history of depression, compared with 4.0% of the control population odds ratio (OR) for a history of depression for these patients was 2.4; 95% CI: 2.1–2.7). However, the fact that symptoms of depression may precede the onset of the motor symptomatology calls for caution in the interpretation of these data.

Alzheimer's Dementia

In a meta-analysis of 20 studies that included 102,172 subjects in eight countries, data from 19 studies supported an increased risk of AD in subjects with primary depression.[10] The early clinical manifestation of the dementia as depressive symptoms could not account for the findings of this study, as the risk correlated with a longer timing between depressive episodes and the onset of AD. A second study consisting of a case-register study of almost 23,000 patients with an affective disorder found an association between the risk of developing AD and the severity of the mood disorder, expressed as the number of major depressive episodes leading to an inpatient admission.[43] Thus, patients with three admissions had close to a three-fold increased risk of dementia (95% CI: 0.64–13.2), compared to patients with only one admission.

Depressive disorders are also relatively frequent among patients with mild cognitive impairment (MCI). In a recently published meta-analysis that included 57 studies involving 20,892 patients, an overall pooled prevalence of depression was 32%.[44] However, the prevalence rates differed between studies performed in the community, which yielded a prevalence of 25%, in contrast in studies conducted in clinics, in which the prevalence of depression was 40%.

Migraine

While a bidirectional relationship between migraine and depression has been reported, it does hold true for other types of headaches. For example, in a prospective study of 496 subjects aged 25–55 years with migraine, 151 subjects with other types of headaches of comparable severity, and 539 healthy controls, who were followed for a two-year period, subjects with a major depression at baseline had more than a three-fold higher risk of developing a new-onset migraine during the two-year follow-up period (OR = 3.4; 95% CI = 1.4–8.7) but no other type of severe headache (OR = 0.6; 95% CI = 0.1–4.6). Likewise, patients with a history of migraine at baseline had almost a six-fold higher risk at baseline of developing a new-onset major depression during follow-up (OR = 5.8; 95% CI = 2.7–12.3).[12]

CLINICAL MANIFESTATIONS OF DEPRESSIVE DISORDERS IN NEUROLOGICAL PATIENTS

The clinical manifestations of depressive disorders in neurological patients are often identical to those of primary depressive disorders. However, in certain neurological disorders, they may display atypical clinical manifestations, which fail to meet diagnostic criteria of the DSM. Furthermore, patients with neurological disorders often exhibit symptoms seen in depressive disorders that can be the expression of the underlying neurological disorder and of iatrogenic effects caused by therapies for the neurological disorder. Accordingly, reaching a diagnosis of depression in these cases may often be challenging.

The sharing of signs and symptoms by depressive and certain neurological disorders can limit the usefulness of screening instruments to identify depression disorders, as their scores may yield a false positive diagnosis. Accordingly, great caution is necessary in the interpretation of screening instrument scores, which may need to be adjusted to enhance their specificity for depression in these patients. For example, patients with epilepsy may report neurovegetative symptoms that are typical of a depressive disorder, such as excessive sleepiness, decreased appetite, poor concentration and memory, and fatigue. All of these symptoms may be the expression of iatrogenic effects caused by the antiepileptic drugs (AEDs) topiramate and zonisamide.[45] In one study of patients with MS, the exclusion of confounding symptoms of fatigue and cognitive symptoms resulted in a decrease in overall prevalence rates of depression in both MS from 15.7–6.8%.[46] These observations may be also applicable to stroke, PD, and AD, in which cognitive deficits, apathy, and neurovegetative symptoms are pivotal symptoms of these neurological disorders.

Atypical clinical manifestations of depression in neurological patients are identified in certain forms of depressive episodes in epilepsy, vascular dementia and AD, and PD. In the next sections, we review the atypical manifestations of depressive disorders in these neurological disorders.

Epilepsy

Psychiatric symptoms in epilepsy patients are defined by their temporal relationship to the actual seizure into *interictal* (symptoms occur independently of seizure occurrence) and *peri-ictal symptoms*, which are divided into *pre-ictal* (symptoms that precede the seizure by several hours to three days), *ictal* (symptoms that are the expression of the seizure), and *postictal* symptoms (symptoms that occur several hours to up to seven days after the ictal event). Distinguishing peri-ictal from interictal symptomatology is of the essence, as interictal symptoms/episodes respond to psychotropic medication, while peri-ictal symptoms do not.

Interictal Dysphoric Disorder

Interictal dysphoric disorder represents an atypical type of an interictal depressive episode. It was initially described by Kraepelin in the beginning of the 20th century,[47] and 20 and 30 years later, its existence was confirmed by Bleuler[48] and Gastaut,[49] respectively, but it was Blumer, in the second half of the 20th century, who brought it to the attention of the epilepsy community.[50] It is estimated that about one-third of the depressed patients with epilepsy may present this type of depressive episode.[50] It has a chronic course and includes a pleomorphic cluster of symptoms of depression, hypomania, anxiety, irritability, and pain that waxes and wanes in severity and is interrupted by symptom-free periods ranging from days to weeks.[50] Recently, interictal dysphoric disorder was also recognized in patients with migraine.[51]

Postictal Depressive Symptoms and Episodes

Postictal depressive symptoms and episodes are rarely investigated by clinicians, despite the fact that they are relatively frequent in patients with treatment-resistant focal epilepsy. In one of the few studies that investigated the presence of habitual postictal psychiatric symptoms among 100 patients with treatment-resistant focal epilepsy, 43 patients endorsed postictal symptoms of depression, which included 13 patients with habitual postictal suicidal symptoms and 22 patients who reported hypomanic symptoms[60]; 45 patients endorsed postictal symptoms of anxiety; seven, psychotic symptoms; and 62 experienced postictal neurovegetative symptoms. Of note, there was a high correlation in the occurrence of depressive, anxiety, psychotic, and neurovegetative symptoms. The median duration of these symptoms was 24 hours, with ranges between one and 208 hours. Among the 43 patients with postictal symptoms of depression, 18 experienced a minimum of six postictal symptoms of depression for a period of at least 24 hours with a semiology that mimicked a typical MDE, with the exception that the duration of the event was significantly shorter than the required two weeks of such episodes. Nonetheless, patients may at times experience postictal depressive episodes of one to three weeks' duration.

Stroke

While the clinical semiology of PSD is similar to that of primary late-onset depression, psychomotor retardation may be more frequent among patients with PSD.[61] These patients are also more likely to display "catastrophic depressive reactions," hyperemotionalism, and diurnal mood variation than patients with idiopathic depression.[62]

Of note, the severity of PSD has been found to correlate with the degree of impairment of activities of daily living (ADL), during both its acute and chronic phases, and it can worsen the severity of vegetative symptoms presenting as disturbances of sleep, libido, and level of energy from the time of the initial evaluation, and persisting at three, six, 12, and 24 months.[63]

Vascular Depression

Vascular depression is another type of depressive episode associated with cerebrovascular disease, consisting of symptoms of depression beginning after the age of 65 years that include abnormal mood, cognitive disturbances with impairment of executive functions, a greater tendency to psychomotor retardation, poor insight, and impaired activities of daily living.[64] In these patients, there is clinical and/or neuroradiological evidence of diffuse, bilateral, white-matter small vessel disease associated with chronic cerebrovascular risk factors such as hypertension, diabetes, carotid stenosis, atrial fibrillation, and hyperlipidemia; they may have never suffered from an overt stroke, or may have only experienced a transient ischemic attack.[65]

Parkinson's Disease

Depression precedes the onset of motor symptoms in 2.5–37% of PD patients.[66,67] The symptom profile differs slightly from primary depressive disorders by exhibiting less guilt, self-reproach, and feelings of failure.

Alzheimer's Dementia

The most common symptoms of depression in AD include dysphoria, loss of interest, indecisiveness, and diminished ability to concentrate, but with limited depressive ideation. These symptoms are often associated with apathy and altered activity, low energy, decreased libido, appetite, and altered sleep.[68] Older depressed patients tend to complain about somatic symptoms and deny feeling sad, or fail to acknowledge a lack of interest or pleasure in activities, which has been referred as "depression without sadness."[69]

There is a general consensus that depression in dementia is less severe than in non-demented patients, with specific symptoms often failing to meet DSM IV or *International Classification of Diseases 10th ed.* (ICD 10) criteria of a discrete mood disorder. The diagnosis of depression in these patients can be often challenging, as the impaired cognitive functions of these patients limit them from verbally expressing their symptoms. In order to overcome these limitations, the National Institute of Mental Health (NIMH) published "Provisional Diagnostic Criteria for Depression of Alzheimer's Disease."[70] These criteria require at least three of the typical symptoms of depression listed in the primary major depressive episodes, of at least two weeks' duration, and causing clinically significant distress or disruption in functioning. These symptoms have to occur in the setting of AD. Yet these specific criteria still fail to reflect the importance of somatic complaints and "depression without sadness."

SCREENING INSTRUMENTS OF DEPRESSION IN NEUROLOGICAL DISORDERS

The limited availability of psychiatrists and mental health care providers in neurology clinics has limited the access of these patients to an appropriate evaluation and treatment of their psychiatric comorbidities. The use of screening instruments allows neurologists to identify patients with depression and anxiety disorders. However, as stated, caution is of the essence in the interpretation of these instruments to avoid making false positive diagnoses of depression.

Epilepsy

Among the available screening instruments developed for patients with primary depressive disorders, three have been validated in patients with epilepsy: The Beck Depression Inventory (BDI-II),[71] the Center for Epidemiological Studies–Depression (CES-D),[72] and the Hamilton Depression Rating Scale (HAM-D).[73] One self-rating instrument, the Neurological Disorders Depression Inventory for Epilepsy (NDDI-E), was developed to identify major depressive episodes specifically in people with epilepsy.[74] This instrument has the advantage of not including any somatic and cognitive item that can be confounded with adverse events of AEDs or from symptoms associated with the epileptic syndrome and/or the underlying neurological disorder. Another self-rating instrument, the Interictal Dysphoric Disorder Inventory (IDDI), was developed to identify interictal dysphoric disorder (IDD),[75] and one questionnaire was developed to identify postictal psychiatric symptoms: the Rush Postictal Psychiatric Symptoms Questionnaire.[60]

Stroke

The commonly used screening instruments in primary depressive disorder have been used in the screening of PSD and have included the BDI,[76] the Hospital Anxiety Depression Scale (HADS),[77] the Zung Scale ZS,[78] the Geriatric Depression Scale (GDS),[79] and the CES-D,[80] while the HAM-D[81] is one of the most frequently used examiner-rating scales.

The Post-Stroke Depression Scale (PSDS)[82] and the Stroke Aphasic Depression Questionnaire (SADQ)[83] are two instruments developed specifically for PSD, the latter for patients with aphasia. The PSDS includes items intended to identify symptoms associated with PSD such as hyperemotionalism and catastrophic reactions. Furthermore, the PSDS has been shown to demonstrate a continuum between major and minor forms of PSD.

Dementia

The HAM-D is one of the commonly used instruments that have been considered to reliably identify depression in patients with AD.[84] The Cornell Scale for Depression and Dementia (CSDD) is an instrument developed for demented patients with depression,[85,86] but a reliable informant is needed to complete this instrument.

Parkinson's Disease

Screening instruments commonly used in primary depression that have been also used in patients with PD include the BDI, HADS, GDS, and the Montgomery-Asberg Depression Rating Scale.[87–89] However, the presence of somatic symptoms resulting from PD may yield a false-positive diagnosis of depression, increasing the sensitivity and lowering their specificity, requiring higher cut-off scores to increase the specificity.[90]

Multiple Sclerosis

Standard screening instruments like the BDI, CES-D, and the abbreviated version of the Patient Health Questionnaire (PHQ-2) have been used successfully in various studies of multiple sclerosis.[91]

A COMORBID DEPRESSION IS ASSOCIATED WITH A WORSE COURSE OF THE NEUROLOGICAL DISORDER

Typically, clinicians have focused on the impact of depression and other psychiatric comorbidities on quality-of-life health measures. However, there are significant data that suggest that depression can have a directly negative impact on the course and overall management of several neurological disorders, including epilepsy, stroke, migraine, PD, AD, and MCI. Unfortunately, neurologists and psychiatrists alike have paid little attention to this literature. These data are briefly reviewed in the following discussion.

Epilepsy

Two studies have suggested that a history of depression preceding the onset of epilepsy or identified at the time of diagnosis of the seizure disorder is associated with a worse response to pharmacotherapy. The first study included 780 patients with newly diagnosed epilepsy followed over a median period of 79 months.[92] Univariate and multivariate logistical regression analyses demonstrated that a history of depression preceding the diagnosis of epilepsy was associated with a two-fold higher risk of developing pharmaco-resistance to AEDs. In the second study, the presence of symptoms of depression and anxiety was investigated in 138 patients with new-onset epilepsy before the start of AED therapy[93]; patients who endorsed symptoms of depression at the time of diagnosis were significantly less likely to be seizure-free after a 12-month follow-up period. Likewise, three studies of patients with treatment-resistant temporal lobe epilepsy who underwent an antero-temporal lobectomy found that a lifetime history of depression was associated with a decreased likelihood of reaching complete freedom from seizure.[93–95]

Furthermore, a lifetime history of depression increases the risk of neurological and psychiatric adverse events to AEDs; the latter have been associated with exposure to certain AEDs known to have negative psychotropic properties, such as barbiturates, benzodiazepines, levetiracetam, topiramate, zonisamide, vigabatrin, and perampanel.[96] Conversely, discontinuation of AEDs with mood-stabilizing properties such as carbamazepine, oxcarbazepine, valproic acid, and lamotrigine can result in the recurrence of depressive episodes in patients with a prior history of mood disorders who had been in remission on these AEDs.[97]

Stroke

PSD has been found to have a negative impact at several levels, including: (1) recovery of cognitive deficits, (2) the ability to perform activities of daily living (ADL), and (3) increased mortality risks. For example, in one study, patients with major PSD had significantly more cognitive deficits than non-depressed patients who experienced a similar location and size of left-hemisphere (but not right-hemisphere) stroke,[98] while in a second study, of 140 patients, the presence of major PSD was associated with greater cognitive impairment two years after a stroke.[99] One study found that the development of in-hospital PSD was the most important variable predicting poor recovery in ADL over a two-year period.[100]

The increased mortality risk associated with PSD is illustrated in a population-based study of 10,025 subjects followed over eight years, of whom 1,925 died.[101] Mortality rate per 1,000 person-years of follow-up was highest in the group with a history of both stroke and depression (HR: 1.88; 95% CI: 1.27–2.79) vs. only depression present HR: 1.23 (1.08, 1.40) vs. only stroke: HR: 1.74 (1.06, 2.85). In another study, patients with PSD had a 3.4-fold higher risk of dying during a 10-year follow-up period than non-depressed patients, independently of other stroke risk factors.[102] Finally, a higher mortality risk was found over a three-year follow-up period in patients with PSD, even though these patients were younger and suffered from fewer chronic conditions.[103]

Migraine

Comorbid depression can influence the course and severity of migraine, as illustrated by a study by Breslau and colleagues, in which patients with migraine and lifetime history of MDD reported a significantly higher severity of migraine attacks compared to patients without any past depressive episode.[104] This phenomenon is not restricted to depression. For example, in an eight-year follow-up study of 100 young adults with migraine or tension-type headache, psychiatric comorbidities were associated with a worse course of the migraines and the non-migraine headaches.[105]

In addition, the comorbid occurrence of depression and migraine with aura can increase the risk of epileptic seizures. Indeed, Hesdorffer and colleagues[106] found that the co-occurrence of MDE and migraine with aura significantly increased the risk for developing unprovoked seizures more than did either MDE or migraine with aura alone. In contrast, migraine without aura was not associated with an increased risk of unprovoked seizures. Conversely, migraine with aura has been found to increase the suicidal risk, as suggested by two epidemiological studies of people aged 12–28 years in which patients diagnosed with migraine with aura had a higher suicidal risk, independent of the psychiatric comorbidities.[107,108]

Parkinson's Disease

Comorbid depression in PD patients has been associated with a more rapid deterioration of motor and cognitive functions, especially executive functions.[109] For example, investigators compared neuropsychological functions among patients with PD and MDD, patients with PD without depression, patients with MDD but without PD, and age-comparable healthy controls. More severe cognitive deficits were identified in patients with MDD, with or without PD, than in both healthy controls and patients with PD without depression, on tests of verbal fluency and auditory attention.[110] In addition, more severe deficits on tasks of abstract reasoning and set alternation were found in patients with PD and MDD than in the other three groups. In a separate study, cognitive functions were compared between 45 PD patients with current depression and 45 patients without depression matched for age, education, gender, age at disease onset, disease duration, and disease severity; patients with depression were significantly more impaired cognitively. While cognitive functions were impaired in both groups, impaired memory was found only in the depressed PD patients.[111]

Alzheimer's Dementia

A history of depression can impact the course of AD when preceding the onset of AD, as well as when it occurs as a comorbid disorder. For example, in a study of 43 patients with AD with mild-to-moderate cognitive impairment, 22 had a history of an MDD preceding the onset of any cognitive impairment, but not at the time of the cognitive evaluation.[112] After controlling for age, education, duration of illness, gender, and medication status, subjects with a history of MDD had significantly lower scores on several neuropsychological tests, which included the Mini-Mental State Exam, Wechsler Adult Intelligence Scale Full-Scale and Verbal Scale IQ, and the Initiation/Perseveration subscale of the Mattis Dementia Rating Scale. These subjects also developed symptoms of dementia at a significantly earlier age than the subjects without a prior history of a depressive disorder.

Furthermore, the presence of comorbid depressive disorders in patients with AD is associated with a faster cognitive deterioration, worse deterioration in ADL,[113] an earlier placement in a nursing facility,[114] and it is also associated with a faster decline in cognitive functions.[115]

Mild Cognitive Impairment

A history of depression in individuals with MCI has been found to be associated with an increased risk of developing AD. For example, 41 of 114 patients with MCI followed for a three-year period had a depressive disorder at baseline.[116] At follow-up, 35 (85%) of these patients had developed AD, in comparison with 32% of the non-depressed subjects, yielding a relative risk of developing AD of 2.6 (95% CI: 1.8–3.6).

WHAT ACCOUNTS FOR THE NEGATIVE IMPACT OF DEPRESSION ON THE COURSE OF THE NEUROLOGICAL DISORDER?

The negative impact of depression on the course of neurological disorders should serve as a wake-up call to neurologists and internists with respect to the need for early identification and management of psychiatric comorbidities in these patients. Some authors have explained these findings by suggesting that depressed patients have difficulty following the treatment recommendations, therefore affecting their compliance with pharmacological treatments and/or prescribed diets.[117] While this may well be one of the potential explanations, it is unlikely to be the only answer.

Neurobiological changes associated with a depressive disorder have to be postulated as possible culprits of this phenomenon. Furthermore, we cannot ignore the close and complex relationship between depression and neurological disorders illustrated in the bidirectional relationship identified between depression and several neurological disorders, including epilepsy, migraine, stroke, PD, and AD. The bidirectional relationship between the depression and some of the neurological disorders does not imply causality; that is, neurological disorders are not the cause of the depressive disorders, nor vice-versa. The existence of common pathogenic mechanisms operant in depressive and neurological disorders is the most likely explanation of such bidirectional relationships. These pathogenic mechanisms, in turn, may facilitate the worse course of neurological disorders. In fact, there are data supporting this hypothesis.

Some of the important pathogenic mechanisms operant in mood disorders that can potentially explain the negative impact of depression on neurological disorders include: (1) neurotransmitter disturbances of serotonin (5HT), norepinephrine (NE), gamma-aminobutyric acid (GABA), and glutamate; (2) neuroendocrine disturbances, manifested by a hyperactive hypothalamic-pituitary-adrenal axis (HPA-A); and (3) inflammatory disturbances. These data are reviewed in detail in other manuscripts by this author.[119,120] Some of the data are summarized in the following discussion.

Neurotransmitter Disturbances

Abnormal serotonergic, noradrenergic, and dopaminergic transmission in the brain of depressed patients is a pivotal pathogenic mechanism of mood disorders.[118] In some animal models of epilepsy, a decreased serotonergic and noradrenergic activity has been shown to facilitate the kindling of seizures, exacerbate seizure severity, and intensify seizure severity,[119] while increments of either NE and/or 5HT transmission with the selective serotonin-reuptake inhibitors (SSRIs) resulted in a dose-dependent seizure-frequency reduction.[120] In humans, abnormal binding of 5-HT-_{1A} receptors has been found to be abnormal in the same neuroanatomical structures of patients with temporal lobe epilepsy (TLE) and patients with primary MDD, as demonstrated in studies carried out with positron emission tomography (PET). These structures included the hippocampus, amygdala, cingulate, and raphe nuclei.[121-124]

Conversely, abnormalities in the GABAergic (decreased) and glutamatergic (increased) systems have been identified as pivotal pathogenic mechanisms in animal models and humans with epilepsy.[125-128] Low GABA-ergic and high glutamatergic activity has also been found in patients with MDD.[129-133]

Decreased serotonergic, dopaminergic, and noradrenergic functions are known to play a role in the pathogenesis of PD,[134] and abnormal serotonergic functions have been identified in migraine[135] and stroke.[136]

Disturbances of Inflammatory Functions

Disturbances of inflammatory functions have been identified in depression, epilepsy, migraine, AD, and stroke,[137-141] manifested by increased inflammatory cytokines and chemokines in the blood of these patients, including proinflammatory cytokines, interleukin-1β (IL-1β), IL-2, IL-6, interferon-γ (IFN-γ), and tumor necrosis factor-α (TNF-α). Among the various cytokines, interleukin-1β (IL-1β) has been found to display proconvulsant properties and to be overexpressed in human brains of patients with TLE, cortical dysplasias, and tuberous sclerosis.[142-145] The mechanisms responsible for IL-1β proconvulsant properties involve a reduction in glutamate uptake by glial cells or an enhanced release of glutamate from these cells, mediated by TNF-α.[146]

Hyperactive Hypothalamic-Pituitary-Adrenal axis

Hyperactive HPA-A is a biological marker of MDD, which consists of excessive cortisol secretion and is clinically demonstrated with a failure of the adrenal gland to suppress the secretion of cortisol to a dose of dexamethasone (also known as the dexamethasone suppression test [DST]).[147] An abnormal DST has been identified in about 50% of patients with MDD, and has been also reported in patients with TLE.[148] Neuropathological consequences attributed to excessive cortisol have included:

1. decreased glial density and neuronal size in the cingulate gyrus;
2. decreased neuronal sizes and neuronal density in layers II, III, and IV in the rostral orbito-frontal cortex, resulting in a decrease of cortical thickness;
3. decrease of glial density in cortical layers V and VI, associated with decreases in neuronal sizes in the caudal orbito-frontal cortex; and
4. a decrease of neuronal and glial density and size in all cortical layers of the dorsolateral prefrontal cortex.[149-154]

Finally, elevated levels of glucocorticoids have been associated with reduced astrocytes' activity and interference with their function. Since recapturing synaptic glutamate is one of the major functions of glial cells, a loss of this type of cell is likely to favor an increase in glutamate in the central nervous system, potentially facilitating a hyperexcitable state in patients with MDD and epilepsy. In addition to the neuropathological changes, structural changes in the temporal and frontal lobes have been identified, including significant hippocampal atrophy, ranging from 8–19%, in depressed patients compared with non-depressed controls.[155-157] Moreover, an inverse relationship between duration of depression and total hippocampal volume has been demonstrated.[158]

Coupled with the decreased GABA-ergic tone associated with MDD, the combination of an increased glutamatergic and decreased GABA-ergic activity may provide a possible explanation for the increased risk that patients with a lifetime history of depression have of developing treatment-resistant epilepsy. Likewise, neuronal cell loss diffusely could facilitate the cognitive deterioration associated with MDD and stroke, PD, AD, and MCI, while hippocampal atrophy may also account for the bidirectional relationship between MDD and AD and MCI. Clearly, these data yield hypotheses that need to be confirmed in future research.

CONCLUSION

The data reviewed in this chapter illustrate the very complex relationship between depressive and neurological disorders, which has significant clinical implications, as patients with a history of a primary depression may be at increased risk of developing several neurological disorders, and/or these neurological disorders have a higher risk of having a severe course and worse response to treatment. As stated herein, common pathogenic mechanisms operant in depression and neurological disorders are the most likely explanation of their complex relationships, and their identification would be expected to yield important therapeutic strategies. This is illustrated by the use of several AEDs with mood-stabilizing and antidepressant properties for the treatment of epilepsy and mood disorder, or the use of antidepressant drugs for the prevention of migraines.

Unfortunately, the complex relationship between depression and neurological disorders and their clinical implications are yet to be recognized by neurologists and psychiatrists, in both academic and clinical domains alike, which is illustrated by the scarce and, in some disorders like epilepsy, the nonexistent evidence-base data of the management of depression in the various neurological disorders. The next question also begs to be answered and yet remains unaddressed: "Given the stated negative impact of a comorbid depressive disorder in patients with epilepsy, stroke, migraine, PD, MCI, and AD, would its early recognition and effective management prevent and/or mitigate their negative course and poor response to treatment?"

Any clinician and neuroscientist would have expected to see this question addressed in experimental and clinical research as well as in clinical practice. Furthermore, this unanswered question should raise great intellectual curiosity in neurologists and psychiatrists alike, while the neuroradiological, neuropathological, and neurochemical changes identified in the brains of patients with a primary depressive disorder should be a red flag to neurologists that depression is in fact a neurological disorder with psychological symptoms.

So what is the reason for the lack of clinical data? The poor communication between neurologists and psychiatrists explains (at least to a large degree) this bizarre phenomenon. The lack of communication between the two disciplines results, in turn, in the failure to properly train neurologists and psychiatrists on the psychiatric aspects of neurological disorders, and vice-versa. Until this phenomenon is corrected, nothing will change. As Goethe stated in his novel *Faust*: "You see what you know."

REFERENCES

1. Akiskal H. Mood disorders. In: Sadock B, Sadock V, eds. *Comprehensive textbook of psychiatry*. New York: Lippincott Williams & Williams; 2005:1559–1575.
2. Kanner AM. Management of psychiatric and neurological comorbidities in epilepsy. *Nat Rev Neurol*. Feb 2016;12(2):106–116.
3. Larson SL, Owens PL, Ford D, Eaton W. Depressive disorder, dysthymia, and risk of stroke. Thirteen-year follow-up from the Baltimore Epidemiological Catchment Area Study. *Stroke*. 2001;32:1979–1983.
4. Pan A, Sun Q, Okereke OI, Rexrode KM, Hu FB. Depression and risk of stroke morbidity and mortality: a meta-analysis and systematic review. *JAMA*. 2011;306(11):1241–1249.
5. Breslau N, Lipton RB, Stewart WF, et al. Comorbidity of migraine and depression: investigating potential etiology and prognosis. *Neurology*. 2003;60(8):1308–1312.
6. Hesdorffer DC, Hauser WA, Annegers JF, Cascino G. Major depression is a risk factor for seizures in older adults. *Ann Neurol*. 2000;47:246–249.
7. Hesdorffer DC, Hauser WA, Ludvigsson P, Olafsson E, Kjartansson O. Depression and attempted suicide as risk factors for incident unprovoked seizures and epilepsy. *Ann Neurology*. 2006;59:35–41.
8. Ownby RL, Crocco E, Acevedo A, et al. Depression and risk for Alzheimer disease: systematic review, meta-analysis, and metaregression analysis. *Arch Gen Psychiatry*. 2006;63(5):530–538.
9. Modrego PJ, Fernandez J. Depression in patients with mild cognitive impairment increases the risk of developing dementia of Alzheimer's type: a prospective cohort study. *Arch Neurol*. 2004;61:1290–1293.
10. Nilsson FM, Kessing LV, Bowlig TG. Increased risk of developing Parkinson's disease for patients with major affective disorder: a register study. *Acta Psychiatr Scand*. 2001;104:380–386.
11. Kanner, AM, Kozak AM, Frey M. The use of sertraline in patients with epilepsy: Is it safe? *Epilepsy Behav*. 2000;1(2):100–105.
12. American Psychiatric Association. *Diagnostic and Statistical Manual of Mental Disorders*. 4th ed. Washington, DC: American Psychiatric Press; 2000.
13. Tellez-Zenteno JF, Patten SB, Jetté N, Williams J, Wiebe S. Psychiatric comorbidity in epilepsy: a population-based analysis. *Epilepsia*. 2007;48:2336–2344.
14. Ettinger A, Reed M, Cramer J. Epilepsy Impact Project Group: Depression and comorbidity in community-based patients with epilepsy or asthma. *Neurology*. 2004;63:1008–1014.
15. Beghi E, Spagnoli P, Airoldi L, et al. Emotional and affective disturbances in patients with epilepsy. *Epilepsy Behav*. 2002;3:225–261.
16. Jacoby A, Baker GA, Steen N, Potts P, Chadwick DW. The clinical course of epilepsy and its psychosocial correlates: findings from a U.K. community study. *Epilepsia*. Feb 1996;37(2):148–161.
17. Serafin DJ, Weisbrot D, Ettinger AB. Multiple sclerosis. In: Kanner AM, ed. *Treatment of depression in neurologic disorders*. New York: Wiley; 2014:157–176.
18. Patten SB, Beck CA, Williams JV, et al. Major depression in multiple sclerosis: a population-based perspective. *Neurology*. 2003;61(11):1524–1527.
19. Sadovnick AD, Remick RA, Swartz E, et al. Depression and multiple sclerosis. *Neurology*. 1996;46(3):628–632.
20. Joffe RT, Lippert GP, Gray TA, et al. Mood disorder and multiple sclerosis. *Arch Neurol*. 1987;44(4):376–378.

21. Schiffer RB, Lippert GP, Gray TA. Depression in neurological practice: diagnosis, treatment, implications. *Semin Neurol.* 2009;29(3):220–233.
22. Robinson RG. Poststroke depression: prevalence, diagnosis, treatment and disease progression. *Biol Psychiatry.* 2003;54:376–387.
23. Burvill PW, Johnson GA, Jamrozik KD, Anderson CS, Stewart-Wynne EG, Chakera TMH. Prevalence of depression after stroke: The Perth Community Stroke Study. *Br J Psychiatry.* 1995;166:320–327.
24. Kotila M, Numminen H, Waltimo O, Kaste M. Depression after stroke. Results of the FINNSTROKE study. *Stroke.* 1998;29:368–372.
25. Wade DT, Legh-Smith J, Hewer RA. Depressed mood after stroke, a community study of its frequency. *Br J Psychiatry.* 1987;151:200–205.
26. Singh A, Black SE, Herrmann N, et al. Functional and neuroanatomic correlations in poststroke depression. The Sunnybrook Stroke Study. *Stroke.* 2000;31:637–644.
27. Robinson RG, Starr LB, Kubos KL, Price TR. A two year longitudinal study of post-stroke mood disorders: findings during the initial evaluation. *Stroke.* 1983;14:736–744.
28. Ebrahim S, Barer D, Nouri F. Affective illness after stroke *Br J Psychiatry.* 1987;151:52–56.
29. Eastwood MR, Rifat SL, Nobbs H, Ruderman J. Mood disorder following cerebrovascular accident. *Br J Psychiatry.* 1989;154:195–200.
30. Folstein MF, Maiberger R, McHugh PR. Mood disorder as a specific complication of stroke. *J Neurol Neurosurg Psychiatry.* 1977;40:1018–1020.
31. Schwartz JA, Speed NM, Brunberg JA, Brewer TL, Brown M, Greden JF. Depression in stroke rehabilitation. *Biol Psychiatry.* 1993;33:694–699.
32. Huff W, Steckel R, Sistzer M. Poststroke depression: risk factors and effects on the course of the stroke. *Nervenarzt.* 2003;74:104–114.
33. Jørgensen T, Wium-Andersen IK, Wium-Andersen MK, et al. Incidence of depression after stroke, and associated risk factors and mortality outcomes in a large cohort of Danish patients. *JAMA Psychiatry.* Oct 1 2016;73(10):1032–1040.
34. Reijnders JS, Ehrt U, Weber WE, Aarsland D, Leentjens AF. A systematic review of prevalence studies of depression in Parkinson's disease. *Mov Disord.* Jan 2008;30;23(2):183–189; quiz 313.
35. Mentis MJ, Delalot D. Depression in Parkinson's disease. *Adv Neurol.* 2005;96:26–41.
36. Starkstein SE, Petracca G, Chemerinski E, et al. Depression in classic versus akinetic-rigid Parkinson's disease. *Mov Disord.* Jan 1998;13(1):29–33.
37. Starkstein SE, Mizrahi R, Power BD. Depression in Alzheimer's disease: phenomenology, clinical correlates and treatment. *Int Rev Psychiatry.* 2008;20(4):382–388.
38. Jette N, Patten S, Williams J, et al. Comorbidity of migraine and psychiatric disorders—a national population-based study. *Headache.* 2008;48(4):501–516.
39. Saaman Z, Farmer A, Craddock N, et al. Migraine in recurrent depression: case-control study. *Br J Psychiatry.* 2009;194(4):350–354.
40. Breslau N, Davis GC, Andreski P. Migraine, psychiatric disorders, and suicide attempts: an epidemiologic study of young adults. *J Psychiatry Res.* 1991;37(1):11–23.
41. Wang Sj, Juang KD, Fuh JL, et al. Psychiatric comorbidity and suicide risk in adolescents with chronic daily headache. *Neurology.* 2007;68:1468–1473.
42. Lewis A. Melancholia: a historical review. *J Ment Sci.* 1934;80:1–42.
43. Kessing LV, Andersen PK. Does the risk of developing dementia increase with the number of episodes in patients with depressive disorder and in patients with bipolar disorder? *J Neurol Neurosurg Psychiatry.* 2004;75:1662–1666.

44. Modrego PJ, Fernandez J. Depression in patients with mild cognitive impairment increases the risk of developing dementia of Alzheimer's type: a prospective cohort study. *Arch Neurol.* 2004;61:1290–1293.

45. Brown RF, Valpiani EM, Tennant CC, et al. Longitudinal assessment of anxiety, depression, and fatigue in people with multiple sclerosis. *Psychol Psychother.* 2009;82(Pt 1):41–56.

46. Mula M, Jauch R, Cavanna A, et al. Clinical and psychopathological definition of the interictal dysphoric disorder of epilepsy. *Epilepsia.* Apr 2008;49(4):650–656.

47. Kraepelin E. *Psychiatrie.* Vol 3. Leipzig: Johann Ambrosius Barth; 1923.

48. Bleuler E. *Lehrbuch der Psychiatrie.* 8th ed. Berlin: Springer; 1949.

49. Gastaut H, Morin G, Lesèvre N. Étude du comportement des épileptiques psychomoteurs dans l'intervalle de leurs crises: les troubles de l'activité globale et de la sociabilité. *Ann Med Psychol (Paris).* 1955;113:1–27.

50. Blumer D, Altshuler LL. Affective disorders. In: Engel J, Pedley TA, eds. *Epilepsy: a comprehensive textbook.* Vol. II. Philadelphia, PA: Lippincott-Raven; 1998:2083–2099.

51. Mula M, Trimble MR. What do we know about mood disorders in epilepsy? In: Kanner AM, Schachter S, eds. *Psychiatric controversies in epilepsy.* San Diego, CA: Academic Press; 2008: pp. 49–66.

52. Kanner AM, Soto A, Gross-Kanner H. Prevalence and clinical characteristics of postictal psychiatric symptoms in partial epilepsy. *Neurology.* 2004;62:708–713.

52. Lipsey JR, Robinson RG, Pearlson GD, Rao K, Price TR. Nortriptyline treatment of post-stroke depression. A double-blind study. *Lancet.* 1984;1(8372):297–300.

54. Gainotti G, Azzoni A, Marra C Frequency, phenomenology and anatomical-clinical correlates of major post-stroke depression. *Br J Psychiatry.* 1999;175:163–167.

55. Fedoroff JP, Starkstein SE, Parikh RM, Price TR, Robinson RG. Are depressive symptoms non-specific in patients with acute stroke? *Am J Psychiatry.* 1991;148:1172–1176.

56. Alexopoulos GS, Meyers BS, Young RC, Campbell S, Silbersweig D, Charlson M. Vascular depression hypothesis. *Arch Gen Psychiatry.* 1997;54:915–922.

57. Mast BT, MacNeill SE, Lichtenberg PA. Poststroke and clinically-defined vascular depression in geriatric rehabilitation patients. *Am J Geriatr Psychiatry.* 2004;12:84–92.

58. O'Sullivan SS, Williams DR, Gallagher DA, Massey LA, Silveira-Moriyama L, Lees AJ. Nonmotor symptoms as presenting complaints in Parkinson's disease: a clinicopathological study. *Mov Disord.* Jan 2008;23(1):101–106.

59. Starkstein SE, Mizrahi R, Power BD. Depression in Alzheimer's disease: phenomenology, clinical correlates and treatment. *Int Rev Psychiatry.* 2008;20(4):382–388.

60. Gallo JJ, Rabins PV. Depression without sadness: alternative presentations of depression in late life. *Am Fam Physician.* 1999;60:820–826.

61. Olin JT, Katz IR, Meyers BS, et al. Provisional diagnostic criteria for depression of Alzheimer disease: rationale and background. *Am J Geriatr Psychiatry.* 2002;10(2):129–141.

62. Beck AT, Ward CH, Mendelson M, et al. An inventory for measuring depression. *Arch Gen Psychiatry.* 1961;4:561–571.

63. Jones JE, Herman BP, Woodard JL, et al. Screening for major depression in epilepsy with common self-report depression inventories. *Epilepsia.* 2005;46(5):731–735.

64. Hamilton M. The assessment of anxiety states by rating. *Br J Med Psychol.* 1959;32:50–55.

65. Gilliam FG, Barry JJ, Meador KJ, Hermann BP, Vahle V, Kanner AM. Rapid detection of major depression in epilepsy: a multicenter study. *Lancet Neurol.* 2006;5(5):399–405.

66. Zigmond AS, Snaith RP: The Hospital Anxiety and Depression Scale. *Acta Psychiatr Scand.* 1983;67:361–370.

67. Zung WW. A self-rating depression scale. *Arch Gen Psychiatry*. 1965;12:63–70.
68. Yesavage JA, Brink TL, Rose TL. Development and validation of the Geriatric Depression Screening Scale. A preliminary report. *J Psychiatr Res*. 1982;17:37–49.
69. Van Dam NT, Earleywine M. Validation of the Center for Epidemiologic Studies Depression Scale-Revised (CESD-R): pragmatic depression assessment in the general population. *Psychiatry Res*. 2011;186(1):128–132.
70. Gainotti G, Azzoni A, Razzano C, Lanzillotta M, Marra C, Gasparini F. The Post-Stroke Depression Rating Scale: a test specifically devised to investigate affective disorders of stroke patients. *J Clin Exp Neuropsychol*. Jun 1997;19(3):340–356.
71. Sutcliffe LM, Lincoln NB. The assessment of depression in aphasic stroke patients: the development of the Stroke Aphasic Depression Questionnaire. *Clin Rehabil*. Dec 1998;12(6):506–513.
72. Alexopoulos GS, Abrams RC, Young RC et al. Cornell scale for depression in dementia. *Biol Psychiatry*. 1988; 23:271–284.
73. Leentjens AF, Verhey FR, Lousberg R, et al. The validity of the Hamilton and Montgomery-Asberg depression rating scales as screening and diagnostic tools for depression in Parkinson's disease. *Int J Geriatr Psychiatry*. 2000;15:644–649.
74. Mohr DC, Hart SL, Julian L. Screening for depression among patients with multiple sclerosis: two questions may be enough. *Mult Scler*. 2007;13:215–219.
75. Hitiris N, Mohanraj R, Norrie J, et al. Predictors of pharmacoresistant epilepsy. *Epilepsy Res*. 2007;75:192–196.
76. Petrovski S, Szoeke CEI, Jones NC, et al. Neuropsychiatric symptomatology predicts seizure recurrence in newly treated patients. *Neurology,*. 2010;75:1015–1021.
77. Kanner AM, Byrne R, Chicharro A, et al. A lifetime psychiatric history predicts a worse seizure outcome following temporal lobectomy. *Neurology*. 2009;72:793–799.
78. Mast BT, MacNeill SE, Lichtenberg PA. Poststroke and clinically-defined vascular depression in geriatric rehabilitation patients. *Am J Geriatr Psychiatry*. 2004;12:84–92.
79. Robinson RG, Starr LB, Kubos KL, Price TR A two-year longitudinal study of post-stroke mood disorders: findings during the initial evaluation. *Stroke*. 1983;14:736–744.
80. Starkstein SE, Robinson RG, Price TR. Comparison of patients with and without post-stroke major depression matched for age and location of lesion. *Arch Gen Psychiatry*. 1988;45:247–252.
81. Ellis C, Zhao Y, Egede LE. Depression and increased risk of death in adults with stroke. *J Psychosom Res*. Jun 2010;68(6):545–551.
82. Morris PL, Robinson RG, Andrzejewski P, Samuels J, Price TR. Association of depression with 10-year poststroke mortality. *Am J Psychiatry*. 1993;150:124–129.
83. Williams LS, Ghose SS, Swindle RW. Depression and other mental health diagnoses increase mortality risk after ischemic stroke. *Am J Psychiatry*. 2004;161:1090–1095.
84. Breslau N, Lipton RB, Stewart WF, et al. Comorbidity of migraine and depression: investigating potential etiology and prognosis. *Neurology*. 2003;60(8):1308–1312.
85. Guidetti V, Galli F. Psychiatric comorbidity in chronic daily headache: pathophysiology, etiology, and diagnosis. *Curr Pain Headache Rep*. 2002;6(6):492–497.
86. Hesdorffer DC, Lúdvígsson P, Hauser WA, et al. Co-occurrence of major depression or suicide attempt with migraine with aura and risk for unprovoked seizure. *Epilepsy Res*. 2007;75(2–3):220–223.
87. Breslau N, Davis GC, Andreski P. Migraine, psychiatric disorders, and suicide attempts: an epidemiologic study of young adults. *J Psychiatry Res*. 1991;37(1):11–23.

88. Wang Sj, Juang KD, Fuh Jl, et al. Psychiatric comorbidity and suicide risk in adolescents with chronic daily headache. *Neurology.* 2007;68:1468–1473.
89. Starkstein SE, Bolduc PL, Preziosi TJ, Robinson RG. Cognitive impairment in various stages of Parkinson's disease. *J Neuropsychiatry.* 1989;1:243–248.
90. Tröster AI, Paolo AM, Lyons KE, Glatt SL, Hubble JP, Koller WC. The influence of depression on cognition in Parkinson's disease: a pattern of impairment distinguishable from Alzheimer's disease. *Neurology.* Apr 1995;45(4):672–676.
91. Cannon-Spoor HE, Levy JA, Zubenko GS, et al. Effects of previous major depressive illness on cognition in Alzheimer disease patients. *Am J Geriatr Psychiatry.* Apr 2005;13(4):312–318.
92. Lyketsos CG, Steele C, Baker L, Galik E, Kopunek S, Steimberg M. Major and minor depression in Alzheimer's disease: prevalence and impact. *J Clin Neuropsychiatry Clin Neurosci.* 1997;9:556–561.
93. Steele C, Rovener B, Chase GA, Folstein M. Psychiatric symptoms and nursing home placement of patients with Alzheimer's disease. *Am J Psychiatry.* 1990;147:1049–1051.
94. Bassuk SS, Berkman LF, Wypij D. Depressive symptomatology and incident cognitive decline in an elderly community sample. *Arch Gen Psychiatry.* Dec 1998;55(12):1073–1081.
95. Kanner AM, Mazarati A, Koepp M. Biomarkers of epileptogenesis: psychiatric comorbidities(?). *Neurotherapeutics.* Apr 2014;11(2):358–372.
96. Kanner AM. Can neurobiologic pathogenic mechanisms of depression facilitate the development of seizure disorders? *Lancet Neurol.* 2012;11(12):1093–1102.
97. Jobe PC. Affective disorder and epilepsy comorbidity in the genetically epilepsy-prone-rat (GEPR). In: Gilliam F, Kanner AM, Sheline YI, eds. *Depression and brain dysfunction.* London: Taylor & Francis; 2006:121–157.
98. Jobe PC, Mishra PK, Browning RA, et al. Noradrenergic abnormalities in the genetically epilepsy-prone rat. *Brain Res Bull.* 1994;35:493–504.
99. Toczek MT, Carson RE, Lang L, et al. PET imaging of 5-HT1A receptor binding in patients with temporal lobe epilepsy. *Neurology.* 2003;60:749–756.
100. Theodore WH, Giovacchini G, Bonwetsch R, et al. The effect of antiepileptic drugs on 5-HT-receptor binding measured by positron emission tomography. *Epilepsia.* 2006;47(3):499–503.
101. Hasler G, Bonwetsch R, Giovacchini G, et al. 5-HT(1A) receptor binding in temporal lobe epilepsy patients with and without major depression. *Biol Psychiatry.* 2007;62(11):1258–1264.
102. Kugaya A, Sanacora G. Beyond monoamines: glutamatergic function in mood disorders. *CNS Spectr.* 2005;10(10):808–819.
103. Choudary PV, Molnar M, Evans SJ, et al. Altered cortical glutamatergic and GABAergic signal transmission with glial involvement in depression. *Proc Natl Acad Sci U S A.* 2005;102:15653–15658.
104. Chaudhuri KR, Schapira AH. Non-motor symptoms of Parkinson's disease: dopaminergic pathophysiology and treatment. *Lancet Neurol.* May 2009;8(5):464–474.
105. D'Andrea G, Welch K, Riddle J, et al. Platelet serotonin metabolism and ultrastructure in migraine. *Arch Neurol.* 1989;46:1187–1189.
106. Mendelson SD. The current status of the platelet 5-HT(2A) receptor in depression. *J Affect Disord.* 2002;57:13–24.

107. Spalletta G, Bossu P, Ciaramella A, Bria P, Caltagirone C, Robinson RG. The etiology of poststroke depression: a review of the literature and a new hypothesis involving inflammatory cytokines. *Mol Psychiatry*. 2006;11:984–991.

108. Brietzke E1, Mansur RB, Grassi-Oliveira R, Soczynska JK, McIntyre RS. Inflammatory cytokines as an underlying mechanism of the comorbidity between bipolar disorder and migraine. *Med Hypotheses*. 2012;78(5):601–605.

109. Muller N, Myint AM, Schwarz MJ. Inflammatory biomarkers and depression. *Neurotox Res*. 2011;19:308–318.

110. Vezzani A, French J, Bartfai T, Baram TZ. The role of inflammation in epilepsy. *Nat Rev Neurol*. 2011;7:31–40.

111. Ravizza T, Gagliardi B, Noe F, Boer K, Aronica E, Vezzani A. Innate and adaptive immunity during epileptogenesis and spontaneous seizures: evidence from experimental models and human temporal lobe epilepsy. *Neurobiol Dis*. 2008;29:142–160.

112. Sheline YI. Brain structural changes associated with depression. In: Gilliam F, Kanner AM, Sheline YI, eds. *Depression and brain dysfunction*. London: Taylor & Francis; 2006:85–104.

113. Öngür D, Drevets WC, Price JL. Glial reduction in the subgenual prefrontal cortex in mood disorders. *Proc Natl Acad Sci U S A*. 1998;95:13290–13295.

114. Rajkowska G, Miguel-Hidalgo JJ, Wei J, et al. Morphometric evidence for neuronal and glial prefrontal cell pathology in major depression. *Biol Psychiatry*. 1999;45(9):1085–1098.

115. Cotter DR, Pariante CM, Everall IP. Glial cell abnormalities in major psychiatric disorders: the evidence and implications. *Brain Res Bull*. 2001;55:585–595.

116. Cotter D, Mackay D, Landau S, Kerwin R, Everall I. Reduced glial cell density and neuronal size in the anterior cingulate cortex in major depressive disorder. *Arch Gen Psychiatry*. 2001;58:545–553.

117. Cotter D, Mackay D, Chana G, Beasley C, Landau S, Everall IP. Reduced neuronal size and glial cell density in area 9 of the dorsolateral prefrontal cortex in subjects with major depressive disorder. *Cereb Cortex*. 2002;12:386–394.

118. Bremner JD, Narayan M, Anderson ER, Staib LH, Miller HL, Charney DS. Hippocampal volume reduction in major depression. *Am J Psychiatry*. 2000;157(1):115–118.

119. Bremner JD, Vythilingam M, Vermetten E, et al. Reduced volume of orbitofrontal cortex in major depression. *Biol Psychiatry*. 2002;51(4):273–279.

8

Diabetes and Depression

Eduardo A. Colón Navarro

INTRODUCTION

The presence of depression in patients with medical illness has been the subject of attention in the psychiatric and general medical literature over many years,[1] underscoring the impact of stress and physiological correlates of depression as precipitating factors affecting physical disease. Symptoms of depression have a further impact on the burden of disease, as do coping styles and social support. The psychiatrist faced with comorbid medical and psychiatric conditions confronts questions about the relationship between these: Is the psychiatric presentation the direct result of a medical disorder, the exacerbation of a preexisting disorder in the setting of medical illness, or at least a significant contributor to the *initiation* and course of the medical problem? Depression is noted to amplify physical symptoms, increase impairment in function, interfere with adherence, increase unhealthy behaviors, and increase mortality.[2] The impact of biological changes from a depressive disorder, and the physiological consequences of medical illness, provide an opportunity to understand the interaction of medical and physiological factors as drivers, consequences, or facilitators of the course of medical illness and its outcomes.

The presence of psychiatric symptoms in endocrine disorders has been a central focus of psychosomatic medicine for many years,[3] with attention to the possible organic underpinnings of psychiatric disorders, as noted by Asher[4]:

> The fact that recorded case reports of myxedema psychosis have loosely resembled paranoia . . . schizophrenia, melancholia or other orthodox psychoses does suggest that the common psychoses . . . may turn out to be not diagnoses in themselves, but manifestations of underlying organic disease.

This chapter focuses on diabetes, in light of the prevalence of this disorder, as well as the growing literature on the interplay of depression and its pathophysiology. Diabetes afflicts 29.1 million people, or 9.3% of the United States population.[5] The worldwide prevalence of diabetes was estimated to be 2.8% in 2000 and anticipated to be 4.4% in 2030.[6] Diabetes requires lifelong adaptation, chronic management, and is often accompanied by complications and comorbidity. It is therefore crucial to understand the interplay of physiological factors and their relationship to the onset and course of the illness.

DEPRESSION RATES IN DIABETES

Early studies identified significant rates of depression in patients with type 1 diabetes[7] and type 2 diabetes.[8] In an early meta-analysis, Anderson et al.[9] confirmed the association, noting that patients with type 2 diabetes were twice as likely to have depression as patients without diabetes, as well as higher depression scores (11% and 31%). A subsequent meta-analysis of cross sectional studies by Ali et al.[10] showed elevated rates of depression in type 2 diabetes (17.6% vs. 9.8%).

In the comprehensive, systematic review of the literature through the Dialogue in Diabetes and Depression,[11] the overall rate of depression is noted to be at least double, with most studies focused on type 2 diabetes, and limited data indicating similar rates in type 1.[7,12] The presence of comorbidities and complications,[13] especially vascular complications,[11] perceived burden of diabetes, smoking, and obesity,[14,15] have been noted as possible contributors. A number of studies suggest that the increased rates are not present if the study controls for complications and the burden of diabetes.[16,11]

Variable rates are noted with the nature of the population, as well as the method of ascertainment. Most epidemiological studies are cross-sectional, and do not allow exploration of the nature of this association over time. Anderson reported higher rates of depression in clinical settings versus community, diagnoses based on self-report versus *Diagnostic and Statistical Manual* (DSM) interviews, and greater rates in uncontrolled versus controlled studies.[9] The correlation has at times been noted as negative, while larger reviews continue to support the association.[10] Difficulties have centered on selection bias, ascertainment methods for both diabetes and depression, the cross-sectional nature of many of the studies, and sample sizes. Most studies reveal higher rates in women; ethnic differences also need closer attention.[11] Higher rates of depression were found in Latinos and African Americans in a study by Katon,[17] but not in a study by Lin et al.[18] In light of the higher prevalence of diabetes in American Indians/Alaskan natives,[19] non-Hispanic blacks,[18,20,21] Hispanic[22] and Asian Americans[23] in the United States, as well as international data indicating variable rates in other ethnic groups, attention to differences in prevalence of depression and its impact on illness across ethnic groups warrants attention and further study.

A follow-up study of patients who developed diabetes in the Diabetes Prevention Program[24] did not find an increase in diagnosis of depression or use of antidepressants.[25] However, this outcome study found a relationship between higher blood glucose levels and the rise in depression ratings. Patients with preexisting depression or antidepressant medication use were not included in this study. Previous studies examining the direct relationship of depressive symptoms to glycemic control have been mixed.[25,26] Other work has suggested an association based on diabetes-related distress, with glycemic control and depression.[14]

In spite of the variability in these studies, depression is recognized as a possible precipitant of diabetes and a significant factor in the management of patients with diabetes, while the role and impact of clinical interventions remain largely unclear. Depression is known to impact function and self-care, and generate a significant illness burden.[27,28] The presence of depression is associated with increased death rates in cardiovascular disease and is associated with added complications in patients with diabetes.[18,21]

DIABETES AS A RISK FACTOR FOR DEPRESSION

Several authors have described depression as a possible risk factor for type 2 diabetes.[29] In a follow-up of the Epidemiologic Catchment Area study, Eaton et al. controlled for various factors and concluded that major depression predicted the onset of diabetes with an estimated relative risk of 23%.[30] In a related commentary, Freedland[31] raised concern about the absence of statistical power in this study. However, a number of subsequent studies have provided additional data to support this association,[31,32,33] with elevated risks of diabetes and glucose deregulation up to 65%.[34] Possible behavioral changes related to depression have been proposed as contributors to this relationship, including poor self-care behavior, higher body mass index, and the presence of unhealthy behaviors.[35] In addition, early speculation raised questions about the possible biochemical changes induced by depression as precipitants of diabetes,[36] a thesis of this volume.

Conversely, the association of depression with diabetes has been postulated to reflect the burden of diabetes management, the impact of emergence of complications, or the presence of biological risk factors in diabetes predisposing to depression, such as dysregulation of the HPA (hypothalamic-pituitary-adrenal) axis, and the presence of inflammatory responses.[26,11]

A systematic review of studies linking the onset of depression to the presence of diabetes in a meta-analysis by Nowen et al.[37] indicated that type 2 diabetes was associated with a 24% increased risk of depression, while subsequent reports have indicated that this risk is less than the risk of depression leading to diabetes,[29] underscoring the significance of depression as a trigger of diabetes.

DATA FOR A BIDIRECTIONAL RELATIONSHIP

The observation of depression as a possible antecedent to diabetes, and the potential impact of diabetes leading to depression, has led to the discussion of a bidirectional relationship.[11] Mezuk et al.'s meta-analysis[29] indicates that depression is associated with a 60% increased risk of type 2 diabetes, while type 2 diabetes is only associated with a modest increase in rates of depression (15%), in a study that excluded patients with diagnosed depression from the longitudinal study. A longitudinal study of 65,381 women between 50 and 75 years of age over a 10-year period by Pan[38] also provides direct data for the bidirectional relationship. The relative risk of type 2 diabetes in women with depression was elevated (odds ratio [OR] 1.17). Those using antidepressant medications were at a higher risk. Women with type 2 diabetes, in follow-up, had a higher risk of developing depression, even after controlling for diabetes-related comorbidity.

INFLAMMATION, DIABETES, AND DEPRESSION

Depression has been recognized as a risk factor for cardiovascular complications, including coronary artery disease.[39,40] Diabetes is frequently present in patients with cardiac illness, and is associated with negative outcomes: decreased modification of factors such as diet and exercise, poor cardiac rehabilitation outcomes, reduced quality of life, and increased morbidity and mortality. In addition, depression has also been associated with increased rates of strokes[38] (see chapters 4 and 5 in this volume for further discussion). While associated risk factors probably play a major role, such as poor adherence, smoking, and lack of lifestyle modifications, the presence of increased inflammatory response in depression and stress has been postulated as a potential pathophysiological mediator.[41] Early work raised awareness of elevations of C-reactive protein (CRP) in depression.[42,43] The awareness and understanding of the presence of inflammatory markers and mediators in this process continue to grow, suggesting complex interactions.

A cross-sectional review of the relationship of elevated CRP levels and depression in the National Health and Nutrition Examination Survey noted a strong association in men, but not in women.[41] Subsequent studies have examined other inflammatory markers. A meta-analysis by Howren et al.[44] examined associations with CRP, interleukin-1 (IL-1), and IL-6, noting a positive association. The association was stronger for depression established by clinical interviews, potentially related to the identification of true clinical depression. Of interest, body mass index (BMI) is noted to be a mediating factor, as obesity is linked with increased inflammation. When BMI is controlled for, the association with CRP and IL-6 was weaker. As in other studies, the potential role of this association in the emergence of cardiovascular disease is raised.

In a comprehensive review of the role of stress in the activation of inflammation, and a hypothesis paper regarding these interactions, Black notes the role of catecholamines and corticosteroids in the induction of the acute phase response to stress, with the stress hormones interacting with IL-6, including facilitation of CRP and fibrinogen.[45] He describes the role of stress response in generating insulin resistance. Proinflammatory cytokines also induce insulin resistance. The author hypothesizes that stress-induced inflammatory changes in the visceral fat and vasculature eventually result in cardiovascular morbidity. It should be noted that depression affects the HPA axis, cortisol, cytokines, activation of platelets, and glycogen metabolism, among other physiological changes (Chapter 4).

A meta-analysis of this data by Dowlati et al.[46] examined reports in patients without other major medical illnesses or antidepressant treatment. This analysis revealed elevation of proinflammatory cytokines TNF (tumor-necrosis-factor)-alpha and IL-6, with no support for elevations of various interleukins (IL-1-beta, IL-2, IL-8), and interferon gamma (IFN-gamma). There was also no elevation of anti-inflammatory cytokines IL-10 and IL-4. While the role of many of these inflammatory mediators, like TNF-a, continues to be noted, their direct role needs further clarification.[47]

In essence, negative moods result in stimulation of inflammation, while inflammatory reactions' effect on the brain induces changes that result in mood and cognitive changes consistent with depression.[48] Therefore, depression induces inflammatory responses with physiological consequences, while inflammation itself can induce depressive symptoms and depressive disorders.

Along with these data, the link between inflammation and diabetes, particularly type 2 diabetes, has received growing attention. Longitudinal studies have raised the possibility that inflammatory processes precede the onset of diabetes, including elevated CRP, IL-6, and fibrinogen levels.[49] In addition, cross-sectional studies describe higher inflammatory markers in metabolic syndrome and diabetes. An association with visceral adipose tissue is also noted. The association of cytokines with insulin resistance and glucose in overweight subjects also points to this association, while questions of cause and effect need further clarification.[50]

The interaction of depression, inflammation, and diabetes, in a complex fashion, provides fertile ground for understanding and underscores the role of depression as a risk factor for diabetes (and other diseases), as well as the interactions that potentially lead to complications and morbidity.

HYPOTHALAMIC-PITUITARY-ADRENAL AXIS

Following the description of abnormal dexamethasone suppression tests (DST) in a subgroup of patients with depression,[51] the association of HPA-axis function with depression became a focus of interest, and provides a window into the physiological substrates of depression and stress.[52,53] Elevations in cortisol levels have been suggested by findings of adrenal gland enlargement, 24-hour urine free cortisol levels, and the DST abnormalities.[49,54,55] The presence of elevated free nocturnal cortisol in a small cohort of adolescents with a family history of depression was associated with development of depression.[56] Studies regarding dexamethasone-growth releasing hormone (GRH) testing have been variable.[49] Other measures have included a lower cortisol awakening response (CAR), and blunted diurnal variation. In spite of limitations regarding sample sizes, use of medications, and heterogeneity of samples, there is overall concern about the presence of cortisol deregulation in patients with depression and how that may affect medical disorders.

In patients with diabetes and metabolic syndrome, there are observations of alterations in awakening cortisol, as well as HPA abnormalities in obesity.[57] In addition, further observations suggest that elevated cortisol levels result in greater visceral fat and insulin resistance.[58] The likelihood of visceral fat promotion by low-grade cortisol stimulation or cycle deregulation suggests a possible role of depression in promoting the emergence of type 2 diabetes,[57] underscoring the physiological nature and impact of depression and its physiological correlates.

The association between all these factors is complex and will help create a reciprocal physiological understanding of depression and diabetes,[54] i.e., its bidirectionality. The presence of depression can result in increased inflammation, alterations of sympathetic and parasympathetic activity, and behavioral changes, which lead to elevation of CRP and IL-2.[44,49] Inflammatory cytokines result in depressive or illness-like behaviors.[44,59] Depression leads to decreased parasympathetic activity, which stimulates increased inflammation,[44,60] while proinflammatory cytokines stimulate release of corticotrophin-releasing hormone (CRH).[44,61] Increased HPA activity, in turn, can result in depression.[62]

TREATMENT

In spite of the prevalence and impact of depression in diabetes, controlled data regarding treatment are relatively limited. Most data support the role of psychological interventions on depressive symptomatology.[62] Pharmacological trials in the treatment of depression in diabetes are few. An early trial of nortriptyline versus placebo demonstrated a beneficial effect on mood, but a potentially negative impact on glycemic control.[63] A subsequent trial of fluoxetine also demonstrated a positive effect after two months, but no significant impact on glycemic control over that limited period of time.[64] A trial of sertraline in a mixed type 1 and type 2 group demonstrated a beneficial effect on relapse prevention. In an open-faced portion of the study, 43% of patients demonstrated remission. Those patients were then randomized to sertraline or placebo and followed for 12 months. Rates of recurrence were significantly lower in patients treated with sertraline.[65]

Treatment of minor depression in a group of elderly patients with paroxetine did not demonstrate any significant benefits.[66] In light of the impact of depression on mortality in elderly patients, more data regarding the potential benefits and risks of pharmacological interventions for depression in patients with diabetes are required.

The recognition of the impact of depression on diabetes has led to increased interest in the delivery of care for depression within primary care.[67] This includes models and interventions for collaborative care, including direct and ongoing nursing intervention, involvement of psychiatrists and psychologists in a consulting fashion, and the utilization of interventions such as problem-solving strategies. The early studies have focused on depression, showing small to moderate effect sizes,[68,69] followed by trials involving depression in diabetes.[68] These studies highlight the feasibility of direct care of depression by the primary care physician and subsequent referral to psychiatric care for complex or refractory patients.

PSYCHOLOGICAL TREATMENTS

In light of the significant impact of diabetes on functioning and well-being, the importance of psychological interventions directed at symptom management and lifestyle changes cannot be overlooked. The ability to manage diabetes and the capacity to cope with the burden of chronic illness are diminished in patients with depression.[73] Depression has a significant impact on social and physical functioning,[1] and impacts lifestyle, including adherence, diet and increased smoking prevalence.[74]

A review of randomized controlled trials[62] provides evidence for the potential utility of psychological interventions in patients with diabetes and depression. An early cognitive behavioral therapy (CBT) trial in 52 patients with type 2 diabetes and depression demonstrated a significant benefit of this intervention over diabetes education, with a significant difference in remission rates at six months, and positive impact on hemoglobin A1C (HgA1C) measurements.[75]

Group counseling and supportive psychotherapy have been reported as beneficial, but evidence is limited by short-term trials and small samples. Mixed interventions, with problem solving and interpersonal therapy, as well as combinations with medication therapy, have yielded positive psychological improvement, but no dramatic medical changes.[62]

A comprehensive meta-analysis of six databases up to January 2015[76] indicates that most lifestyle and diabetes self-management and support programs for diabetic patients, but without focusing on the presence of depression, have a positive impact on glycemic control, but those without support did not. The report indicates that best effect is noted with services delivered in persons with more than 10 contact hours.

Larger sample studies with larger numbers of patients will help delineate which factors are most important in providing care for the subgroup of diabetic patients with depressive symptoms, especially in combination with support and management interventions, to maximize impact on mood along with glycemic control.

CONCLUSION

Endocrine disorders have long been recognized as conditions closely linked with psychiatric illness and central to psychosomatic medicine.[3] The evaluation and understanding of the links between hormonal and other physiological changes, and their correlation with psychiatric symptoms and syndromes, provides a window into the complex interactions between the regulation of physiological systems and their impact on behavior.

Depression is a complex illness, which highlights the interaction of genetic predisposition, psychosocial stressors, and medical illness. While the stress of coping with the challenge of acute or chronic illness, along with changes in functional capacity, provide a rich substrate for the emergence of depressive symptoms, the physiological changes induced by illness must be understood as a trigger or cause for the emergence of depressive symptoms. Recent data enrich this complex picture, by describing physiological changes that may serve as the cause or trigger for medical illness such as diabetes, and play a major role in the emergence of complications and negative outcomes. Depression may not only be a precipitant or causative factor in the onset of diabetes, it may also have a significant impact on the management of this chronic illness. The understanding of the involvement of depression in diabetes must extend beyond the crucial knowledge of its effect on well-being and functional status, to the exploration of its influence on the development of diabetes as well as its effect on the course of this chronic and disabling disease.

REFERENCES

1. Moussavi S, Chatterji S, Verdis E, et al. Depression, chronic diseases, and decrements in health: results from the World Health Surveys. *Lancet.* 2007;370:851–858.
2. Katon WJ. Clinical and health services relationships between major depression, depressive symptoms, and general medical illness. *Biol Psychiatry.* 2003;54:216–226.
3. Leigh HKS. The psychiatric manifestations of endocrine disease. *Advance Intern Med.* 1984;29:413–445.
4. Asher R. Myxedematous madness. *BMJ.* 1949;22:555–562.
5. Cowie CC, Eberhardt MS, American Diabetes Association. *Diabetes 1996 Vital Statistics.* Alexandria, VA: American Diabetes Association;1996:51–59.
6. Wild S, Green G, Sicree A, et al. Global prevalence of diabetes: Estimates for the year 2000 and projections for 2030. *Diabetes Care.* 2004;27:1047–1053.

7. Popkin MK, Callies A, Lentz RD, et al. Prevalence of major depression, simple phobia, and other psychiatric disorders in patients with long-standing type 1 diabetes mellitus. *Arch Gen Psychiatry.* 1988;45:64–68.

8. Gavard JA, Lustman PJ, Clouse RE. Prevalence of depression in adults with diabetes: an epidemiological evaluation. *Diabetes Care.* 1993;16:1167–1178.9.

9. Anderson RJ, Freedland KE, Clouse RE, et al. The prevalence of comorbid depression in adults with diabetes: a meta-analysis. *Diabetes Care.* 2001;24:1069–1078.

10. Ali S, Stone MA, Peters JL, et al. The prevalence of co-morbid depression in adults with Type 2 diabetes: a systematic review and meta-analysis. *Diabetes Med.* 2006;23:1165–1173.

11. Roy T, Lloyd CE. Epidemiology of depression and diabetes: a systematic review. *J Affect Disord.* 2012;142S1:S8–S21.

12. Pouwer F, Geelhoed-Duijvestijn PH, Tack CJ, et al. Prevalence of comorbid depression is high in out-patients with Type 1 or Type 2 diabetes mellitus. Results from three outpatient clinics in the Netherlands. *Diabetes Med.* 2010;27:217–224.

13. Gendelman N, Snell-Bergeon JK, McFann K, et al. Prevalence and correlates of depression in individuals with and without Type 1 diabetes. *Diabetes Care.* 2009;32:575–579.

14. Fisher L, Skaff MM, Mullan JT, et al. A longitudinal study of affective and anxiety disorders, depressive affect, and diabetes distress in adults with Type 2 diabetes. *Diabetes Med.* 2008;25:1096–1101.

15. Champaneri S, Wand GS, Malhotra SS, et al. Biological basis of depression in adults with diabetes. *Curr Diabetes Rep.* 2010;10:396–405.

16. Brown LC, Majumdar SR, Newman SC, et al. Type 2 diabetes does not increase risk of depression. *CMAJ.* 2006;175:42–46.

17. Katon W, Fan MY, Unutzer J, et al. Depression and diabetes: a potentially lethal combination. *J Gen Intern Med.* 2008;23:1571–1575.

18. Lin EH, Heckbert SR, Rutter CM, et al. Depression and increased mortality in diabetes: unexpected causes of death. *Ann Fam Med.* 2009;7:414–421.

19. Barnes PM, Adams PF, Powell-Griner E. Health characteristics of the American Indian or Alaska Native adult population: United States, 2004–2008. *Natl Health Stat Report.* 2010;(20):1–22.

20. American Diabetes Association. *Vital Statistics* 1996:51–59.

21. de Groot M, Lustman PJ. Depression among African-Americans with diabetes. *Diabetes Care.* 2001;24:407–408.

22. Colon EA, Giachello A, McIver L, Pacheco G, Vela L. Diabetes and depression in the Hispanic/Latino community. *Clin Diabetes.* 2013;31:43–45.

23. Nanditha A, Ma RC, Ramachandran AS, et al. Diabetes in Asia and the Pacific: implications for the global epidemic. *Diabetes Care.* 2016;39:472–485.

24. Diabetes Prevention Program Research Group. Reduction in the incidence of Type 2 diabetes with lifestyle intervention or metformin. *NEJM.* 2002;346:393–403.

25. Marrero DG, Ma Y, De Groot M, et al. Depressive symptoms, antidepressant medication use, and new onset of diabetes in participants of the Diabetes Prevention Program, and the Diabetes Prevention Program Outcomes Study. *Psychosom Med.* 2015;77:303–310.

26. Lustman P, Anderson R, Freedland KE, et al. Depression and poor glycemic control: a meta-analytic review of the literature. *Diabetes Care.* 2000;23:934–942.

27. Egede LE, Nietert PJ, Zheng D. Depression and all-cause and coronary mortality in adults with and without diabetes. *Diabetes Care.* 2005;28:1339–1345.

28. Katon W, Rutter C, Simon G, et al. The association of comorbid depression with mortality in patients with Type 2 diabetes. *Diabetes Care.* 2005;28:2668–2672.

29. Mezuk B, Eaton WW, Albrecht S, Golden SH. Depression and type 2 diabetes over the lifespan: a meta-analysis. *Diabetes Care.* 2008;31:2383–2390.
30. Eaton W, Armenian H, Gallo J, et al. Depression and risk for onset of type II diabetes. A prospective population-based study. *Diabetes Care.* 1996;19:1097–11102.
31. Freedland KE. Section II: The research: Article summaries and commentaries hypothesis 1. Depression is a risk factor for the development of Type 2 diabetes. *Diabetes Spect.* 2004;7:150–152.
32. Carnethon M, Kinder L, Fair J, et al. Symptoms of depression as a risk factor for incident diabetes: findings from the National Health and Nutrition Examination Epidemiologic Follow-Up Study. *Am J Epidemiol.* 2003;158:416–423.
33. Kawakami N, Takatsuka N, Shimizu H, et al. Depressive symptoms and occurrence of type 2 diabetes among Japanese men. *Diabetes Care.* 1999;22:1071–1076.
34. Campayo A, de Jonge P, Roy JF, et al. Depressive disorder and incident diabetes mellitus: the effect of characteristics of depression. *Am J Psychiatry.* 2010;167:580–588.
35. Lloyd CE, Pambianco G, Orchard TJ. Does diabetes related distress express the presence of depressive symptoms and/or poor self-care in individuals with Type 1 diabetes? *Diabetes Med.* 2010;27:234–237.
36. Finkelstein FO, Finkelstein SH. Depression in chronic dialysis patients: assessment and treatment. *Nephrol Dialys Transpl.* 2000;15:1911–1913.
37. Nowen A, Winkley K, Twisk J, et al. Diabetes mellitus as a risk factor for the onset of depression: a systematic review and meta-analysis. *Diabetologia.* 2010;53:2480–2486.
38. Pan A, Lucas M, Sun Q, et al. The bidirectional relationship of depression and diabetes: a systematic review. *Clin Psychol Rev.* 2011;31:1239–1246.
39. Frasure-Smith N, Lespérance FA. Depression and anxiety as predictors of 2-year cardiac events in patients with stable coronary artery disease. *Arch Gen Psychiatry.* 2008;65:62–71.
40. Lichtman JHJ, Bigger T, Blumenthal JA, et al. Depression and coronary heart disease recommendations for screening, referral, and treatment: a science advisory from the American Heart Association Prevention Committee of the Council on Cardiovascular Nursing, Council on Clinical Cardiology, Council on Epidemiology and Prevention, and Interdisciplinary Council on Quality of Care and Outcomes Research: endorsed by the American Psychiatric Association. *Circulation.* 2008;118:1768–1775.
41. Ford DE, Erlinger TP. Depression and c-reactive protein in US adults- data from the Third National Health and Nutrition Examination Survey. *Arch Intern Med.* 2014;164:1010–1014.
42. Maes M. Evidence for an immune response in major depression: a review and hypothesis. *Prog Neuropharmacol Biol Psychiatry.* 1995;19:11–38.
43. Maes M, Bosmans E, DeJongh R, et al. Increased serum IL-6 and IL-1 receptor antagonist concentrations in major depression and treatment resistant depression. *Cytokine.* 1997;9:853–858.
44. Howren BE, Lamkin DM, Suls J. Association of depression with C-reactive protein, IL-1, and IL-6: a meta-analysis. *Psychosom Med.* 2009;71:171–186.
45. Black PH. The inflammatory consequences of psychologic stress: relationship to insulin resistance, obesity, atherosclerosis and diabetes mellitus, type II. *Med Hypotheses.* 2006;67:879–891.
46. Dowlati Y, Herrmann N, Swardfager W, et al. A meta-analysis of cytokines in major depression. *Biol Psychiatry.* 2010;67:446–457.
47. Postal M, Appenzeller S. The importance of cytokines and autoantibodies in depression. *Autoimmunity Rev.* 2015;14:30–35.

48. Messay B, Lim A, Marsland AL. Current understanding of the bi-directional relationship of major depression with inflammation. *Biol Mood Anxiety Disord.* 2012;2:4. https://doi.org/10.1186/2045-5380-2-4

49. Champaneri S, Wand GS, Malhotra SS, et al. Biological basis of depression in adults with diabetes. *Curr Diabetes Rep.* 2010;10:396–405.

50. Rubin DA, McMurray RG, Harrell JS, et al. The association between insulin resistance and cytokines in adolescents: the role of weight status and exercise. *Metabolism.* 2008;57:683–690.

51. Carroll BJ. The dexamethasone suppression test for melancholia. *Br J Psychiatry.* 1982;140:292–304.

52. McEwen B. Protective and damaging effects of stress mediators. *NEJM.* 1998;338:171–179.

53. Selye H. Stress and the general adaptation syndrome. *BMJ.* 1950;1:1383–1392.

54. Golden SH. A review of the evidence for a neuroendocrine link between stress, depression and diabetes mellitus. *Curr Diabetes Rev.* 2007;3:252–259.

55. Sachar EJ, Hellman L, Fukushima DK, et al. Cortisol production in depressive illness—a clinical and biochemical clarification. *Arch Gen Psychiatry.* 1970;23:289–298.

56. Rao U, Hammen CL, Poland RE. Risk markers for depression in adolescents: sleep and HPA measures. *Neuropsychopharmacology.* 2009;34:1936–1945.

57. Gutt M, Davis CL, Spiter SB, et al. Validation of the insulin sensitivity index: a comparison with other measures. *Diabetes Res Clin Pract.* 2000;47:177–184.

58. Purnell JQ, Kahn SE, Samuels MH, et al. Enhanced cortisol productions rates, free cortisol, and 11 beta HSD 1 expression correlate with visceral fat and insulin resistance in men: effect of weight loss. *Am J Physiol.* 2009;296:E351–E357.

59. Dantzer R, O'Connor JC, Freund GG, et al. From inflammation to sickness and depression: when the immune system subjugates the brain. *Nature Rev Neurosci.* 2008;9:46–56.

60. Kop WJ, Gottdiener JS. The role of immune system parameters in the relationship between depression and coronary artery disease. *Psychosom Med.* 2005;67:S37–S41.

61. Pennix BW, Kritchevsky SB, Yaffe K, et al. Inflammatory markers and depressed mood in older persons: results from the health, aging, and body composition study. *Biol Psychiatry.* 2003;54:566–572.

62. Petrak F, Herpertz S. Treatment of depression in diabetes: an update. *Curr Opin Psychiatry.* 2009;22:211–217.

63. Lustman PJ, Griffith LS, Clouse RE, et al. Effects of nortriptyline on depression and glycemic control in diabetes: results of a double-blind, placebo-controlled trial. *Psychosom Med.* 1997;59:241–250.

64. Lustman PJ, Freedland KE, Griffith LS, et al. Fluoxetine for depression in diabetes: a randomized, double-blind, placebo-controlled trial. *Diabetes Care.* 2000;23:618–623.

65. Lustman PJ, Clouse R, Nix BD, et al. Sertraline for prevention of depression recurrence in diabetes mellitus. *Arch Gen Psychiatry.* 2006;63:521–529.

66. Paile-Hyvärinen M, Wahlbeck K, Eriksson JG. Quality of life and metabolic status in mildly depressed women with type 2 diabetes treated with paroxetine: a single-blind randomised placebo controlled trial. *BMC Fam Pract.* 2003;4:7.

67. Katon WJ, Lin EHB, Von Korff M, et al. Collaborative care for patients with depression and chronic illnesses. *NEJM.* 2010;363:2611–2620.

68. Johnson JA, Al Sayah F, Wozniak L, et al. Collaborative care versus screening and follow-up for patients with diabetes and depressive symptoms: results of a primary care-based comparative effectiveness trial. *Diabetes Care.* 2014;37:320–3226.

69. Thota AB, Sipe TA, Byard GJ, et al. Collaborative care to improve the management of depressive disorders: a community guide systematic review and meta-analysis. *Am J Prev Med.* 2012;42:525–538.

70. Van der Feltz-Cornelis CM, Nuyen J, Stoop C, et al. Effects of interventions for major depressive disorder and significant depressive symptoms in patient with diabetes mellitus: a systematic review and meta-analysis. *Gen Hosp Psychiatry.* 2010;32:380–395.

71. Pan A, Lucas M, Sun Q, et al. The bidirectional relationship of depression and diabetes: a systematic review. *Clin Psychol Rev.* 2011;31:1239–1246.

72. Pennix BW, Kritchevsky SB, Yaffe K, et al. Inflammatory markers and depressed mood in older persons: results from the health, aging, and body composition study. *Biol Psychiatry.* 2003;54:566–572.

73. Hermanns N, Kulzer B, Krichbaum M, et al. How to screen for depression and emotional problems in patients with diabetes: comparison of screening characteristics of depression questionnaires, measurement of diabetes-specific emotional problems and standard clinical assessment. *Diabetologia.* 2006;49:469–477.

74. Gonzalez J, Delahanty L, Safren S, et al. Differentiating symptoms of depression from diabetes-specific distress: relationship with self-care in type 2 diabetes. *Diabetologia.* 2014;51:1822–1825.

75. Lustman PJ, Griffith LS, Freedland KE, et al. Cognitive behavior therapy for depression in type 2 diabetes mellitus. A randomized, controlled trial. *Ann Intern Med.* 1998;129:613–621.

76. Pillay J, Armstrong MJ, Butalia S, et al. Behavior programs for Type 2 diabetes mellitus: a systematic review and network meta-analysis. *Ann Intern Med.* 2015;163:848–860.

9

Wound Healing and Depression

Frederick J. Stoddard, Jr. and Robert L. Sheridan

Depression and wound healing are bidirectional processes for adults and children, consistent with the conception of depression as systemic. This systemic interaction is similar to the "bidirectional impact of mood disorder on risk for development, progression, treatment, and outcomes of medical illness" generally (Januzzi et al. 2000; Evans et al. 2005). Scientific evidence is expanding on the etiological role of stress on disease, with the first translational study linking brain (PET/CT) amygdala activity robustly predicting cardiovascular events, providing insight into the mechanism through which emotional stressors can lead to disease in human beings (Tawakol et al, 2017). And evidence is growing that the bidirectional impact of mood disorder may be true for injuries and for surgery (Stoddard, Sheridan et al. 2015; Upton et al. 2014). Depression is highly prevalent in U.S. households (Pratt, Brody 2014), and worldwide in 2010, it was the second leading cause of life-years lived with disability and the leading cause of disability-adjusted life-years (DALYs; Ferrari et al. 2013). The 2013 update of the *Global Burden of Disease* reported that, while injuries continue as an important cause of morbidity and mortality worldwide, the decline in rates from 1990–2013 was so dramatic that "the world is becoming a safer place to live in" related to most but not all injuries (Haagsma et al. 2015). Nevertheless, a new National Academies of Sciences, Engineering and Medicine report, "A National Trauma Care System to Achieve Zero Preventable Deaths after Injury" sets a higher bar for the United States, including civilians and military, based on many advances that have saved lives on the battlefields in Afghanistan and Iraq (Berwick et al. 2016).

Developmentally, the clinical problems associated with depression and wounds vary across the life span, and the case studies that follow illustrate similarities and differences throughout the life cycle. One key similarity is that patients from backgrounds of poverty are at increased risk for depression, nonadherence to care, and poor wound outcomes. A second similarity is that in acute care, delirium after injury may precede depression, requiring diagnosis and management. And a third similarity is that interpreters play a critical role, since communicating and being understood in the patients', parents', or caretakers' language is essential—poorer outcomes occur with patients whose wounds and treatments are painful, shocking, and not understood by the patient or family. A fourth similarity is that patients with neurodevelopment disabilities of all ages require special care. The fifth similarity is assuring that safety comes first, since many injured patients of all ages are survivors of neglect, abuse, or (for refugees) may be victims of political violence and still at risk.

Others have injured themselves and may be at risk of further self-harm. Differences across the age span are described here for infants, children and adolescents, young and middle-aged adults, and the elderly. In the care of infants (Stoddard 2002), interventions for the depressed child healing from wounds are centered on supporting the mother–infant dyad, recognition and enhancement of parental resilience, lessening of stress and guilt, and pediatric dosing of analgesic and anxiolytic medications. Each biopsychosocial intervention may improve wound healing via neurohumoral and immunological mechanisms, as will be discussed later. Years ago, Anna Freud spoke of the importance of bodily illness in the mental lives of children (Freud 1952). For injured older children and adolescents, parental and pharmacological interventions may be similar to those for younger children, adapted to the cognitive, affective, and behavioral stages of older children, with the addition of antidepressants or mood stabilizers. Young and middle-aged adults' wounds often are associated with comorbid developmental or psychiatric risks such as impulsivity, workplace hazards, pre-existing mental disorder, or substance abuse complicating the assessment process. For the injured geriatric patient, assessing their stage in the aging process, determining what will enhance restoration of function, providing evidence-based psychotherapy and pharmaco-therapy for the elderly patient, and assessing the availability of responsible caretakers or the lack of them, are all essential to planning the next steps in their care. A last similarity across the life span, but with differences developmentally, too, is end-of-life care for the depressed patient with wounds that may occur in any care setting. Wounds do not always heal, and some patients die at varying stages of wound treatment, depending on wound severity and complications. Responding therapeutically with empathic end-of-life care to the needs of the dying patient with depression and wounds, and the grieving family, including palliative and hospice care, continues to the end of life and beyond (O'Malley et al. 2015).

Patients who are injured may be at risk of depression, including suicide risk, especially with painful, disfiguring, disabling, or large injuries such as amputations (Stoddard, Saxe 2001; Stoddard, Sheridan, et al. 2011; Maytal et al. 2010; Stoddard et al. 2014b; Thombs et al. 2006, 2007). Injured children and adolescents are particularly at developmental risk for psychopathology that may emerge later in their lives (Stoddard 2014a; Stoddard et al. 2017). Following injury or trauma, depression is more common than post-traumatic stress disorder (PTSD) in studies that examine both. Often both are present, which may be associated with inadequately treated acute pain (Bryant et al. 2009; Holbrook et al. 2010; Sheridan et al. 2014) or the need for early treatment of PTSD and/or depression with follow-up (Stoddard et al. 2011; Stoddard, Luthra et al. 2011), particularly "stepped" collaborative treatment (Zatzick et al. 2011), which can also be done through collabora-tive telecare technologies (Engel et al. 2016).

In turn, patients with depression and comorbid disorders such as learning disabilities, substance abuse, or PTSD may be at increased risk for incurring injuries due to symptoms of depression such as inattention or lack of self-care, at which point their depression may complicate their healing and recovery from injury. In either case, treatment of depression, once diagnosed, is indicated, since depression is a risk factor for poorer outcomes, and treatment of it may improve outcomes from injury and/or illness.

Wound healing is a complex biochemical, cellular, and systemic phenomenon tradition-ally divided into three phases: inflammation (angiogenesis and inflammation), prolifera-tion (epithelialization, angiogenesis, and provisional matrix formation), and remodeling (maturation and remodeling) (Broughton et al. 2006), which may involve any bodily tissue or system. Healing varies related to the age of the person, the extent of the wound(s), the organ(s) affected, the nature of the lesion(s), the time since injury, pain, the inflammatory response, infection, and psychosocial adversity. The neurohumoral milieu has a very important impact on the systemic response to trauma and wound healing (Weber et al. 2010). Physiological stress activates the hypothalamic-pituitary-adrenal axis (HPA-A) and the sympathetic-adrenal-medullary axis (SAM-A), and increased cortisol and catecholamines directly affect components of the process of healing (Gouin, Kiecolt-Glaser 2011). Stress also affects oxytocin, vasopressin, local cytokines, and susceptibility to infection, and higher oxytocin and vasopressin levels in marital couples were found to correlate with faster wound healing (Gouin, Kiecolt-Glaser 2011; Kiecolt-Glaser et al. 1998; Broadbent, Koschwanez 2012; Gouin et al. 2010). The systemic effects of depression may impact these responses by altering this neurochemistry, including through epigenetic regulation of the oxytocin system (Simons et al. 2017). Microbial symbionts, through upregulation of oxytocin, contribute a multidirectional gut microbe-brain-immune axis output affecting wound healing capability (Poutahidis et al. 2013). Also important are prior protective or risk factors, and their interactions, such as how early or late treatment is instituted, genetics, nutritional status, medications, and prior injury, illness, or substance abuse. For instance, depression has an impact on nutritional health, which in turn has a very profound impact on wound repair (Molnar et al. 2016). Observations of depressed patients with injuries, postoperatively or in rehabilitation, have led clinicians to become curious about the relationship of depression to impaired wound healing.

The relationship between depression and medical illness was the subject of a major review that led to clinical and research recommendations (Evans et al. 2005). It concluded, from workgroups on cardiovascular disease (Celano, Huffman 2011; Baumeister et al. 2011); on cancer and HIV (Ciesla, Roberts 2001); on stroke, Parkinson's disease (PD), Alzheimer's disease (AD), and epilepsy; and on diabetes (Nouwen 2010), osteoporosis, obesity, and pain:

> Mood disorders are prevalent in patients with chronic medical illnesses and are more than simply a consequence of medical comorbidity. Presence of depression considerably worsens medical prognosis, because it hinders adherence to treatment regimens, impairs physical and cognitive function, diminishes quality of life, increases morbidity, and in some cases, decreases survival. Depression might be an etiologic factor for incident disease (e.g., cardiac disease, stroke, cancer, epilepsy), which has important implications for prevention and early intervention for both depression and the medical illness itself. Depression also might affect the course of medical diseases (e.g., cardiac, cerebrovascular, neurological disorders, diabetes, cancer, and HIV/AIDS). Depression in medically ill patients is treatable. Preliminary data on treatment of depression in patients with comorbid medical conditions are encouraging, but additional studies are needed to confirm that treating depression improves overall medical outcomes. (Evans et al. 2005, p 181)

These conclusions address some but not all types of wound healing, notably excluding wounds due to injuries, trauma, and surgery.

CASE EXAMPLE

Depression impairing healing of burns wounds in a child: A seven-year-old girl, Maria, was admitted for 60% total body-surface-area burn injuries due to an explosion. Her survival was not assured, and her mother, with a history of depression, was very depressed and unable to accept treatment for herself. Maria manifested extreme sensitivity to mild to moderate pain associated with dressing changes and with physical therapy. Her wounds were grafted but slow to heal. She manifested depressive and post-traumatic symptomatology, and resisted participation in physical therapy and rehabilitation. Psychotherapy through an interpreter, combined with a slow increase in sertraline, was associated with improved mood, wound healing, and more active engagement in rehabilitation.

Psychological factors play a critical role in healing, including from depression; for instance, as a result of the placebo effect. It therefore is likely that positive psychological factors may enhance wound healing. Placebo treatment of depression has been shown to be effective by functional neuroimaging, which demonstrated metabolic increases associated with recovery from depression in the prefrontal cortex, posterior insula, inferior parietal cortex, and dorsal anterior cingulate cortex (ACC), thalamus, and hypothalamus (Mayberg 2002). While a small study found no effect, it is unclear whether or not placebo treatment also can improve wound healing (Vits et all 2013).

CASE EXAMPLE

Psychiatric treatment facilitating healing of wounds and amputations, and psychosocial recovery (Sheridan, Schaefer et al. 2012): A 16-year-old girl, a highly competitive soccer player, with a highly organized, very supportive family, was in a severe vehicular accident. She presented initially in severe pain, with a traumatic brain injury with small subarachnoid hemorrhages and temporary ventriculostomy, 70% total body-surface-area burns including her face, and inhalation injury with tracheostomy (Sheridan 2016). She was sedated and treated with infusions of fentanyl, midazolam, and vecuronium, and required bilateral below-knee amputations, and amputation of most of her dominant right hand. She was evaluated psychiatrically during acute treatment, especially after extubation, and during rehabilitation, and she had typical mixed symptomatology over the course of recovery. She had acute and neuropathic pain at healing wound sites, transient agitation and delirium, depression in part related to her bodily injuries and disfigurement and rehabilitation, and PTSD from her traumatic experiences. She responded very well to skillful and empathic treatment with psychotherapy and sequential pharmacotherapy (morphine, midazolam, risperidone, lorazepam, and sertraline) during her acute care and rehabilitation. These specific treatments appeared to facilitate wound healing, energy, and tolerance of pain for physical therapy; psychological adaptation to her scars and multiple amputations; her seven-month hospital stay; and her gradual social reintegration. She recovered well over two years and was fitted with prosthetic legs, which allowed her to resume many activities, including completing high school and beginning college.

There is evidence that family health and function, as in this case, has a strong impact on pediatric injury recovery, but it might be adversely affected by depression (Sheridan, Lee et al. 2012). Psychiatric intervention was integral to this patient's experience of emotional and physical healing from the wounds of a mutilating multisystem injury, and her recovery was similar to those of recent military casualties in Afghanistan and Iraq (Sheridan et al. 2014).

An area of increasing clinical and research interest involves possible linkages between clinical depression and impaired wound healing, with increased morbidity and mortality. Clinical and research observations of patients with coronary artery bypass surgery, burns and other trauma, orthopedic procedures, diabetic ulcers, and related animal studies, tend to support the hypothesis that biologically driven factors associated with depression (e.g., cortisol) slows the healing of both wounds from trauma, and similarly from surgery, involving incising and closing wounds therapeutically with the goal of postoperative healing (Doering et al. 2005; Grace et al. 2005; Terrier et al. 2005; Williams et al. 2011; Milani, Lavie 1996). Postoperative pain management has been found to improve postoperative immune response and in turn may reduce stress and improve wound healing (Kohler et al. 2016; Beilin et al. 2003; Walburn et al. 2009; Broadbent et al. 2003; Solowiej et al. 2009, 2010a, 2010b). Depression may be associated with increased mortality, as well as morbidity in these patients (Rosenberger et al. 2006), but one study of healing of diabetic foot ulcers did not support this (Vedhara et al. 2010). If the hypothesis that depression impairs wound healing gains further support, it would further indicate the importance of diagnosing depressive states, and investigating further to what extent and how treatment of depression improves wound healing and outcomes.

CASE EXAMPLE

Worsening depression in a 63-year-old woman with bipolar disorder and multiple medical conditions, including a history of lung cancer and early-stage breast cancer (Irwin et al. 2016): A 63-year-old woman was admitted to the inpatient psychiatry service of the Massachusetts General Hospital for electroconvulsive therapy (ECT) but was only partially treated with it during that admission and required outpatient ECT. Due to depression, she had earlier disengaged from medical and psychiatric care, and after discharge she refused surgery, further delaying her cancer and psychiatric care. Her psychiatrist engaged this patient in her own care, including home visiting, and the psychiatric and cancer center team leveraged the cancer center resources with system navigators, unfamiliar with severe mental illness, to help her negotiate the complex health care systems and access cancer care. Paroxetine was prescribed for her depression in addition to outpatient ECT. With the biological treatments of her depression, combined with persistence, flexibility, and proactive communication of the team, she completed outpatient ECT and had her lumpectomy five months after her breast cancer diagnosis.

Basic science research has enhanced understanding of how the allostatic load of stress from wounds can contribute to depression and the growth of several sectors of the amygdala and reduction of the hippocampus and prefrontal cortex. Brain plasticity affecting those brain regions may shape and be shaped, too, by the counterweight of resilient behavioral and physiological response systems, and allostasis (the active process of adaptation and maintaining homeostasis) (McEwen et al. 2015). These tend to support physical healing and adaptation to stress through central regulation of processes such as inflammatory cytokines, oxidative stress, glucocorticoids, and autonomic, immune, and metabolic systems that may be triggered by many stressors, including wounds or injury (Ebrecht et al. 2004; McEwen, Gianaros 2011; Davidson, McEwen 2013).

CASE EXAMPLE

Depression in an elderly man with early dementia, impairing healing of a wound and hip fracture: A 85-year-old Spanish-speaking widower who retired at 75 from his construction business, with early dementia, fell in the bathroom of his home, resulting in a laceration to his leg and right hip fracture. He was hospitalized, and on psychological evaluation was diagnosed with major depression, which began during his grieving for his wife of 60 years who had died three years earlier. Although depressed, with early memory impairment, he reluctantly consented to wound closure and hip replacement, but he ate and slept little, was non-adherent to care, and his leg and hip wounds were healing poorly. He was referred for mental health evaluation.

With the help of an interpreter, he described to his psychologist whom he felt was helpful, his loneliness, loss of appetite, and insomnia, and how he lost the meaning in his life after his wife's death, caring only for his daughter and her family in a nearby city. Memantine was considered for his memory impairment but not begun, since his dementia was at an early stage. He was not aware that he had symptoms of clinical depression that could be treated, and willingly engaged in psychotherapy and utilized meditation oriented toward positive emotions (Derubeis 2008; Hofmann et al. 2011) and, although hesitant, began escitalopram at low doses, which were effective in the biological treatment of his depression, improving his memory somewhat, and facilitated his motivation to participate in rehabilitation and home care. Medication and/or psychotherapy may alter the neurochemistry of depression, reducing symptoms.

Animal models have provided some support to the proposition that treatment of depression may improve wound healing. An established biological model for a mechanism delaying wound healing is increased cortisol secretion secondary to depression and/or stress, and impaired immune response, (Kiecolt-Glaser and Glaser 2002) in addition to or along with the other factors such as genetic or epigenetic risks for depression. Cellular models relate both to wound healing and to depression include cytokines, the inflammatory response (Miller et al. 2009), and cellular aging (Telgenhoff, Shroot 2005) reflected in shorter leukocyte telomere length (LTL) (Verhoeven et al. 2015). Another model of stress impacting wound healing investigated genetic correlates—immediate early gene (IEG) expression from the medial prefrontal cortex, and locomotion, in isolation-reared juvenile rats. Levine et al. (2007) compared isolation-reared to group-reared samples, and found that immediate gene expression in the medial prefrontal cortex (mPFC) was reduced, and behavioral hyperactivity increased, in juvenile rats with 20% burn injuries. Wound healing in the isolation-reared rats was significantly impaired. They concluded that these results provide candidates for behavioral biomarkers of isolation rearing during physical injury; i.e., reduced immediate mPFC gene expression and hyperactivity. They suggested that a biomarker such as IEGs might aid in demarcating patients with resilient and adaptive responses to physical illness from those with maladaptive responses (McEwen 1998).

Treatment choices, as summarized here, for depression associated with wounds center on psychotherapies and psychopharmacology, but they also include electric shock treatment and transcranial magnetic stimulation (TMS) (O'Reardon et al. 2007). For each type of treatment, research evidence for improved wound healing does not yet adequately support specific psychotherapies or biological therapies, and further research is needed. Among psychotherapies in use with some success to treat depression and enhance wound healing are psychodynamic therapy, and, with children and adolescents, psychodynamic play therapy, and cognitive therapy, including digital technology, for example, video games and virtual reality (Meersand, Gilmore 2018), cognitive behavior therapy (Clark, Beck 2010), hypnosis (Spiegel, Spiegel 2004), group therapy, family therapy, and meditation (Derubeis et al. 2008; Hofmann et al. 2011). Innovative online interventions are progressing rapidly, such as one that is a brief, web-based, with six one-hour sessions of a self-help intervention for primary prevention of major depression or secondary prevention for those with prior depressive episodes (Buntrock et al. 2016). However, many treatments for depression that could improve healing are not always well adhered to (Wang et al. 2007; Ghio et al. 2014), and digital health is not reaching most seniors 65 and older and is also associated with socioeconomic disparities (Levine et al. 2016).

Religion and spirituality have been associated with healing in the teachings and sacred texts of all major religions from ancient times, and pastoral care and hospital chaplaincy are accepted services benefiting those who are ill and who desire them in the community and in hospital care. This has become the subject of great scientific interest and improved research in recent times (Koenig 1997). Many studies show health benefits, as in a major review on the topic (Powell et al. 2003) that found a 25% reduction in overall mortality in those attending church services, but some also find evidence that religion or spirituality may interfere with recovery, and be maladaptive as well as adaptive, in terms of its impact on health (Jarvis, Northcott 1987). Throughout history, the destructive effects of punitive rigidity, prejudice, and guilt, especially of certain religious cults, are well known. Fricchione and Peteet (2015) concluded that more studies find health benefits from religion and spirituality than problems, but highlights that "Spirituality is not a substitute for adherence to mainstream medical and surgical management."

Mind–body medicine, formerly termed *complementary and alternative medicine* (CAM), has a growing role in medical treatment (Fricchione 2015). Complementary and alternative treatments are widely used, some of them promising, but they are also little studied in relation to wound healing (Freeman et al. 2010). These include physical exercise (Silveira et al. 2013), yoga (Louie 2014), mindfulness (Piet, Hougaard 2011), acupuncture (Smith et al. 2010), and cannabinoids (Whiting et al. 2015) and other agents. "The greatest risk of pursuing a CAM therapy is the possible delay of other well-established treatments. Clinical, research, and educational initiatives designed to focus on CAM in psychiatry are clearly warranted due to the widespread use of these therapies" (Freeman et al. 2010, p. 678).

CONCLUSION

Depression and other mood disorders are common in patients with wounds associated with injuries and surgical procedures. They may be triggered by the pain and stress of the injury or surgery, or be preexisting. The relationship of depression and wound healing is bidirectional, with the course of each influencing the other. When depressive or other mood disorders are diagnosed, the overall medical prognosis for child and adult patients is worse because it interferes with their adherence to aftercare interventions, impairs physical and cognitive functioning, reduces quality of life, and increases morbidity and mortality. Depression is a risk factor for incurring some types of injuries, particularly those associated with alcohol, self-injury or suicide, and abuse. This indicates directions for the prevention of injuries and a need for trauma surgery through treatment of depression and mood disorders. Based on epidemiological, clinical, and basic science research on wound healing, depression is also likely to affect the course of wound healing following injuries, surgery, and medical illness. In patients with these conditions, depression may be both diagnosed and treated, and treatment guidelines are available (American Psychiatric Association 2010). Nevertheless, studies examining the relationship between clinical depression and wound healing are few, and more are needed to further identify the best treatments to optimize wound healing and treat depression.

REFERENCES

1. Evans DL, Charney DS, Golden RN, et al. Mood disorders in the medically ill: scientific review and recommendations. *Biol Psychiatry*. 2005;23:175–189.
2. Celano CM, Huffman JC. Depression and cardiac disease: a review. *Cardiol Rev*. 2011;19:130–142.
3. Baumeister H, Hutter N, Bengel J. Psychological and pharmacological interventions for depression in patients with coronary artery disease. *Cochrane Database Syst Rev*. 2011;(9):CD00812.
4. Ciesla JA, Roberts JE. Meta-analysis of the relationship between HIV infection and risk for depressive disorders. *Am J Psychiatry*. 2001;158:725–730.
5. Nouwen A, Winkley K, Twisk J. Type 2 diabetes mellitus as a risk factor for the onset of depression: a systematic review and meta-analysis. *Diabetologia*. 2010;53:2480–2486.
6. Ferrari AJ, Charlson FJ, Norman RE, et al. Burden of depressive disorders by country, sex, age, and year: findings from the Global Burden of Disease study 2010. *PLoS Med*. 2013 Nov;10(11):e1001547. http://dx.doi.org/10.137/journal.pmed.1001547
7. Pratt LA, Brody DJ. Depression in the U.S. household population. *Natl Cent Health Stats Data Brief*. 2014;172:1–8.
8. Haagsma JA, Graetz N, Bolliger I, et al. The global burden of injury: incidence, mortality, disability-adjusted life years and time trends from the Global Burden of Disease study 2013. *Inj Prev*. 2015;0:1–16. doi:10.1136/injuryprev-2015-041616
9. Berwick DM, Downey AS, Cornett EA. A national trauma care system to achieve zero preventable deaths after injury: recommendations from a National Academies of Sciences, Engineering, and Medicine report. *JAMA*. 2016;316(9):927–928.
10. Stoddard FJ. Care of infants, children and adolescents with burn injuries. In: Lewis M, ed. *Child and adolescent psychiatry*, 3rd ed. Baltimore, MD: Lippincott Williams & Wilkins; 2002:1188–1208.

11. Freud A. The role of bodily illness in the mental life of children. *Psychoanal Study Child.* 1952;7:69.
12. O'Malley PJ, D'Amato HG, Stoddard FJ. Death and grief counseling in children and adolescents. In: Fogel BS, Greenberg DB, eds. *Psychiatric care of the medical patient*, 3rd ed. New York, Oxford University Press; 2015:1564–1577.
13. Stoddard FJ, Saxe G. Ten-year research review of physical injuries. *J Am Acad Child Adolesc Psychiatry.* 2001;40(10):1128–1145.
14. Stoddard FJ, Sheridan R, Selter L. General surgery: basic principles. In: Fogel BS, Greenberg DB, eds. *Psychiatric care of the medical patient*, 3rd ed. New York, Oxford University Press; 2015:1367–1388.
15. Maytal G, Rabinowitz T, Stewart TD, et al. Chronic medical illness and rehabilitation. In: Stern TA, Fricchione GL, Cassem NH, Jellinek MS, Rosenbaum JF, eds. *Massachusetts General Hospital handbook of general hospital psychiatry*, 6th ed. London, Elsevier Health Sciences; 2010: 397–399.
16. Stoddard FJ. Outcomes of traumatic exposure. In: SJ Cozza, JA Cohen, JG Doherty, eds. *Disaster and trauma. Child and adolescent psychiatric clinics of North America.* 2014;23(2):243–256.
17. Stoddard FJ, Sorrentino E, Drake JE, et al. Posttraumatic stress disorder diagnosis in young burned children. *J Burn Care Res.* 2017;38(1):e343–e351. doi:10.1097/BCR.0000000000000386
18. Thombs BD, Bresnick MG, Magyar-Russell G. Depression in survivors of burn injury: a systematic review. *Gen Hosp Psychiatry.* 2006;28:494–502.
19. Thombs BD, Haines JM, Bresnick MG, et al. Depression in burn reconstruction patients: symptom prevalence and association with body image dissatisfaction and physical function. *Gen Hosp Psychiatry.* 2007;29:14–20.
20. Stoddard FJ, Simon NM, Pitman RK. Trauma- and stressor-related disorders. In: Hales RE, Yudofsky S, Roberts L, eds. *American Psychiatric Publishing textbook of psychiatry: DSM-5 Edition*, Arlington, VA: American Psychiatric Press; 2014b:455–498.
21. Upton D, Solowiej K, Woo KY. A health professional perspective of the prevalence of mood disorders in patients with acute and chronic wounds. *Int Wound J.* 2014 Dec;11(6):627–635. doi: 10.1111/iwj.12018. Epub Jan 4, 2013.
22. Stoddard FJ, Sheridan RL, Martyn JAJ, et al. Pain management. Chapter 23. In: Ritchie EC, ed. *Combat and operational behavioral health.* In: Lenhart MK, ed. *The textbooks of military medicine.* Washington, DC: Department of the Army, Office of The Surgeon General, Borden Institute; 2011:339–358.
23. Bryant RA, Creamer M, O'Donnell M, et al. A study of the protective function of acute morphine administration on subsequent posttraumatic stress disorder. *Biol Psychiatry.* 2009;65(5):438–440.
24. Holbrook TL, Galarneau MR, Dye JL, et al. Morphine use after combat injury in Iraq and posttraumatic stress disorder. *NEJM.* 2010;362(2):110–117.
25. Stoddard FJ, Luthra R, Sorrentino EA, et al. A randomized controlled study of sertraline to prevent posttraumatic stress disorder in burned children. *J Child Adolesc Psychopharmacol.* 2011;21:469–477.
26. Sheridan RL, Stoddard FJ, Kazis LE, et al. Multi-Center Benchmarking Study. Long-term post-traumatic stress symptoms vary inversely with early opiate dosing in children recovering from serious burns: effects durable at four years. *J Traum Acute Care Surg.* Mar 2014;76(3):828–832.

27. Zatzick D, Rivera F, Jurkovich G, et al. Enhancing the population impact of collaborative care interventions: mixed method development and implementation of stepped care targeting posttraumatic stress disorder and related comorbidities after acute trauma. *Gen Hosp Psychiatry*. 2011;33(2):123–134.

28. Engel CC, Jaycox LH, Freed MC, et al. Centrally assisted collaborative telecare for posttraumatic stress disorder and depression among military personnel attending primary care: a randomized clinical trial. *JAMA Intern Med*. 2016;176(7):948–956. doi:10.1001/jamainternmed.2016.2402

29. Broughton G, Janis JE, Attinger GE. The basic science of wound healing. *Plast Reconstr Surg*. 2006;117(75 Suppl)125S–134S.

30. Weber KT, Bhattacharya SK, Newman KP, et al. Stressor states and the cation crossroads. *J Am Coll Nutr*. Dec 2010;29(6):563–574.

31. Gouin JP, Kiecolt-Glaser JK. The impact of psychological stress on wound healing: methods and mechanisms. *Immunol Allerg Clin N Am*. 2011;31(1):81–93.

32. Kiecolt-Glaser JK, Page GG, Marucha PT, et al. Psychological influences on surgical recovery: perspectives from psychoimmunology. *Am Psychol*. 1998;53:1209–1218.

33. Broadbent E, Koschwanez HE. The psychology of wound healing. *Curr Opin Psychiatry*. 2012;25(2):135–140. doi:10.1097/YCO.0b013e32834e1424

34. Gouin JP, Carter CS, Pournajafi-Nazarloo H, et al. Marital behavior, oxytocin, vasopressin, and wound healing. *Psychoneuroendocrinology*. Aug 2010;35(7):1082–1090. doi:10.1016/j.psyneuen.2010.01.009. Epub. Feb 9, 2010.

35. Simons RL, Lei MK, Beach SR, et al. Methylation of the oxytocin receptor gene mediates the effect of adversity on negative schemas and depression. *Dev Psychopathol*. 2017 Aug:29(3):725–736. doi: 10.1017/S0954579416000420.

36. Poutahidis T, Kearney SM, Levkovich T, et al. Microbial symbionts accelerate wound healing via the neuropeptide hormone oxytocin. *PLoS One*. 2013;30;8(10):e78898. doi:10.1371/journal.pone.0078898

37. Molnar JA, Vlad LG, Gumus T. Nutrition and chronic wounds: improving clinical outcomes. *Plast Reconstr Surg*. Sep 2016;138(3 Suppl):71S–81S.

38. Doering LV, Moser LK, Lemankiewicz W, et al. Depression, healing and recovery from coronary artery bypass surgery. *Am J Crit Care*. 2005;14:316–324.

39. Grace SL, Abbey SE, Kapral MK, et al. Effect of depression on five-year mortality after an acute coronary syndrome. *Am J Cardiol*. 2005;96(9):1179–1185.

40. Milani RV, Lavie CJ. Impact of cardiac rehabilitation on depression and its associated mortality. *Am J Med*. 1996;120(9):799–732.

41. Januzzi JL, Stern TA, Pasternak RC, et al. The influence of anxiety and depression on outcomes of patients with coronary artery disease. *Arch Int Med*. 2000;160(13):1913–1921.

42. Kohler O, Gasse C, Petersen L, et al. The effect of concomitant treatment with SSRIs and statins: a population-based study. *Am J Psychiatry*. 2016;173(8):807–815.

43. Beilin B, Shavit V, Mordashev B, et al. Effects of postoperative pain management on immune response to surgery. *Anesth Analg*. 2003;97:822–827.

44. Walburn J, Vedhara K, Hankins M, et al. Psychological stress and wound healing in humans: a systematic review and metanalysis. *J Psychosom Res*. 2009;67(3):253–271.

45. Broadbent E, Petrie KJ, Booth RJ. Psychological stress impairs early wound healing following surgery. *Psychosom Med*. 2003;65:865–869.

46. Rosenberger PH, Jokl P, Ickovics J. Psychosocial factors and surgical outcomes: an evidence-based literature review. *J Am Acad Orthop Surg*. 2006;14(7):397–405.

47. Vedhara K, Miles JNR, Wetherell MA, et al. Coping style and depression influence the healing of diabetic foot ulcers: observational and mechanistic evidence. *Diabetologia*. 2010;53(8):1590–1598.

48. Miller AH, Maletic V, Raison CL. Inflammation and its discontents: the role of cytokines in the pathophysiology of major depression. *Biol Psychiatry*. 2009 May 1;65(9):732–741.

49. Ebrecht M, Hextall J, Kirtley LG, et al. Perceived stress and cortisol levels predict speed of wound healing in healthy male adults. *Psychoneuroimmunology*. 2004;29(6):798–809.

50. Kiecolt-Glaser JK, Glaser R. Depression and immune function: central pathways to morbidity and mortality. *J Psychosom Res*. 2002;53(4):873–876.

51. Tarrier N, Gregg L, Edwards J, et al. The influence of pre-existing psychiatric illness on recovery in burn injury patients: the impact of psychosis and depression. *Burns*. 2005;31(1):45–49.

52. Thombs BD, Bresnick MG, Magyar-Russell G. Depression in survivors of burn injury: a systematic review. *Gen Hosp Psychiatry*. 2006;28:494–502.

53. Irwin KE, Freudenreich O, Peppercorn J, et al. Case records of the Massachusetts General Hospital. Case 30-2016. A 63-year-old woman with bipolar disorder, cancer, and worsening depression. N Engl J Med. 2016 Sep 29;375(13):1270–1281. doi: 10.1056/NEJMcpc1609309.

54. Williams LH, Miller DR, Fincke G, et al. Depression and incident lower limb amputations in veterans with diabetes. *J Diabetes Complications*. 2011;25(3):175–182.

55. Levine JB, Leeder AD, Parekkadan B, et al. Isolation rearing impairs wound healing and is associated with increased locomotion and decreased early gene expression in the medial prefrontal cortex of juvenile rats. *J Neurosci*. 2007;151(2):589–603.

56. O'Reardon JP, Solvason HB, Janicak PG, et al. Efficacy and safety of transcranial magnetic stimulation in the acute treatment of major depression: a multisite randomized controlled trial. *Biol Psychiatry*. 2007;62(11):1208–1216. http://dx.doi.org/10.1016/j.biopsych.2007.01.018

57. Meersand P, Gilmore KJ. Chapter 4: Play in the digital age. In: Play Therapy: a Psychodynamic Primer for the Treatment of Young Children. Arlington, VA: American Psychiatric Association Publishing; 2018:91–122.

58. Mayberg HS, Silva JA, Brannan SK, et al. The functional neuroanatomy of the placebo effect. *Am J Psychiatry*. 2002;159:728–737.

59. Vits S, Dissemond J, Schadendorf D, et al. Expectation-induced placebo responses fail to accelerate wound healing in healthy volunteers: results from a prospective controlled experimental trial. *Int Wound J*. 2015;12(6):664–668. doi:10.1111/iwj.12193. Epub. Dec 30 2013.

60. McEwen BS, Gray JD, Nasca C. Recognizing resilience: learning from the effects of stress on the brain. *Neurobiol Stress*. 2015(1):1–11.

61. McEwen BS, Gianaros PJ. Stress- and allostasis-induced brain plasticity. *Annu Rev Med*. 2011;62:431–445.

62. Davidson RJ, McEwen BS. Social influences on neuroplasticity: stress and interventions to promote well being. *Nat Neurosci*. 2013;15(5):689–695. doi:10.1038/nn.3093

63. Sheridan RL, Schaefer PW, Whalen M, et al. Case records of the Massachusetts General Hospital. Case 36-2012. Recovery of a 16-year-old girl from trauma and burns after a car accident. *NEJM*. 2012 Nov;367(21):2027–2037. doi:10.1056/NEJMcpc1200088

64. Sheridan RL, Lee AF, Kazis LE, et al. Multi-Center Benchmarking Study Working Group. The effect of family characteristics on the recovery of burn injuries in children. *J Trauma Acute Care Surg*. Sep 2012;73(3 Suppl 2):S205–S212.

65. Sheridan RL, Shumaker PR, King DR, et al. Case records of the Massachusetts General Hospital. Case 15-2014. A man in the military who was injured by an improvised explosive device in Afghanistan. *NEJM*. 2014 May;370(20):1931–1940.

66. Sheridan RL. Fire-related inhalation injury. *NEJM*. 2016;375:464–469. doi:10.1056/NEJMra1601128

67. Clark D, Beck AT. Cognitive theory and therapy of anxiety and depression: convergence with neurobiological findings. *Trend Cogn Sci*. 2010;14:418–424.

68. Derubeis RJ, Siegle GJ, Hollon SD. Cognitive therapy versus meditation for depression: treatment outcomes and neural mechanisms. *Nature Rev Neurosci*. 2008;9:788–796.

69. Hofmann SG, Grossman P, Hinton DE. Loving-kindness and compassion meditation: potential for psychological interventions. *Clin Psychol Rev*. 2011;31:1126–1132.

70. Buntrock C, Ebert DD, Lehr D, et al. Effect of a web-based guided self-help intervention for prevention of major depression in adults with subthreshold depression: a randomized clinical trial. *JAMA*. 2016;315(17):1854–1863.

71. Levine DM, Lipsitz SR, Linder JA. Research Letter. Trends in seniors' use of digital health technology in the United States, 2011–2014. *JAMA*. 2016;316(5):538–540.

72. Koenig HG. *Is religion good for your health? Effects of religion on physical and mental health*. New York: Haworth Press; 1997.

73. Powell LH, Shahabi L, Thoresen CE. Religion and spirituality: linkages to physical health. *Am Psychologist*. 2003;58:36–52.

74. Jarvis GK, Northcott HC. Religion and differences in morbidity and mortality. *Soc Sci Med*. 1987;25:813–824.

75. Fricchione GL, Peteet JR. Spiritual and religious issues in medical illness. In: Fogel BS, Greenberg DB, eds. *Psychiatric care of the medical patient*, 3rd ed. New York, Oxford University Press; 2015:322–339.

76. Fricchione GL. Mind-body medicine. In: Fogel BS, Greenberg DB, eds. *Psychiatric care of the medical patient*, 3rd ed. New York, Oxford University Press; 2015:305–321.

77. Telgenhoff D, Shroot B. Cellular senescence mechanisms in chronic wound healing. *Cell Death Differ*. 2005;12:695–698.

78. Verhoeven JE, van Oppen P, Revesz D, et al. Depressive and anxiety disorders showing robust, but not dynamic, 6-year longitudinal association with short leukocyte telomere length. *Am J Psychiatry*. 2015;173:617–624; doi:10.1176/appi.ajp2015.15070887

79. Spiegel H, Spiegel D. *Trance and treatment*. Washington, DC: American Psychiatric Press; 2004.

80. McEwen BS. Protective and damaging effects of stress mediators. *NEJM*. 1998;153:171–179.

81. Solowiej K, Mason V, Upton D. Review of the relationship between stress and wound healing, part 1. *J Wound Care*. 2009;18:(9):357–366.

82. Solowiej K, Mason V, Upton D. Psychological stress and pain in wound care, part 2: a review of pain and stress assessment tools. *J Wound Care*. 2010a;19(3):110–115.

83. Solowiej K, Mason V, Upton D. Psychological stress and pain in wound care, part 3: management. *J Wound Care*. 2010b;19(4):153–155. doi:10.1097/TA.0b013e3182ab111c

84. Stoddard FJ, Schneider JC, Ryan CM. Physical and psychiatric recovery from burns. *Surg Clin North Am*. 2014;94(4):863–878. And *Psychiatr Clin North Am*. 2015;38(1):105–120.

85. Freeman MP, Fava M, Lake J, et al. Complementary and alternative medicine in major depressive disorder: the American Psychiatric Association Task Force report. *J Clin Psychiatry*. 2010;71:669–681.

86. Piet J, Hougaard E. The effect of mindfulness-based cognitive therapy for prevention of relapse in recurrent major depressive disorder: a systemic review and meta-analysis. *Clin Psychol Rev.* 2011;31:1032–1040.
87. Louie L. The effectiveness of yoga for depression: a critical literature review. *Issues Ment Health Nurs.* 2014;35:265–276.
88. Silveira H, Moraes H, Oliveira N, et al. Physical exercise and clinically depressed patients: a systematic review and meta-analysis. *Neuropsychobiology.* 2013;67:61–68.
89. Smith CA, Hay PP, Macpherson H. Acupuncture for depression. *Cochrane Database Syst Rev.* 2010;(1): Art. No. CD004046.
90. Whiting PF, Wolff RF, Deshpande S, et al. Cannabinoids for medical use: a systematic review. *JAMA.* 2015;313:2456–2473. doi:10.1001/jama.2015.6358
91. Wang PS, Angermeyer M, Borges G, et al. Delay and failure in treatment seeking after first onset of mental disorders in the World Health Organization's World Mental Health Survey Initiative. *World Psychiatry.* 2007;6(3):177–185.
92. Ghio L, Gotelli S, Marcenaro M, et al. Duration of untreated illness and outcomes in unipolar depression: a systematic review and meta-analysis. *J Affect Disord.* 2014;152–154:45–51.
93. Gelenberg AT, Freeman MP, Markowitz JC, Rosenbaum JF, Thase ME, Trivedi MH, van Rhoads RS. American Psychiatric Association, Working Group on Major Depressive Disorder. *Practice guideline for treatment of patients with major depressive disorder*, 3rd ed. 2010. http://www.psychiatryonline.com/pracGuide/pracGuideTopic_7.aspx.
94. Fred Tawakol A, Ishai A, Takx RA, Figueroa AL, Ali A, Kaiser Y, Truong QA, Solomon CJ, Calcagno C, Mani V, Tang CY, Mulder WJ, Murrough JW, Hoffmann U, Nahrendorf M, Shin LM, Fayad ZA, Pitman RK. Relation between resting amygdalar activity and cardiovascular events: a longitudinal and cohort study. *Lancet.* 2017;389:834–845

10

Psychopharmacology of Depression as a Systemic Illness for Primary and Specialty Care Clinicians
Focus on Adverse Drug Reactions and Drug–Drug Interactions

Kelly L. Cozza, Rita Rein, Gary H. Wynn, and Eric G. Meyer

The opinions or assertions contained herein are the private views of the authors and are not to be construed as official or as reflecting the views of the Unite States Department of the Army, Department of the Navy, Uniformed Services University of the Health Sciences, or the Department of Defense.

INTRODUCTION

Drug–drug interactions (DDIs) are an important, but often overlooked and under-recognized clinical issue in psychosomatic medicine. The frequency of DDIs, especially with polypharmacy, has been well documented (Davies et al. 2004). Most of the details of how drugs interact with each other have been well elucidated, most notably the pharmacokinetic interactions involving the major cytochrome P450 (CYP450) hepatic enzymes. In fact, DDIs attributed to the antidepressant fluoxetine (Vaughan 1988, Von Ammon Cavanaugh 1990) spearheaded the need for increasing practical clinical knowledge of DDIs in medical practice.

The bench and clinical research has been translated into many pharmacy program databases, books, articles, and "apps" to aid clinicians in predicting and/or determining potential DDIs in their patients (Cozza et al. 2003, Strain et al. 2004). Improvements in clinical pharmaceutical software and revised FDA oversight have helped, but they are far from perfect (Cavuto et al. 1996). Without knowledge of underlying DDI principles, DDI apps and software may lead to "prescribing paralysis," or avoidance of a potentially useful drug for fear of a forewarned interaction. Conversely, many warn of every possible and insignificant interaction, which may lead to "alert-fatigue" or ignoring the too-frequent warnings (Zorina et al. 2013).

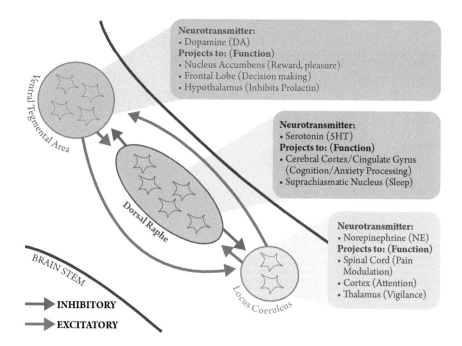

Neurotransmitter:
• Dopamine (DA)
Projects to: (Function)
• Nucleus Accumbens (Reward, pleasure)
• Frontal Lobe (Decision making)
• Hypothalamus (Inhibits Prolactin)

Neurotransmitter:
• Serotonin (5HT)
Projects to: (Function)
• Cerebral Cortex/Cingulate Gyrus
  (Cognition/Anxiety Processing)
• Suprachiasmatic Nucleus (Sleep)

Neurotransmitter:
• Norepinephrine (NE)
Projects to: (Function)
• Spinal Cord (Pain
  Modulation)
• Cortex (Attention)
• Thalamus (Vigilance)

Ventral Tegmental Area

Dorsal Raphe

BRAIN STEM

Locus Coeruleus

→ INHIBITORY

→ EXCITATORY

Figure 10.1 The monoamine hypothesis is a mainstay in the theory of depression and the use of antidepressants. The above image depicts a cross section of the brain stem, where the majority of the monoamines are produced. Each neurotransmitter has it's own function, as described in the boxes on the right. These three neurotransmitters can excite or inhibit the release of the other transmitters. Notably, serotonin is inhibitory of norepinephrine and dopamine, which may be related to the feelings of depression patients report when started on an SSRI for anxiety (Schatzberg and Nemeroff 2009, ElMansari, Guiard et al. 2010, Hamon and Blier 2013, Stahl 2013).

BRIEF REVIEW OF MONOAMINE HYPOTHESIS AND PSYCHOTROPIC MECHANISMS OF ACTION FOR DEPRESSION

The monoamine hypothesis is a mainstay in the theory of depression and the use of antidepressants (see Figure 10.1). Three neurotransmitters comprise the system: dopamine, serotonin, and norepinephrine. These neurotransmitters are synthesized through a multistep process from amino acids, which is comparatively more difficult than other neurotransmitters (GABA, glutamate, acetylcholine), which are made via glucose metabolism (Abdallah et al. 2014). As such, recovery of the monoamines after they have been released into synaptic cleft is crucial. The monoamines are thus captured by re-uptake pumps, which allow the neurotransmitter to be reused, decreasing the need for synthesis. Drugs that block reuptake (selective serotonin reuptake inhibitors [SSRIs] and serotonin-norepinephrine reuptake inhibitors [SNRIs]), or reduce the breakdown of neurotransmitters (monoamine oxidase inhibitors [MAOIs]) increase the amount of time these neurotransmitters have in the synaptic cleft, thereby increasing the signal from that neuron. It is for this reason that monotherapy with

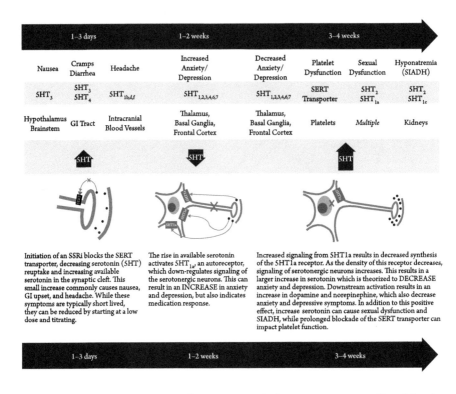

Figure 10.2 SSRI mechanism of action, effects, receptors, and effects over time. (2006, Stahl 2013) (2011).

an SSRI, a typical first-line treatment for depression, may worsen depression in those with deficiencies in norepinephrine and/or dopamine (Andrews et al. 2015, Fried and Nesse 2015). Clinically, providers may recognize this phenomenon in patients presenting with a melancholic type depression. They endorse no symptoms of anxiety, but do report an inability to concentrate and/or feel joy (Belzer and Schneier 2004). Thus, the use of medications that block the reuptake of serotonin and norepinephrine (SNRI) might be required, as an SSRI would only further decrease their dopamine and norepinephrine levels (Outhred et al. 2013, Blier 2013). Conversely, those patients with an anxious depression (Alpert et al. 2008) may report more anxiety when started on bupropion, as it doesn't modulate serotonin but does increase norepinephrine and dopamine. Indeed, when considering the use of medications to reduce symptoms, providers are wise to carefully consider which symptoms they are attempting to target (Wiseman 2012).

Figure 10.2 delineates some of the cellular and receptor alterations caused by SSRIs, the most commonly prescribed antidepressants, and includes time course, side effects, and potential toxicities of SSRI treatment. Importantly, when using an SSRI, it is critical to understand its pharmacodynamic and downstream effects, which can greatly improve the quality of informed consent, as patients will know what to expect and when. Initially, there is a brief surge of serotonin in the synaptic cleft, which may cause brief gastrointestinal (GI) upset, nausea and headache. These symptoms typically resolve

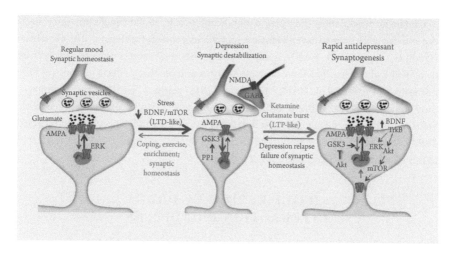

Figure 10.3 Glutamate Hypothesis: Stress and depression decrease, while rapid-acting antidepressants (e.g., ketamine) increase, synaptic connections. Under normal, nonstress conditions, synapses of glutamate terminals are maintained and regulated by circuit activity and function, including activity-dependent release of brain derived neurotrophic factor (BDNF) and downstream signaling pathways. Stress and depression are associated with neuronal atrophy and decreased synaptic connections in the prefrontal cortex and hippocampus. This is thought to occur via decreased expression and release of BDNF as well as increased levels of adrenal glucocorticoids. This decrease has been compared with long-term depression (LTD). Rapid-acting antidepressants, notably ketamine, cause a burst of glutamate that results in an increase in synaptogenesis that has been compared with long-term potentiation (LTP). The increase in glutamate is thought to occur via blockade of N-methyl-Daspartate (NMDA) receptors located on inhibitory γ-aminobutyric acid (GABA)-ergic neurons, resulting in disinhibition of glutamate transmission. The burst of glutamate increases BDNF release and causes activation of mammalian target of rapamycin (mTOR) signaling, which then increases the synthesis of synaptic proteins required for new spine synapse formation. These new connections allow for proper circuit activity and normal control of mood and emotion. However, the new synapses are unstable and are lost after about 10 days, which coincides with depression relapse in patients.

Akt, protein kinase b; AMPA, α-amino-3-hydroxy-5-methyl-4-isoxazolepropionicacid; ERK, extracellular signal-regulated kinases; GABA, γ-aminobutyric acid; GSK, glycogen synthase kinase; PP1, phosphoprotein phosphatase 1; TrkB, tropomyosin receptor kinase B. Duman RS. Pathophysiology of depression and innovative treatments: remodeling glutamatergic synaptic connections. *Dialogues Clin Neurosci.2014;16(1):11-27* © AICH. *Image and legend reproduced with the permission of the publisher Association La Conférence Hippocrate – Servier Research Group, Suresnes, France.*

after a few days, allowing for further titration of the medication to an effective dose. After one to two weeks, the increase in serotonin stimulates 5HT1A, an autoreceptor, which decreases the firing rate of serotonergic neurons (Albert et al. 2014). It is purportedly due to this auto-downregulation that patients may report an increase in anxiety or depression (Köhler et al. 2016). Educating patients about these side effects through high-quality informed consent and shared decision making is helpful for patient adherence (Lee and Emanuel 2013) and even treatment (Rutherford et al. 2016). Increased signaling from 5HT1A over one to two weeks induces a homeostatic drive that reduces the synthesis of the 5HT1A autoreceptor, which ultimately results in a surge in serotonin signaling and the reduction of depressive and anxiety related symptoms.

Glutamate modulation may play a significant role in mood regulation since some depressed patients seem to have glutamatergic excitotoxic activity (see Figure 10.3, "Glutamate Hypothesis Overview"). NMDA receptor antagonists may exert antidepressant activity by affecting glutamate, but the exact mechanisms and feedback effects are not yet fully delineated (Newport et al. 2015). Miller et al. (2016) suggest, "NMDA receptor antagonism initiates protein synthesis and increases excitatory synaptic drive in corticolimbic brain regions, either through selective antagonism of inhibitory interneurons and cortical disinhibition, or by direct inhibition of cortical pyramidal neurons." The reader is referred to this excellent review for more complete details.

BRIEF REVIEW OF DRUG INTERACTION PRINCIPLES

To better understand medications for the treatment of depression, it is important to have a working knowledge of how drugs may interact with each other. We provide a brief review of pharmacodynamics, pharmacokinetics and the relevant issues associated with medications used for depression in this section. For a full explanation of pharmacology, metabolism, and drug interactions, the reader is referred to texts on the subject (Schatzberg and Nemeroff 2011, Wynn et al. 2009, Stahl 2013),

Pharmacodynamic Drug–Drug Interactions

Pharmacodynamic (PD) interactions are those that occur because of disruptions to a drug's intended mechanism of action at the intended receptor site (in the case of antidepressants, generally in the brain). Serotonin syndrome (sweating, autonomic dysfunction, etc.), is a pharmacodynamic drug interaction caused by the additive receptor-mediated effects of MAOI and SSRI co-administration. Most pharmacodynamic effects and interactions are intuitive and easily predictable. Another example of a pharmacokinetic interaction can occur with the MAOI phenelzine and the beta-blocker metoprolol, which may lead to postural hypotension with a subsequent fall and potential injury. In this case, phenelzine is used as an antidepressant but has the common side effect of lowering blood pressure, which is additive to the antihypertensive effect of metoprolol. This chapter will only briefly reference PD effects, since most of these interactions are readily predictable or apparent if the clinician is aware of the drug's mechanism of action.

Pharmacokinetic Principles

Pharmacokinetics (PK) is the study of how a drug moves through the body, particularly with regard to the time course of drug absorption, distribution, elimination, and metabolism. PK drug interactions occur when one drug interferes with another drug's absorption, distribution, elimination, or metabolism. The absorption of many drugs can be adversely affected by co-administration with food or buffers, and these absorption-based pharmacokinetic drug interactions are also relatively predictable. Metabolic interactions are more complex, as they are affected by metabolic inhibition, induction, and pharmacogenetics (an individual's genetically determined metabolic activity) at metabolic sites such as the gut wall and liver. The majority of drug interactions are metabolism related, and are described in the most detail in the following sections.

Absorption

Absorption is the movement of a drug into the blood stream. The complexity of the absorption process varies by the route of administration of a drug (e.g., oral, transversal/topical, intravenous, intramuscular). The primary route of administration for most psychotropics is oral administration. Absorption of these ingested drugs can be easily altered. These alterations can result in significant changes to a drug's bioavailability. Overall, most medications are absorbed more slowly with food. This can be an advantage if side effects occur when peak plasma levels rise too quickly on an empty stomach (e.g., acetylcholinesterase inhibitors are often are prescribed during or right after meals to avoid peak levels that can cause nausea). Most psychotropics are absorbed more rapidly on an empty stomach, which can be a beneficial trait for treating acute symptoms. A few psychotropics, however, such as ziprasidone, need to be taken with food in order for consistent and sufficient drug absorption to occur (Miceli et al. 2007). GI and hepatic blood flow, pH levels, and the amount of food consumed can also change the absorption of drugs. In addition, if a drug is a substrate of P-glycoprotein in the gut wall, then absorption will be decreased. P-glycoproteins act as "bouncers" at the villi of enterocytes, pushing drugs out from the enterocytes back into the gut lumen before they can be absorbed into the hepatic circulation (Terada and Hira 2015). If a second drug inhibits or induces the P-glycoprotein, then the first drug's absorption and serum levels may change.

Distribution

Distribution is the movement of the drug from one area of the body to another and is primarily affected by an individual's physical volume, drug removal rate, and the ratio of protein-bound versus free drug. Free drug is the non–protein-bound portion of circulating drug, and this is the portion with pharmacological effect. Changes in protein binding may alter the concentration of non–protein-bound drug and lead to DDIs. Albumin is the major serum protein that binds to drugs. Most psychotropics are highly protein-bound (venlafaxine is an exception). If two or more drugs compete for protein-binding sites on serum proteins, displacement may occur and more free drug will be available. Increased free drug could result in adverse effects. Even judicious use of therapeutic drug monitoring may overlook this interaction since most drug levels measure the total (free and bound) levels. Some drugs that are highly protein-bound, such as phenytoin (von Wincklemann et al. 2008), are notorious for this problem. Measuring of free and bound drug is available but often requires a special lab request.

Excretion

Excretion is the removal of drug and metabolites from the body primarily through the kidneys, and is a step which generally occur after metabolism (although some drugs are excreted unchanged without being metabolized, such as digoxin). Drugs that impact kidney function may alter the excretion of other drugs. Examples include thiazide diuretics, angiotensin-converting enzyme (ACE) inhibitors, non-steroidal anti-inflammatory drugs (NSAIDs), and furosemide that can raise serum lithium levels (Grandjean and Aubry 2009). This interaction may be due in part to an increase in the tubular reabsorption of lithium (Imbs et al. 1997). Alternatively, drugs such as caffeine, mannitol, acetazolamide, and theophylline may lower lithium levels (Grandjean and Aubry 2009).

Metabolism

Pharmacokinetic metabolism is the enzymatic alteration of a drug through the attachment or detachment of small components (e.g., a hydroxyl group) in order to further process the drug towards elimination. Overall, there are three ways that drugs are cleared from the body. Two of these processes are enzymatic (phase 1 and 2 metabolism) while the third and final occurs via elimination. (e.g., renal). None of these processes is mutually exclusive for a particular drug's clearance, because many use combinations of all three. Most drugs go through phase 1 and/or phase 2 metabolism (Wynn et al. 2009). This metabolism occurs at gut wall enterocytes and liver hepatocytes. Most of the metabolic enzymes are located in the endoplasmic reticulum of cells at these two locations.

Phase 1 Metabolism

Phase 1 metabolism is an oxidative process and usually detaches a small moiety from the molecule (i.e., a methyl or alkyl group) or simply oxidizes a portion of the molecule (i.e., RCH3 to RCH2OH). This process creates a more polar compound by exposing a hydroxyl group where the metabolism occurred, and makes the new compound more water soluble. In addition, the new hydroxyl group may act as a "handle" for the phase 2 enzymes to conjugate a moiety to the compound. As a rule, phase 1 enzymes alter compounds from their active form to an inactive or less active metabolite, but there are numerous exceptions to this rule. For example, the analgesic agent tramadol provides mild analgesia through monoaminergic activity but exerts more significant analgesia through its 2D6 metabolite O-desmethyltramadol that has mu-opioid receptor activity (Laugesen et al. 2005). In other cases the active parent compound is transformed into a similar or less active compound (e.g., fluoxetine to norfluoxetine by 2D6, Mandrioli et al. 2006). The enzymes that do most of the oxidative phase 1 drug metabolism are the P450 enzymes. The P450 enzymes are located throughout the body, but their highest concentration is in the endoplasmic reticulum of hepatocytes and gut wall enterocytes (Galetin et al. 2010).

Many drugs are metabolized by several P450 enzymes, depending on their drug concentration levels, the combination with other drugs, and genotype(s) (see inhibition, induction, and pharmacogenetics later in this chapter). For example, 3A4/5 is often considered a low-affinity/high-capacity enzyme; many drugs will be metabolized by 3A4 even if it is not the preferred metabolic site for a particular drug. 2D6 on the other hand is a high-affinity/low-capacity enzyme; it binds to some drugs very tightly, but can easily be saturated. Some metabolic activity may need to be carried by or "taken up" by other enzymes that have high capacity and low affinity, such as 3A4/5 if 2D6 is incapacitated or full, either by genetic default, or by a drug interaction. An example of this is risperidone, which is preferentially metabolized by 2D6 to an active metabolite, 9-hydroxy risperidone (9-OHR). 3A4 also metabolizes risperidone to the 9-OHR, just not as efficiently. More specifically, an individual's 2D6 polymorphism explains over half of the inter-individual variation in risperidone plasma concentration (Vandenberghe et al. 2015), given that 2D6 is low capacity and often relies on 3A4 for overflow metabolism. When compounds are metabolized by enzymes other than their preferred metabolism site, there are often higher rates of adverse drug reactions (ADRs) and increased discontinuation of the drug due to these ADRs.

Another CYP450 enzyme of importance is 1A2. This enzyme is found exclusively in the liver and metabolizes polycyclic aromatic hydrocarbons (PAHs). Cigarette smoke contains many PAHs. Chronic smoking ultimately leads to induction (see following) of 1A2, so that 1A2 has enhanced activity. Clozapine, and to some extent olanzapine, are dependent on 1A2 for their metabolism (Sagud et al. 2009). There is also evidence that suggests smoking increases the clearance of fluphenazine and haloperidol. Therefore, the starting or cessation of smoking could have significant effects on drug levels and efficacy. There are other oxidative phase 1 enzymes such as alcohol dehydrogenase, various esterases, and monoamine oxidases. Most of these enzymes are located throughout the body. A general review of the non-P450 phase 1 enzymes was written by Strolin and Tipton (Strolin Benedetti 2007).

Pharmacokinetic DDIs involving metabolism are the most important DDI mechanisms to understand. Although metabolic pharmacokinetic interactions can be complicated, with proper knowledge they can be straightforward and often predictable.

Metabolic pharmacokinetic interactions occur under two conditions: inhibition and induction, and they are influenced by genetics, discussed in a later section of this chapter.

Phase 2 Metabolism

Phase 2 metabolism involves adding a moiety to the drug, usually rendering it inactive and more water-soluble for excretion. The workhorses of phase 2 conjugating enzymes are the Uridine 5'-diphospho-glucuronosyltransferases (UGTs). These enzymes are found co-located with the CYP450 enzymes in the endoplasmic reticulum of hepatocytes. The UGT enzymes add a glucuronic acid molecule to the drug, often at the hydroxyl site that the CYP450 enzymes created. Acetylation, methylation, and sulfation are carried out by other phase 2 enzymes. Because phase 2 metabolism adds a moiety to a drug, it nearly always deactivates the drug to an inert substance ready for rapid excretion and elimination. Similarly to the CYP450 enzymes, there are many UGT enzymes: the major ones are UGT1A1, UGT1A3, UGT1A4, UGT1A6, UGT1A9, and UGT2B15. UGT1A3 and UGT2B7 have the most identified substrates (drugs that are metabolized by the enzyme).

Throughout the rest of this chapter, all UGT enzymes will be named with the prefix UGT to prevent confusion with CYP450 enzymes.

Interactions may also occur with phase II enzymes (e.g., glucuronidation via UGTs and sulfation). UGT enzymes are the most numerous and clinically important phase II enzymes. They are found in the endoplasmic reticulum and the nuclear membrane of liver, kidney, brain, and placental cells (Radominska-Pandya et al. 2002). Many drugs are metabolized first by phase I metabolism (P450 and others) and then by glucuronidation, but some drugs are directly conjugated by UGTs, such as lorazepam, temazepam, and oxazepam. Drugs primarily metabolized by UGTs include lamotrigine, valproate, nonsteroidal anti-inflammatory drugs, zidovudine, and many opioids. Most glucuronide metabolites are inactive, so inhibition or induction of these enzymes produces no clinically relevant effects. A few drugs are known to produce active metabolites via glucuronidation, such as morphine to morphine-6-glucuronide (DePriest 2015), a metabolite of morphine that is about 20 times more potent as an analgesic compound than morphine. Beyond glucuronidation via UGT2B7, morphine also undergoes glucosidation via 2B7 in a complementary metabolism performed by the same enzyme (Chau 2014). Inhibition of UGT2B7 glucuronidation by ketamine (or other UGT2B7 inhibitors) may result in clinically significant interactions, even at anesthetic level doses of ketamine (Uchaipichat et al. 2011).

Transporters: "Phase 0"

Membrane transporters may also be inhibited or induced via drug interactions, and exhibit genetic polymorphisms. The membrane-bound transporters are sometimes called "Phase 0" or Phase III" of the metabolic system. They were first called "p-glycoproteins" and are still commonly referred to in the literature that way or as "P-gps." Transporters are present in the blood–brain barrier, placenta, intestine, hepatocytes, renal tubule cells, and many other sites. They regulate the transfer of exogenous and endogenous compounds into and out of organs and other target cells. Transporters play a large role in the penetration of drugs like antiretrovirals (ART) and psychotropics into the brain. Functioning membrane transporters play a role in treatment-resistant depression by blocking transport of psychotropics into the brain. Importantly, if a membrane transporter is inhibited by a transport inhibitor, then the concentration of drugs that are "dependent upon," or substrates of, that transporter will get through the membrane to the other side, increasing transport across the membrane. Many drugs, including a number of psychotropics, are inhibitors of membrane transporters. A full explanation of the importance of transporters may be found elsewhere (Oesterheld 2009, O'Brien et al. 2012), and where known, transporter activity of drugs mentioned in this chapter is indicated in the tables.

Drug Variability

Drug serum concentration levels can vary tremendously from individual to individual. The following section will discuss the major reasons for this variability, including the mechanisms of DDIs and their role in variability.

Age and Gender Drug variability is dependent to some extent on age and gender. For the most part, enzymatic activity is stable from the teenage years through adult life until enzymatic activity begins to decline in much later years of life. Other changes, such as reduced hepatic blood flow, poorer absorption, and decreased renal function, may also alter serum drug levels in older adults. Generally, lower doses and frequent therapeutic drug monitoring (TDM), if possible, are recommended in the geriatric population. The ability to predict gender differences in drug metabolism and distribution is less clear, with more external factors (such as age, genetics, and personal habits [e.g., smoking or alcohol use]) confounding the study of gender differences. Research into this issue has shown that women may have slightly more activity than men at 2A6, 3A4, and 2B6; lower activity at 1A2, 2E1, and some UGT; and no difference in 2D6 and 2C9 (Anderson 2008). So, although size, age, and gender have something to do with variability in drug effectiveness, why is there so much variability given two people of similar size, gender, age, and race and medical illness? The pharmacokinetic reasons for drug variability are metabolic inhibition and induction and patient genetics. A review of metabolic inhibition, induction, and pharmacogenetics follows.

Inhibition Inhibition (Figure 10.4) occurs when a second drug interferes with the metabolism of the first drug. An example would be fluoxetine's inhibition of 2D6. If fluoxetine is added for a patient taking tamoxifen (primarily metabolized by 2D6 to its active metabolite), then tamoxifen levels will rise, sometimes dramatically (Binkhorst et al. 2013). This is because fluoxetine (which is also metabolized by 2D6

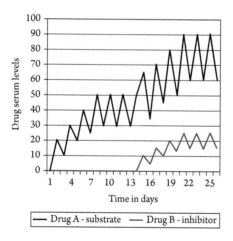

Figure 10.4 Drug–drug interaction—inhibition. Drug A develops steady-state concentrations after 4 half- lives (t1/2). Its peak levels are 50 and trough levels 30 at steady state. Drug B is introduced sometime later after drug A is in steady-state concentrations. Drug B develops its own steady-state after 4 half -lives. Drug B, however, is a competitive inhibitor of the enzyme(s) that drug A uses for its metabolism. Drug A develops a new steady state, with peak levels at 90 and trough levels at 60. Reproduced with permission of the editors: Cozza, KL; Armstrong, SG; Oesterheld, JR, Armstrong, NB; Wynn, GH: Overview of drug interactions in psychosomatic medicine, in. Psychosomatic Medicine, Michael Blumenfield, M; Strain, JJ (Eds), 2006.

to norfluoxetine) is competitively inhibiting tamoxifen's metabolism to its active metabolite endoxifen. Importantly, inhibition of the metabolism of a pro-drug not only *increases* the plasma level of the parent compound but significantly *decreases* the active metabolite and can have very grave consequences. Inhibition occurs immediately once the inhibitor is introduced, and it ceases once the inhibitor is withdrawn, as long as the half-life of the inhibitor is relatively short. In the preceding example, since fluoxetine has a long half-life (Shi et al. 2010), 2D6 will still be inhibited for one to two weeks after its discontinuation. In addition, inhibition generally is competitive like the previous example, but there are many exceptions. In particular, the morphology of the 3A4 enzyme allows for many sites of action, and some drugs inhibit 3A4 through noncompetitive inhibition. Inhibition may not be a problem if the drug that has its metabolism inhibited has a wide safety margin and few side effects. Inhibition can create significant side effects or toxicity of a drug that has a relatively narrow safety margin (e.g., tricyclic antidepressants, clozapine, or pimozide) by raising the serum level of the potentially toxic parent drug, or it may drastically reduce effectiveness of pro-drugs, which rely on the inhibited metabolic enzyme to produce the therapeutic active compound.

Figure 10.4 presents what happens to serum levels of drug A when a potent inhibitor of drug A's metabolic enzyme (usually in the gut wall or the liver) is present. Inhibition of metabolism is immediate and generally causes the serum level of the parent drug to increase. If that parent drug (for example, a tricyclic antidepressant) has a narrow margin of safety, then toxicity may result. Inhibition slows the metabolism of a drug dependent on the inhibited enzyme. Inhibition may occur at cytochrome P450 enzymes in the liver and gut wall (phase I metabolism), and/or during phase II metabolism (glucuronidation [UGTs], sulfation [SULTs], methylation, etc.) in the liver. P450 enzymes that metabolize current medications include cytochromes 3A4, 2D6, 1A2, 2C9, 2C19, 2E1, and 2B6, among others. 3A4 and 2D6 and glucuronidation are affected by commonly used medications, to include most psychotropics. Table 10.1, "Common Substrates, Inhibitors and Inducers of Cytochrome P450 Enzymes," presents many of the most common inhibitors of 3A4 and 2D6, as well as the drugs with narrow margins of safety that are dependent on those enzymes for metabolism.

Induction Induction is not quite the opposite of inhibition, despite its name (Figure 10.5). Induction involves the gradual increase in enzymatic activity brought on by a drug that stimulates the production of more metabolic enzymes. This process takes time, on the order of one to two weeks, as the drug stimulates second-messenger systems. This leads to increased mRNA synthesis and then more protein/enzyme production. Once the inducer is discontinued, the process of "un-induction" also takes one to two weeks, as the cells return gradually to homeostasis without the inducer in the environment. An example of induction would be adding carbamazepine for a woman on a low ethinyl estradiol (EE) oral contraceptive (OC). EE is metabolized by 3A4, and carbamazepine induces 3A4. After several weeks on carbamazepine, the patient's EE level will decrease due to its enhanced metabolism from the induced 3A4, creating the possibility of breakthrough bleeding or an unwanted pregnancy (Davis et al. 2011). If homeostasis

Table 10.1 Common Substrates, Inhibitors, and Inducers of Cytochrome P450 Enzymes

P450 Enzyme	Common Substrates*	Common Inhibitors	Common Inducers
1A2	Amitriptyline	Acyclovir	Tobacco smoke
	Caffeine	Amiodarone	Carbamazepine
	Cyclobenzaprine	Cimetidine	Eso/omeprazole
	Fluvoxamine	**Ciprofloxacin/ Fluoroquinolones**	Rifampin
	Olanzapine	**Flutamide**	Ritonavir
	Verapamil	Fluvoxamine	Broccoli/cauliflower
	R-warfarin	Verapamil	
2B6	Bupropion	Clopidogrel	Pan-inducers[†]
	Cyclophosphamide	Fluoxetine	Lopinavir/ritonavir
	Efavirenz	Fluvoxamine	Ritonavir
		Paroxetine	
		Ritonavir	
2D6	Antiarrhythmics	**Bupropion**	Pan-inducers[†] possibly
	Metoprolol	**Diphenhydramine**	
	Oxycodone	**Fluoxetine**	
	SSRIs	**Paroxetine**	
	Tramadol	**Quinidine**	
	Tricyclic antidepressants	**Ritonavir**	
	Typical antipsychotics		
3A4	Antiarrhythmics	**Cimetidine**	**Carbamazepine**
	β-blockers	**Clarithromycin**	Efavirenz
	Buspirone	Diltiazem	Nevirapine
	Carbamazepine	**Efavirenz**	Oxcarbazepine
	Calcium channel blockers	**Erythromycin**	**Pan-inducers[†]**
	Cyclosporine	**Grapefruit Juice**	**Ritonavir**
	Ergots	**Itraconazole**	**St. John's wort**
	Lurasidone	**Ketoconazole**	Topiramate
	Oral contraceptives	**Nefazodone**	
	Methadone	**Ritonavir**	
	Oral contraceptives		
	Protease inhibitors		
	Statins		
	TriazoloBZDs[‡]		
	Zolpidem		

All drugs in **bold** type are potent in their cytochrome P-450 metabolic inhibition or induction.

*A substrate is a drug that must utilize the enzyme for metabolism.

[†]Pan-inducers = Carbamazepine, phenobarbital, phenytoin, rifamycins

[‡]TriazoloBZDs = triazolobenzodiazepines: alprazolam, midazolam, triazolam.

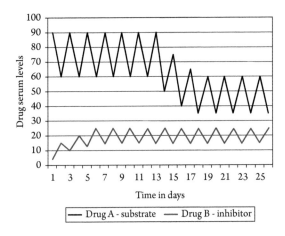

Figure 10.5 Drug–drug interaction—induction. Drug A is in steady state, having been introduced sometime before this graph, with peak levels of 90 and (Court 2009) trough levels of 60. Drug B is started on day 1, and develops steady state after 4 half-lives. After 2 weeks, levels of drug A decrease, as drug B has gradually induced the enzyme(s) involved in metabolizing drug A. Drug A now has a steady state, with peak levels at 60 and trough levels at 35.

is developed with co-administration of EE and carbamazepine and later the carbamazepine is discontinued, the EE levels will gradually rise in one to two weeks (un-induction). This, too, could lead to side effects from higher EE levels (e.g., headaches or a sense of bloating).

Figure 10.5 presents what happens to drug A when a potent inducer of drug A's metabolic enzymes is introduced. Induction of metabolism actually increases the number of sites available for metabolism. This process is not immediate and can take up to two weeks to occur. When more enzymes are available, more drug is metabolized, and the net effect is a lowering of available parent drug, or more rapid metabolism. An inducer may cause the level of a drug dependent on that enzyme to drop below the level needed for clinical effectiveness. In some cases, metabolic induction may increase the production of active and/or toxic metabolites. Table 10.1 presents many of the most common inducers of CYP3A4 and 2D6, as well as some of the medications with narrow therapeutic windows dependent on those enzymes for metabolism.

Genetics A final, but not the least important, reason for drug level variability is due to genetics. The term *pharmacogenetics* (PG) is used to describe the study of these variations. All metabolic enzymes show genetic variability, although the degree of variability of some enzymes can be small and may not be clinically relevant. For example, 3A4 has genetic variability, and some people have 3A5 as well, which seems to have similar activity to 3A4, but the 3A subfamily has no alleles that code for decreased or absent activity. Other enzymes have wide-ranging variability, such as 2D6 or 2C19, with phenotypes that range from the extremes of no activity to ultra-rapid activity when compared to the normal/wild-type. Those with normal/wild-type activity are extensive metabolizers (EMs), those with slow or no function are poor metabolizers (PMs), and those with ultra-rapid activity are called ultra-extensive metabolizers (UEMs). It is important to realize that phenotypic variability can occur due to a variety of allele alterations, including frame shifts, point mutations, splicing defects, and entire missing alleles. For 2D6, there are more than 100 known different variants and subvariants that have been identified (Gaedigk 2013).

Genetic variability can be extremely important for clinicians to understand. For instance, Grasmader et al. (2004) demonstrated that variations in 2D6, and to some extent 2C19, influence the metabolism of secondary tricyclic antidepressants. Similarly, in a study of atomoxetine in adult patients with attention-deficit hyperactivity disorder, the authors report that 2D6 PMs had higher frequencies of dry mouth, erectile dysfunction, hyperhidrosis, insomnia, and urinary retention compared to other metabolizer groups (Fijal et al. 2015). If genotyping is known, it should be used to guide treatment plans either through drug selection or dosing adjustments. Genotyping prior to initiation of pharmacotherapy may result in overall reduction in healthcare-related costs within certain diagnostic categories (e.g., schizophrenia) (Herbild et al. 2013). In cases where genotyping is not known ahead of time, genotyping should be considered when there are severe side effects or ADRs to help guide treatment decisions.

Genetic variability can be measured two ways. A simple method involves giving a "probe" drug to an individual. The probe is a compound that has a known metabolite that is exclusively created by the enzyme activity one wishes to measure. Another way is genetic testing, primarily through microarray chip technology, which can check for multiple alleles from multiple metabolic enzymes (29). This method is widely available, and costs for such testing continue to decline over time. Such testing should be considered for complicated patients with multiple medications, patients with unusual or unexpected responses to medications, or in cases where medication options include drugs with narrow therapeutic windows dependent primarily (or exclusively) on one enzyme for metabolism.

PSYCHOTROPIC MANAGEMENT OF DEPRESSION: POTENTIAL DRUG INTERACTIONS, SIDE EFFECTS, AND ADVERSE REACTIONS

Antidepressants

Effective treatment of psychiatric symptoms is important, since comorbid mood disorders increase the risk of non-adherence to medical care (DiMatteo et al. 2000, Nakimuli-Mpungu et al. 2013, Nel and Kagee 2013), including high-risk populations such as persons with HIV/AIDS or organ transplant, where non-adherence to antiretroviral therapy (ART) medical treatment increases the risk for viral resistance and HIV treatment failure (Gonzalez et al. 2011) or transplanted organ loss. The use of antidepressants for the treatment of mood disorders and/or pain in patients with comorbid illness, and polypharmacy (particularly in geriatric medicine) requires clinicians to select antidepressants based on medication adverse side effect profiles, comorbid symptomatology, and the potential for DDIs, since most are generally equally effective for depression.

Table 10.2, "Antidepressants," contains information about metabolic profiles, common side effects and toxicities, select individual drug clinical issues, and potential drug interactions. Further details, to include important drug-specific differences, clinical issues, supporting research, and detailed referencing, are presented later in this section. Selective serotonin reuptake inhibitors (SSRIs) and SNRIs are presented first both in the table and within the text, as they are used the most in the treatment of depression with comorbid medical illness. The rest of available antidepressants are reviewed by class, not necessarily in order of effectiveness or popularity

Selective Serotonin Reuptake Inhibitors (SSRIs)

The SSRIs have been widely used since the early 1980s because of their simplicity of use (once a day dosing), and reasonable side effect and safety profile, which also resulted in increased primary-care prescribing. Additionally, the combination of tricyclic antidepressants (TCAs; potentially toxic drugs with narrow therapeutic windows, mostly dependent upon 2D6 metabolism) with potent CYP2D6 inhibitors such as the SSRI fluoxetine, ushered in the study of P450-mediated DDIs. Vaughan (1988) was one of the first to describe TCA toxicity in two patients, one receiving nortriptyline and the other receiving desipramine with fluoxetine. Although the unique metabolic profile of the SSRIs has been elucidated over the past 30 years, drug-interaction cases continue to be reported, as seen in a recent report of phenytoin toxicity after fluoxetine initiation (Lance and Ternouth 2015).

Most SSRIs are associated with gastrointestinal symptoms, jitteriness, carbohydrate craving, and sexual dysfunction, although if a patient suffers these side effects on one SSRI, he or she may not on another in this class. Some patients complain of a sense of "apathy" while on an SSRI as well. See Images 1A and 1B for explanations concerning mechanism of action and neurotransmitter–side effect relationships. All SSRIs may cause a "flu-like" withdrawal syndrome, the most significant occurring with paroxetine (Himei and Okamura 2006), and particularly affecting neonates (Pogliani et al. 2010).

SSRIs have been implicated in platelet dysfunction associated with the risk of bleeding, particularly upper GI bleeding in patients taking nonsteroidal anti-inflammatory drugs NSAIDs (Dalton et al. 2003), (Andrade et al. 2010). A recent meta-analysis (Jiang et al. 2015) indicates that the risk of GI bleeding is doubled with SSRI use, especially in patients taking NSAIDS with SSRIs. They suggest this may be mitigated with acid-reducing medications, although there have been no large studies to date, and an earlier meta-analysis concluded that the risk for bleeding was only modestly increased (Anglin et al. 2014). Some SSRIs have been associated with arrhythmias (citalopram and escitalopram), and all may be associated with pathological changes in cardiac tissue (Lusetti et al. 2015).

SSRIs may cause extrapyramidal symptoms (EPS) due to dopamine blockade (Leo 1996, Schillevoort et al. 2002), and they have been known to cause the syndrome of inappropriate antidiuretic hormone secretion (SIADH) (Arinzon et al. 2002). Serotonin syndrome is a potential toxicity with all antidepressants, particularly when combined with other serotonergic medications.

Table 10.2 Antidepressants

Antidepressant	Metabolic Site (s)	Metabolic Enzymes Inhibited	Clinical Considerations	Potential DDIs
SSRIs				
SSRI Common Features	Most metabolized at CYP2D6	No inducers	**Common Side Effects:** Apathy Carbohydrate craving GI upset Jitteriness/tremor Serotonin syndrome Sexual dysfunction Sleep disruption SIADH Withdrawal syndrome	Potent and moderate CYP2D6 inhibitors like duloxetine, quinidine, bupropion, venlafaxine and paroxetine may increase serum levels of SSRIs, increasing side effects
Citalopram (Celexa)	CYP2C19, 2D6, 3A4 Transporter ABCB1	CYP2D6 (minimal) ABCB1	Potential for arrhythmia in doses over 60 mgs (or if inhibited or "boosted" by "pan-inhibitor" like ritonavir)	Lower potential for interactions Keep dosage at/below 40 mgs/day if on CYP2D6 inhibitors
Escitalopram (Lexapro)	CYP2C19, 2D6, 3A4 Transporter ABCB1	CYP2D6 (minimal)	Potential for arrhythmia in doses over 60 mgs (or if inhibited or "boosted" by "pan-inhibitor" PIs like ritonavir)	Lower potential for clinical interactions with other drugs Keep dosage at/below 20 mgs/day if on CYP2D6 inhibitors

(Continued)

Table 10.2 Continued

Antidepressant	Metabolic Site (s)	Metabolic Enzymes Inhibited	Clinical Considerations	Potential DDIs
Fluoxetine (Prozac)	CYP2C9, 2C19, 2D6, 3A4 Transporter ABCB1	**CYP2D6, 2C19,** 2B6, 2C9 3A4, 1A2 ABCB1		Very-long-acting active metabolite Potent CYP2D6 & 2C19 inhibition by fluoxetine may increase serum levels of: *Antiarrhythmics* *Cobicistat* *(in Stribild)* *Metoprolol* *Oxycodone* *Phenobarbitol* *Phenytoin* *SSRIs* *Tamoxifen (prevents metabolism to active drug)* *Tramadol (prevents metabolism to active drug)* *Tricyclic antidepressants* *First-generation antipsychotics*
Fluvoxamine (Luvox)	CYP1A2, 2D6 Transporter ABCB1	**CYP1A2, 2C19,** 2B6, 2C9 3A4b 2D6 ABCB1	Known for many intolerable side effects in PWHA	Potent CYP1A2 and 2C19 inhibition by fluvoxamine may increase serum levels of: *Caffeine* *Olanzapine* *Phenytoin*

Paroxetine (Paxil)	CYP2D6, 3A4	**CYP2D6, 2B6**, 3A4, 2C19, 1A2	Sedating Weight gain Most severe withdrawal syndrome, especially in neonates	Potent CYP2D6 and 2B6 inhibition by paroxetine may increase serum levels of: *Antiarrhythmics* *Bupropion* *Metoprolol* *Oxycodone* *SSRIs* *Tamoxifen (prevents metabolism to active drug)* *Tramadol (prevents metabolism to active drug)* *Tricyclic antidepressants* *Typical antipsychotics* Potent CYP pan-inhibitors[a] may increase serum levels of paroxetine
Sertraline (Zoloft)	CYP2B6, 2C9, 2C19, 2D6, 3A4 UGT2B7, UGT1A1 transporter ABCB1	CYP2D6, 2B6, 2C9, 2C19, 3A4, 1A2, ABCB1		Least potential for clinical interactions Becomes a more potent CYP2D6 inhibitor at doses >200 mgs/day
SNRIs				
Desvenlafaxine (Pristiq)	UGT CYP3A4	CYP2D6	Potential for: HTN, weight gain, sexual dysfunction	CYP2D6 inhibition by desvenlafaxine may increase serum levels of metoprolol and other CYP2D6-dependent meds CYP2D6 inhibition by desvenlafaxine may reduce effectiveness of prodrugs dependent upon CYP2D6 like: *Tramadol* *Tamoxifen*

(Continued)

Table 10.2 Continued

Antidepressant	Metabolic Site (s)	Metabolic Enzymes Inhibited	Clinical Considerations	Potential DDIs
Duloxetine (Cymbalta)	CYP1A2, 2D6	CYP2D6	Potential for: HTN Sexual dysfunction Weight gain	CYP2D6 inhibition by duloxetine may increase serum levels of metoprolol and other CYP2D6-dependent meds CYP2D6 inhibition by duloxetine may reduce effectiveness of prodrugs dependent upon CYP2D6 like: *Tramadol* *Tamoxifen*
Levomilnacipran (Fetmiza)	CYP3A4 (primary), 2C8, 2C19, 2D6	None	Weight neutral Potential for HTN Sexual dysfunction	Potent CYP3A4 inhibitors like PIs may increase serum levels of levomilnacipran Potent CYP3A4 inducers and pan-inducers may reduce serum levels
Milnacipran (Savella)	Renal excretion Unchanged: (50–60%) Conjugation: (20–30%) CYP3A4: (10%)	None	Weight neutral Potential for: HTN Sexual dysfunction	Lower potential for pharmacokinetic CYP450 interactions
Venlafaxine (Effexor)	CYP2D6, 2C19, 3A4	CYP2D6 CYP3A4	Potential for: HTN Sexual dysfunction, Weight gain	Potent CYP pan- inhibitors like ritonavir may increase serum levels of venlafaxine CYP2D6 inhibition by venlafaxine may increase serum levels of metoprolol and other CYP2D6-dependent meds CYP2D6 inhibition by venlafaxine may reduce effectiveness of pro-drugs dependent upon CYP2D6 like: *Tramadol* *Tamoxifen*

MAOIs

Drug	Metabolism	Inhibits	Side effects/notes	Interactions
Isocarboxazid (Marplan) Phenelzine (Nardil) Tranylcypromine (Parnate)			Most common side effect is HYPOtension Tyramine reaction (HTN, serotonin syndrome) when taken with tyramine-containing foods/beverages	All are MAO A and MAO B inhibitors Contraindicated with ALL serotonergic drugs
Selegiline (Emsam)				Selective MAO B inhibitor

"Novel" or atypical

Drug	Metabolism	Inhibits	Side effects/notes	Interactions
Bupropion (Wellbutrin/ Zyban)	CYP2B6 (primary) CYP2D6, 1A2, 2A6, 2C9, 2E1, 3A4 glucuronidation	CYP2D6	May reduce seizure threshold, especially at higher doses Contraindicated if hx of seizures, head injury	Modest CYP2D6 inhibition by bupropion may increase serum levels of metoprolol and other CYP2D6-dependent meds CYP2D6 inhibition by bupropion may reduce effectiveness of pro-drugs dependent upon CYP2D6 like: *Tramadol* *Tamoxifen*
Mirtazapine (Remeron)	CYP1A2, 2D6, 3A4 glucuronidation	None known	Weight gain Anti-nausea Sedating May be protective with JC virus	Least potential for clinical interactions with ART
Nefazodone (Serzone)	CYP3A4, 2D6	**CYP3A4**	Brand Serzone not available in the US	Potent CYP3A4 Inhibitors like nefazodone may increase serum levels of CYP3A4-dependent meds such as: *Cyclosporine* *Protease inhibitors* *Rilpivarine* *Miraviroc*

(Continued)

Table 10.2 Continued

Antidepressant	Metabolic Site (s)	Metabolic Enzymes Inhibited	Clinical Considerations	Potential DDIs
Reboxetine	CYP3A4	CYP2D6, 3A4 Transporters	Not available in the United States	Potent CYP3A4 inhibitors like PIs, clarithromycin, and GFJ may increase serum levels of reboxetine; Potent CYP3A4 inducers may decrease serum levels of reboxetine
Trazodone (Deseryl)	CYP3A4	None known	Sedating, often used as sleep aid	Potent CYP3A4 inhibitors like PIs, clarithromycin, and GFJ may increase serum levels; Potent CYP3A4 inducers may reduce serum levels of trazodone
Vilazodone (Viibryd)	CYP3A4	Mild INDUCTION of CYP2C19	Must take with food for full absorption	Potent CYP3A4 inhibitors like PIs, clarithromycin, and GFJ may increase serum levels; Potent CYP3A4 inducers may reduce serum levels of vilazodone
Vortioxetine (Brintellix)	CYP2D6, 2B6, 3A4, 2C9, 2C19, 2A6, 2C8	None known		Potent CYP pan-inhibitors like fluoxetine and ritonavir may increase serum levels of vortioxetine
Tricyclics				
TCA Common Features	All use CYP2D6, many use 3A4	Most are only mild inhibitors of CYPs	Multiple side effects: Constipation; Drowsiness; Dry mouth; Orthostatic hypotension; Weight gain; Toxicities: Arrhythmia; Potential for anticholinergic delirium	All potent CYP inhibitors of 2D6, as well as pan-inhibitors like ritonavir, may increase TCA serum levels to toxicity; CYP pan-inducers[a] may reduce TCA serum levels; Use therapeutic drug monitoring (TDM)

Drug	Metabolism	Inhibits/Induces	Clinical features	Reference
Amitriptyline (Elavil)	CYP1A2, 2C19, 2D6, 3A4 UGT1A4	CYP1A2, 2C19, 2D6	Active metabolite = nortriptyline Greater weight gain, drowsiness, risk for delirium	See "Common Features," Table 10.3
Clomipramine (Anafranil)	CYP1A2, 2C19, 2D6, 3A4	CYP1A2, 2C19, 2D6, 3A4	Has indication for OCD	See "Common Features"
Desipramine (Norpramin)	CYP2D6	CYP2D6, 2C19	Less risk for weight gain, drowsiness, risk for delirium	See "Common Features"
Doxepin (Adapin, Sinequan)	CYP1A2, 2D6, 2C19, 3A4 UGT1A3, UGT1A4	CYP1A2, 2C19, 2D6	Greater weight gain, drowsiness, risk for delirium	See "Common Features"
Imipramine (Tofranil)	CYP1A2, 2C19, 2D, 3A4 UGT1A3, UGT1A4	CYP2C19, 2D6	Active metabolite = desipramine Greater weight gain, drowsiness, risk for delirium	See "Common Features"
Nortriptyline (Pamelor)	CYP2D6	CYP2D6, 2C19	Therapeutic window = 50–150 ng/dl Less risk for weight gain, drowsiness, risk for delirium	See "Common Features"
Protriptyline (Vivactil)	CYP2D6	unknown		See "Common Features"
Trimipramine (Surmontil)	CYP2C19, 2D6, 3A4	unknown		See "Common Features"

Note: Primary route of metabolism listed first.

Bold CYP indicates **potent** inhibitor or inducer of that cytochrome P450 enzyme.

CYP = cytochrome, DDIs = drug–drug interactions, UGT = uridine 5′-diphosphate glucuronosyltransferase, ABCB = ATP binding cassette B transporter (p-glycoprotein transporter), PWHA = Persons with HIV and AIDS, JC = Jacob-Creutzfeld, HTN = hypertension, GF = grapefruit juice, OCD = Obsessive-Compulsive Disorder, CSF = cerebrospinal fluid

[a]Pan-inducers: drugs that induce many if not all CYPP450 enzymes, and include barbiturates, carbamazepine, ethanol, phenytoin, and rifamycins

Citalopram and escitalopram

Citalopram and escitalopram are generally well tolerated, although citalopram is more sedating than its enantiomer and should be taken at night, which is useful for patients with initial and middle insomnia. Like all SSRIs, GI side effects, jitteriness, and sexual dysfunction may need attention or may lead to discontinuation without prompt attention and support.

Citalopram and escitalopram carry a US Food and Drug Administration (FDA 2012) warning about potential cardiac toxicity at higher doses unrelated to drug interactions. They suggest minimizing risk by maintaining doses below 40 mg/day in general, and below 20 mg/day for geriatric patients, those on polypharmacy, or those with hepatic disease that may affect metabolism, and that citalopram and escitalopram be discontinued or not prescribed at all in those with a QTc >500 msec. Maljuric et al. (2015) found a modest QT prolongation with citalopram use and not with other SSRIs in a large population study. Although no SSRI class effect was observed, use of citalopram was associated with a longer QTc F (corrected with Fridericia), while SSRIs were not associated with clinically relevant QTc F prolongation. Closely monitoring for arrhythmia after citalopram/escitalopram overdose is appropriate (Waring et al. 2010). Citalopram's manufacturer suggests that potent inhibitors of CYP3A4 and potent inhibitors of CYP2C19 such as omeprazole may inhibit the metabolism of citalopram, and raise serum levels (despite no clinically significant elevation when ketoconazole was co-administered with citalopram). Due to the risk of arrhythmia, the manufacturer recommends 20 mg/day as the maximum recommended dose of citalopram when administered with drugs combinations that inhibit both CYP3A4 and 2C19 (Celexa 2014).

Escitalopram oxalate is the S-enantiomer of citalopram; it is considered 30 times more potent than citalopram at the human serotonin transporter, and it has the same metabolic CYP450 profile as citalopram (Sanchez et al. 2004, Rao 2007). Citalopram and escitalopram are very weak inhibitors of CYP2D6 (unlike fluoxetine, paroxetine, and high-dose sertraline, which are potent inhibitors of CYP2D6. Both drugs have a broad metabolic profile and are therefore less likely to participate in DDIs (von Moltke et al. 2001). In vivo studies of citalopram have found no clinically significant CYP450 interactions with trazodone, alprazolam, carbamazepine, clozapine, theophylline, warfarin, imipramine, mephenytoin, tricyclics, cyclosporine, digoxin, risperidone, or clozapine (Brosen and Naranjo 2001, Larsen et al. 2001, Liston et al. 2001, Moller et al. 2001, Hall et al. 2003, Spina et al. 2003, Prapotnik et al. 2004). Citalopram's package insert (PI) indicates that 22 days of administration of 40 mg of citalopram increased the plasma levels of metoprolol twofold, but there were no significant effects on blood pressure or heart rate. The manufacturer also reported that that citalopram increased desipramine levels 52% (Celexa 2014). Despite recent population studies that have found no bradycardia associated with metoprolol use with CYP2D6 inhibiting antidepressants in hospitalized bradycardia patients (Kurdyak et al. 2012), it seems prudent to use caution (to include serum drug monitoring when appropriate) if citalopram and escitalopram are co-administered with CYP2D6-dependent medications with narrow therapeutic windows like metoprolol, TCAs, and some calcium channel blockers.

Fluoxetine

Fluoxetine is commonly activating, and may be useful in patients with fatigue or hyper-somnolence. Like all SSRIs, insomnia, GI side effects, and sexual dysfunction may need attention or may lead to discontinuation without prompt attention. Fluoxetine's active metabolite, norfluoxetine, has a 7–15-day half-life, which may be useful in patients who have difficulty remembering to take their medication on a daily basis, despite its potential to cause drug interactions via inhibition of multiple metabolic cytochromes.

Fluoxetine has a diverse metabolism including CYPs 2C9, 2C19, 2D6, and 3A4 (Ring et al. 2001, Mandrioli et al. 2006). Fluoxetine and its active metabolite norfluoxetine are potent inhibitors of CYP2D6 and 2C19, and mild or moderate inhibitors of many others (Hesse et al. 2000, Liston et al. 2002, Bertelsen et al. 2003, Ohno et al. 2007). Additionally, fluoxetine is both a substrate and an inhibitor of ABCB1 transport (Khairul et al. 2006). Fluoxetine is considered a pan-inhibitor and has significant number of DDIs concerning for use in medically ill and polypharmacy populations, complicated by its extended half-life. Metabolic inhibition by fluoxetine and its metabolite may last for weeks as compared to the other SSRIs (Spina et al. 2003). Serotonin syndrome and Parkinsonism have been reported in patients who were stable on fluoxetine until potent pan-inhibitors (like PIs and cimetidine) were co-administered (DeSilva et al. 2001, Hori et al. 2003). Tricyclic antidepressants were among the first drugs described in the literature whose serum levels were increased by fluoxetine (Cavanaugh 1990), leading to worsened depressive symp-toms, confusion, and other signs of toxicity (Bell and Cole 1988). Fluoxetine also inhib-its the metabolism of trazodone (metabolized by CYP3A4) and its CYP2D6-dependent major metabolite metachlorophenylpiperazine (MCPP) (Maes et al. 1997), increasing the risk of toxicity from this compound. Co-administration of fluoxetine and CYP2D6 substrates with narrow therapeutic windows (like TCAs, antipsychotics, some calcium channel blockers, venlafaxine, methadone, metoprolol, lidocaine, and donepezil) may lead to toxicity of these agents (Preskorn et al.1994, Belpaire et al. 1998, Spina et al. 2002). Potent inhibitors of CYP2D6 like fluoxetine prevent inactive pro-drugs from becoming effective metabolites. Fluoxetine and other CYP2D6 inhibitors are contraindicated with tamoxifen for this reason (Binkhorst et al. 2013).

Fluvoxamine

Fluvoxamine is extensively metabolized by CYPs 1A2 and 2D6, is a potent inhibitor of CYPs 1A2 and 2C19, and is a moderate inhibitor of many others. Fluvoxamine is con-sidered a pan-inhibitor and has significant number of DDIs with many drugs that have narrow margins of safety. In particular, CYP1A2-dependent theophylline, olanzapine, clozapine, lansoprazole, omeprazole, lidocaine, tizanidine, and CYP2C9-dependent war-farin and CYP2C9/and 2C19-dependent phenytoin, and the CYP2D6-dependent ter-tiary tricyclic antidepressants (Granfors et al. 2004, Carrillo and Benitez, 2000).

A careful caffeine history should be obtained prior to initiation of fluvoxamine or in any patient complaining nausea and jitteriness or insomnia once taking fluvoxamine. Fluvoxamine can increase the plasma concentration-versus-time curve of caffeine from 0–24 hours fivefold (Christensen et al. 2002). Caffeine is exclusively metabolized at

CYP1A2, and patients should be warned that they may develop caffeine side effects when fluvoxamine is co-administered (Carrillo and Benitez 2000).

Paroxetine

Patoxetine is associated with the most severe withdrawal syndrome, as well as with pulmonary hypertension in neonatal SSRI withdrawal syndrome (Himei and Okamura 2006, Pogliani et al. 2010). It is a sedating SSRI and generally is administered at night. Paroxetine is primarily metabolized by CYPs 2D6 and 3A4, and is a very potent inhibitor of CYP2D6 and a moderate inhibitor of others (Hemeryck et al. 2001). Its potent inhibition of CYP2D6 has been implicated in causing toxicity of benztropine, clozapine, and TCAs in multiple case reports (Taylor 1995, Armstrong and Schweitzer 1997, Joos et al. 1997). Controlled clinical studies have found that paroxetine significantly increases plasma concentrations of perphenazine, clozapine and norclozapine, risperidone, methadone, tamoxifen, and secondary tricyclics such as nortriptyline and desipramine (Centorrino et al. 1996, Ozdemir et al. 1997, Leucht et al. 2000, Spina et al. 2001, Begre et al. 2002). In a randomized study of paroxetine and sertraline co-administered with desipramine, Alderman et al. (1997) found that paroxetine increased the plasma Cmax of desipramine 358% in healthy volunteers, as well as increasing the paroxetine levels tenfold. Tramadol co-administration with paroxetine has been reported to cause serotonin syndrome, a pharmacodynamic interaction that is enhanced by the pharmacokinetic inhibition of tramadol's metabolism at 2D6 (Egberts et al. 1997, Lantz et al. 1998). Paroxetine co-administration should be avoided with drugs with narrow therapeutic windows that are dependent on CYP2D6, such as metoprolol, calcium channel blockers, and TCAs.

Sertraline

Sertraline has a somewhat better side effect profile than many other antidepressants, and it is very safe in overdose (Hansen et al. 2005). Sertraline has a diverse metabolism, including CYPs 2B6, 2C9, 2C19, 2D6, and 3A4, and is a potent inhibitor of CYPs 1A2 and 2C19, and a moderate inhibitor of many others. Since sertraline is metabolized at several different CYP450 enzymes, it is only subject to inhibition or induction by pan-inhibitors and pan-inducers such as carbamazepine and phenytoin (Pihlsgard and Eliasson 2002). The manufacturer's package insert indicates that co-administration of low-dose pimozide (2 mg) with 200 mg of sertraline increased the serum levels of pimozide 40%, without alterations in electrocardiogram (Roerig 2016). It is important to note that standard doses of pimozide combined with sertraline were not tested, and pimozide (see following) is contraindicated with any CYP3A4 or 1A2 inhibitor. In comparison to other SSRIs, sertraline has the least inhibitory potential at CYP2D6, leading to very modest CYP2D6 interactions, and generally only at higher doses. Sertraline does not seem to have the independent potential for cardiac arrhythmias in higher doses as is seen with citalopram and escitalopram, but at doses >200 mg/d, it acts as a potent inhibitor of CYP2D6, and then carries the same warnings as paroxetine and fluoxetine when co-administered with CYP2D6-dependent medications with narrow therapeutic windows like metoprolol, TCAs, calcium channel blockers. It is prudent to monitor serum levels and side effects of any drug (e.g., TCAs, warfarin) with a narrow therapeutic index when co-administered with sertraline. There has been a small case series indicating that even at low doses (e.g., 25 mg), sertraline's inhibition of UGTs may increase lamotrigine levels (Kaufman and Gerner 1998).

Serotonin-Norepinephrine Reuptake Inhibitors (SNRIS)

SNRIs affect the reuptake of both serotonin and norepinephrine at the target receptor sites, which is the same mechanism of action as TCAs. SNRIs are associated with fewer anticholinergic, antihistaminic, and antimuscarinic symptoms than the TCAs, and are not nearly as toxic in overdose or arrhythmogenicity. SNRIs are associated with GI symptoms, jitteriness, carbohydrate craving, and sexual dysfunction. All SNRIs, like SSRIs, may cause a "flu-like" withdrawal syndrome (Perahia et al. 2005). They are marketed for urinary incontinence and for the treatment of neuropathic pain and diabetic neuropathy in addition to depression.

SNRIs have been implicated in platelet dysfunction associated with the risk of bleeding, and may cause a rise of blood pressure or hypertension. Ghassemi et al. (2014), in a retrospective data-mining study of more than 14, 000 intensive care unit (ICU) admissions, found an association with prolonged hospital stay for patients taking SSRIs and SNRIs prior to admission, and an association with greater mortality associated with greater serotonin reuptake inhibition.

Desvenlafaxine

Desvenlafaxine is mostly metabolized via glucuronidation (uridine diphosphate-glucuronosyltransferase enzymes [UGTs]) and CYP3A4. Desvenlafaxine is a mild inhibitor of CYP2D6 and 3A (von Moltke et al. 1997), and has low potential to increase serum levels of medications dependent on CYP2D6 and 3A4 for metabolism (Spina et al. 2012). See Venlafaxine for side effects/toxicity and specific clinical issues.

Duloxetine

Duloxetine is a potent inhibitor of serotonin and norepinephrine reuptake, with weak inhibition of dopamine (Lantz et al. 2003). It is effective in treating depression in adults. In addition, it has been found to be effective in the treatment of urinary incontinence in women with and without depression, as well as fibromyalgia and diabetic neuropathic pain (Arnold et al. 2004, Cardozo et al. 2004, Brannan et al. 2005). In a recent review (Perahia et al. 2013) of safety data from all placebo-controlled trials of duloxetine and post-marketing reports concerning duloxetine, duloxetine "bleeding-related treatment-emergent adverse events" did not seem associated with increasing duloxetine doses, and was independent of NSAID use.

Duloxetine is metabolized at CYPs 1A2 and 2D6 (Caccia 2004, Lobo et al. 2008), and is a moderate to potent inhibitor of CYP2D6 (Skinner et al. 2003). Co-administration of CYP1A2 inhibitors including fluvoxamine can result in significantly increased serum levels of duloxetine. Similarly, CYP2D6 inhibitors (e.g., ritonavir, paroxetine, fluoxetine, and bupropion) can result in elevated plasma levels of duloxetine (Cymbalta 2016), which is likely to result in elevated incidence or severity of adverse drug reactions. Although duloxetine is metabolized in part by CYP1A2, there are no studies to date to indicate a difference in metabolism between smokers and nonsmokers, or EMs and PMs, at this enzyme. Duloxetine has been shown to increase levels of desipramine, a CYP2D6 substrate (Skinner et al. 2003). There is a possibility that duloxetine could affect the serum levels of other CYP2D6-dependent drugs such as metoprolol, venlafaxine, calcium channel blockers, risperidone, and the TCAs. Since duloxetine may be used extensively in patients with chronic pain, co-administration with tramadol may occur. Although there are no published reports to date, tramadol is a pro-drug that requires activation at CYP2D6 to be effective (Tirkkonen and Laine 2004). Duloxetine may diminish the biotransformation of tramadol to its active metabolite by inhibiting CYP2D6, leading to a less therapeutic effect of tramadol. Duloxetine is metabolized at CYP1A2 and 2D6. Potent 2D6 inhibitors, such as ritonavir, diphenhydramine, and bupropion, have the potential to increase serum levels of duloxetine, although no reports of such interactions have been found to date.

Levomilnacipran

Side effects of levomilnacipran are similar to all SNRIs. Levomilnacipran and milnacipran are mostly cleared by the kidneys, and are minimally metabolized by CYP3A4, little influenced by cytochrome genetic polymorphisms, inhibitors, and inducers (Paris et al. 2009, Spina et al. 2012).

Venlafaxine

Side effects of venlafaxine are similar to desvenlafaxine. Venlafaxine is primarily metabolized to its active metabolite, O-desmethylvenlafaxine, at CYP2D6, and to its less active metabolite at CYP3A4 (Otton et al. 1996, McAlpine et al. 2007). Venlafaxine also appears to be a substrate of ABCB1 transport (Gareri et al. 2008). Venlafaxine is a mild inhibitor of CYPs 2D6 and 3A4 (von Moltke et al. 1997). Inhibitors of CYP2D6 such as quinidine, paroxetine, diphenhydramine, ketoconazole, fluvoxamine, fluoxetine, and bupropion have been shown to increase serum venlafaxine concentrations (Lessard et al. 2001, Kennedy et al. 2002, Lindh et al. 2003, Fogelman et al. 1999). Co-administration with the pan-inhibitor cimetidine increased venlafaxine levels by 13%, which may not be clinically relevant unless the patient has altered hepatic function (Troy et al. 1998). As a mild 2D6 inhibitor, venlafaxine has been shown to increase concentrations of imipramine (Ball et al. 1997), desipramine, haloperidol, and risperidone (Spina et al. 2003). Venlafaxine has reduced the concentration of indinavir, a protease inhibitor (PI) metabolized by CYP3A4, but this reduction is probably due to induction of P-glycoproteins, not pharmacokinetic interaction (Levin et al. 2001).

Novel/Atypical Antidepressants

Bupropion

Bupropion inhibits the reuptake of norepinephrine and dopamine, and is sometimes classified as a norepinephrine-dopamine disinhibitor (NDDI), with little or no effect on serotonin, histamine, muscarinic, acetylcholine or epinephrine receptors, which provides for a rather benign side-effect profile. It has been used for smoking cessation and weight loss as well as for depression. Bupropion's modulation of dopamine pathways seems to result in improved alertness and focus, and has a less negative effect on sexual functioning (Stah et al. 2004).

Bupropion is primarily metabolized at the minor CYP450 enzyme CYP2B6 and is a potent inhibitor of CYP2D6 (Hesse et al. 2000). Since bupropion can lower the seizure threshold at high doses, there is a potential for bupropion to become toxic when co-administered with CYP2B6 inhibitors, such as ritonavir, efavirenz, paroxetine, cyclophosphamide, thiotepa, clopidogrel, and ticlopidine (Hesse et al. 2000, 2001, von Moltke et al. 2001, Richter et al. 2004). A case series by Park-Wyllie & Antoniou examining concomitant use of these agents for as long as two years found no recorded episodes of seizures (Park-Wyllie and Antoniou 2003). Although encouraging, no pharmacokinetic data were available, and none of the patients were on high-dose ritonavir. Bupropion serum concentrations may be reduced by CYP2B6 metabolic induction, as evidenced by both low and high daily doses of ritonavir, and routine doses of efavirenz in healthy volunteers (Robertson et al. 2008, Park et al. 2010). Bupropion dosage may need to be increased (up to the recommended maximum dose) with mixed inhibitor/inducers such as ritonavir. Bupropion co-administration with metoprolol, CYP26 substrate, has been noted to cause sinus bradycardia (McCollum et al. 2004). Guzey et al. (2002) studied bupropion clinically by co-administering it with dextromethorphan, a specific metabolic marker for CYP2D6. Bupropion changed a genotypic extensive metabolizer, (the term used for a normal metabolizer) a phenotypic PM (poor metabolizer) at CYP2D6, but this was a single case report. Bupropion may have also inhibited the metabolism of sertraline and venlafaxine in a patient taking all three antidepressants, leading to serotonin syndrome (bupropion is rarely associated with serotonin syndrome, and when it is implicated, it is generally in co-administration with a CYP2D6-dependent serotonergic antidepressant; Munhoz 2004). Kennedy et al. (2002) combined bupropion with venlafaxine, paroxetine, or fluoxetine in patients with sexual dysfunction on monotherapy. They found that bupropion significantly elevated venlafaxine serum levels. Bupropion's package insert indicates that in a study of 15 CYP2D6 EMs, bupropion increased the peak concentration (C_{max}), area under the concentration curve (AUC), and half-life of desipramine, an effect that was noted for up to seven days. The manufacturer suggests that any drug dependent on CYP2D6 should be dosed at lower dosages and titrated cautiously when co-administered with bupropion. . In addition, they warn that adding bupropion to a regimen already containing a CYP2D6-dependent medication with a narrow therapeutic window may require decreasing the dosage of the CYP2D6-dependent drug to prevent toxicity.

Mirtazapine

Mirtazapine administration results in increased norepinephrine and serotonin activity by antagonizing alpha2-receptors and postsynaptic 5-HT receptors (Timmer et al. 2000). Mirtazapine is very sedating, especially at lower doses.

Mirtazapine is metabolized at multiple CYP450 enzymes, including CYP1A2, 2D6, and 3A4, with glucuronidation into three metabolites one of which, N-desmethylmirtazapine, is active (Störmer et al. 2000, Timmer et al. 2000). Mirtazapine and its active metabolite do not affect the CYP450 system. Mirtazapine's diverse metabolism profile makes it less prone to pharmacokinetic drug interactions, unless co-administered with pan-inhibitors (like PIs, fluconazole, fluvoxamine) or pan-inducers (like carbamazepine). Anttila et al. (2001) report two cases in which co-administration of mirtazapine with fluvoxamine resulted in a threefold and fourfold increase in mirtazapine levels and worsened anxiety, probably due to fluvoxamine's inhibition of all of the cytochromes needed for mirtazapine's metabolism. Cimetidine, a modest CYP450 inhibitor, increases mirtazapine's serum concentration by only 22% (Sitsen et al. 2000). Conversely, the CYP450 "pan-inducer" carbamazepine decreases mirtazapine's serum concentration significantly (Sitsen et al. 2001).

Nefazodone

Nefazodone potently acts as serotonin antagonist and inhibits serotonin and norepinephrine reuptake (Greene and Barbhaiya 1997). Nefazodone has significant risk of hepatotoxicity (Stewart 2002) and was voluntarily removed from the U.S. market in 2004 and eventually the worldwide market by its initial manufacturer due to concerns for hepatotoxicity and DDI profile. Generic preparations are still found in the United States, abroad, and online.

Nefazodone is metabolized into three active metabolites at CYP3A4 and is a potent inhibitor of CYP3A4 (von Moltke et al. 1999, Kalgutkar et al. 2005). Nefazodone's two most active metabolites are CYP3A4-dependent, and the weaker but anxiogenic metabolite, m-chlorophenylpiperazine (m-CPP) is metabolized at CYP2D6 (von Moltke et al. 1999). The concentration of m-CPP may be increased in genetically poor metabolizers (PMs) at CYP2D6 and by potent inhibitors of CYP2D6 like fluoxetine and paroxetine. Nefazodone was found to significantly increase the serum levels of midazolam, alprazolam, carbamazepine, and methylprednisolone in clinical studies (Laroudie et al. 2000, Kotlyar et al. 2003, Lam et al. 2003, DeVane et al. 2004). Nefazodone has been reported to cause rhabdomyolysis when co-administered with lipid-lowering agents like simvastatin (Skrabal et al. 2003). It has also been associated with a tenfold elevation in cyclosporine levels in a cardiac transplant patient, and tacrolimus toxicity in a renal transplant patient (Olyaei et al. 1998, Wright et al. 1999). Nefazodone has been reported to affect clozapine, haloperidol, and zopiclone (Greene and Barbhaiya 1997, Alderman et al. 2001, Khan and Preskorn 2001). Nefazodone co-administration with CYP3A4 substrates requires careful monitoring, especially for drugs with a narrow therapeutic window. Nefazodone is contraindicated with pimozide (Serzone 2005). The discontinuation of a potent CYP3A4 inhibitor like nefazodone can lead to the loss of clinical effectiveness of a co-administered drug whose serum levels were elevated while taking nefazodone. Ninan (2001) presents a case of alprazolam withdrawal when a patient discontinued nefazodone, indicating that alprazolam plasma levels decrease rapidly in the absence of potent CYP3A4 inhibition.

Reboxetine

Reboxetine is an SNRI, yet it has some mild serotonin reuptake inhibition as well. It is currently unavailable in the United States; the data from Europe suggest efficacy in patients without medical comorbidity. It is similar to atomoxatine in norepinephrine receptor and G protein-gated inwardly rectifying potassium (GIRK) channel activity (Kobayashi et al., 2010). Reboxetine is metabolized at CYP3A4, is a weak inhibitor of CYP2D6 and 3A4, and is a moderate inhibitor of transporters/P-glycoprotein (Wienkers et al. 1999, Kobayashi et al. 2010).

Trazodone

Trazodone is a postsynaptic 5-HT2 antagonist and presynaptic 5-HT reuptake inhibitor serotonin antagonist as well as a reuptake inhibitor (Vande Griend and Anderson 2012). Trazodone is primarily metabolized at CYP3A4 to active metabolite m-chlorophenylpiperazine (m-CPP), which is further metabolized at CYP2D6 (Rotzinger et al. 1999). Trazodone and its active metabolite do not affect the CYP450 system. Trazodone is vulnerable to 3A4 and 2D6 inhibition. Co-administration of trazodone with CYP3A4 or CYP2D6 inhibitors have led to elevated serum trazodone levels. PIs and ketoconazole have inhibited trazodone metabolism in vitro, and ritonavir has reduced the clearance of trazodone and worsened side effects and performance in vivo (Zalma et al. 2000, Greenblatt et al. 2003). In a single-dose, blinded, four-way crossover study of healthy volunteers, it was found that ritonavir significantly increased trazodone plasma concentration, which in turn increased sedation and fatigue and impaired performance on the digit-symbol substitution test (Greenblatt et al. 2003). Inhibition of CYP2D6 may lead to preferential accumulation of trazodone's metabolite, m-CPP, which has been linked to neurotoxic and hepatotoxic reactions. Fluoxetine and haloperidol, CYP2D6 inhibitors, have increased serum levels of the anxiogenic m-CPP (Maes et al. 1997, Mihara et al. 1997). Carbamazepine, a known CYP3A4 inducer, can significantly decrease serum concentrations of trazodone when co-administered (Otani et al. 1996). Though of unknown clinical significance, subtherapeutic levels may lead to a return of symptoms (e.g., depression or insomnia) and unnecessary termination of trazodone.

Vilazodone

Vilazodone's mechanism of action is not fully understood, but it affects serotonin reuptake. Its side-effect profile is similar to the SSRIs', and it is considered weight neutral. It must be taken with food to achieve maximum absorption and optimal therapeutic serum levels. Vilazodone is dependent upon CYP3A4 for its metabolism, and dosage reduction to 20 mgs (one-half of usual dosage) is recommended when taken with strong CYP3A4 inhibitors like ketoconazole or PIs, efavirenz and delavirdine (Boinpally et al. 2014). When co-administered with potent CYP3A4 inducers such as St. John's wort or pan-inhibitors, doses up to 80 mgs/day may be necessary. Careful monitoring of effectiveness is warranted when vilazodone is used with mixed inhibitors/inducers such as ritonavir.

Vortioxetine

Vortioxetine is considered a multimodal antidepressant that acts as a serotonin (5¬HT) transporter inhibitor, a 5¬HT3A and 5¬HT7 receptor antagonist, and a 5¬HT1A and

5¬HT1B receptor partial agonist. It may enhance cognition (Boinpally et al. 2014, Orsolini et al. 2016), as well as depression, and is currently the only drug with proven efficacy in elderly patients. Its side effects include nausea, GI distress and vomiting, headache, dizziness, sedation, as well as dry mouth. Vortioxetine is primarily metabolized by CYP2D6, but also utilizes CYP3A4, 2B6, 2C9, 2C19, 2A6, and 2C8, and it is not an inhibitor or inducer of any cytochromes or transporters.

Ketamine

Ketamine is an NMDA antagonist. Ketamine has a direct antagonistic effect on NMDA receptors, resulting in a rapid release of dopamine associated with elevated mood and improved functioning in depressed patients, most likely affecting the glutamate system (see Image 2). Its use may be limited by the potential for psychotomimetic (like psychosis) and dissociative side-effects/adverse effects; it is rather short-acting, and ketamine must be administered intravenously (Harrison et al. 2016). See Image 2, "Glutamate Hypothesis," for overview.

There is a case report of shortened/reduced response to ketamine for depression, which was reversed after the removal of lorazepam. These authors cite animal studies where ketamine-induced release of dopamine was affected by diazepam, and suggest that lorazepam may mute or block release of dopamine in humans (McIntyre et al. 2016). Inhibition of UGT2B7 glucuronidation by ketamine (or other UGT2B7 inhibitors) may result in clinically significant interactions, even at anesthetic-level doses of ketamine with UGT2B7-dependent opiates, resulting in toxicity. Ketamine's use in pain, depression, and in general psychiatry is still under intense study. Although promising, the need for frequent re-administration in most patients, as well as the potential for abuse, requires further study before it becomes a treatment standard.

Tricyclic Antidepressants (TCAs)

The TCAs are toxic in overdose, leading to cardiac arrhythmia. The tertiary amines are "dirtier" or affect more receptors, to include histaminic, cholinergic, and muscarinic, which often leads to dry mouth, constipation, weight gain, sedation, and cognition difficulties far more than occurs with the secondary amines. The routes of metabolism and potential for DDIs are presented in Table 10.2, "Antidepressants." All TCAs are metabolized to some degree by CYP2D6. The tertiary TCAs are metabolized by CYP2C19, 3A4, and 1A2 to secondary amines. Imipramine, clomipramine, and amitriptyline are metabolized to the secondary TCAs desipramine, N-desmethyl-clomipramine, and nortriptyline, respectively. All secondary TCAs are metabolized by CYP2D6 (Newport et al. 2015). Clinicians should be aware that TCAs are CYP450 inhibitors with significant number of potential DDIs reports in literature (Ford et al. 2015). For example, imipramine and nortriptyline can increase concentrations of olanzapine, chlorpromazine, and other phenothiazines (Brosen 2004, Uchaipichat et al. 2011). TCAs have significant DDIs due to their narrow therapeutic windows and potential cardiotoxicity. TCAs are vulnerable to CYP450 inhibition and induction. All TCAs are susceptible to inhibition by potent CYP2D6 inhibitors like paroxetine, fluoxetine, or quinidine, and TCAs will be less efficiently metabolized by CYP2D6 genetic PMs. Significant increases in TCA concentrations can occur when potent CYP2D6 inhibitors are co-administered (Gillman 2007). Baird (2003) reported a case of loss of antidepressant efficacy after oxcarbazepine (CYP3A4 inducer) was co-administered with clomipramine. Serum levels of clomipramine dropped from a total TCA level of 109 ng/mL (49 ng/mL parent plus 60 ng/mL norclomipramine metabolite) to 98 ng/mL total TCA, with a parent:metabolite ratio of 0:98 ng/mL. The patient suffered from worsened depressive symptoms (Loga et al. 1981).

Monoamine Oxidase Inhibitors (MAOIs)

The MAOIs currently in psychiatric use in the United States as antidepressants include tranylcypromine, phenelzine, and isocarboxazid, and they are nonselective, irreversible inhibitors of monoamine oxidase (MAO), a phase 1 non-CYP450 metabolic enzyme system. Selegiline, a selective inhibitor of type B MAO, is an anti-Parkinson's drug as well as an antidepressant available in transdermal formulation. Moclobemide is a reversible type A MAO inhibitor for the treatment of depression and is not so diet-dependent and responsive. The most common side effect of MAOIs is orthostatic hypotension and dizziness, but the most life-threatening complications are those associated with food–drug interactions and DDIs. Tyramine-containing foods need to be avoided with the non-selective MAOIs, and serotonergic medications must not be co-administered with these drugs.

The nonselective, irreversible MAOIs require a two-week washout period before other serotonergic medications can be safely introduced (Rasheed et al. 1994). In reverse, four to five half-lives of serotonergic drugs need to pass before the introduction of the nonselective MAOIs, so that in the case of fluoxetine, a washout of up to five weeks may be necessary. Drugs with serotonergic effects include all antidepressants, antipsychotics, mood stabilizers, and some narcotics like meperidine. Linezolid, an oxazolidinone antibiotic is a relatively weak, nonselective reversible MAOI (Quinn and Stern 2009). Although there were no reports of serotonin syndrome when linezolid was co-administered with serotonergic compounds during phase I, II, and III trials, there have been warnings and reports since that time (Baird 2003, Fiedorowicz and Swartz 2004, Stevens et al. 2004).

Antipsychotics (Neuroleptics) for Depression

The use of antipsychotic (neuroleptic) medications for treatment of mood disorders in patients with comorbid illness or in the elderly, and especially the use of polypharmacy in these populations requires clinicians to select antipsychotics based on medication-adverse side effect profiles, comorbid symptomatology, and the potential for DDIs. Table 10.3 summarizes features common to all typical/first-generation antipsychotics and atypical/second-generation antipsychotics, including side effects, toxicities, and "black box warnings" (BBWs), followed by specifics for all of those available in the United States.

Metabolic syndrome includes diabetes, weight gain, and dyslipidemia and is a common side effect of atypical antipsychotics and other medications, including PIs. In general, atypical/second-generation antipsychotics will have additive metabolic effects when co-administered with PIs and other medications with a similar effect on lipid and glucose

Table 10.3 Antipsychotics (Neuroleptics) for Depression

Antipsychotics	Mechanism of Action	Metabolic Site(s)	Enzymes Inhibited (no inducers)	Clinical Considerations	Potential DDIs with ART
First-Generation Antipsychotics					
Common Features				Increased risk of: cognitive/motor impairment EPS, NMS, TD hyperprolactinemia leukopenia/neutropenia orthostatic hypotension Greater risk for EPS, dystonia, and TD in PWHA Increased risk of death in elderly patients with dementia	Since these are older drugs, there are fewer data about specific metabolic sites and drug interactions Potent CYP pan-inhibitors like ritonavir and lopinavir may increase serum levels Potent CYP "pan-inducers"[a] may reduce serum levels Most are potent inhibitors of CYP2D6, and may increase serum levels of drugs dependent on CYP2D6
Chlorpromazine (Thorazine)		CYP2D6, 1A2, 3A4 UGT1A4, 1A3			See "Common Features"
Fluphenazine (Prolixin)		CYP2D6, 1A2	**CYP2D6**, 1A2		See "Common Features"
Haloperidol (Haldol)		CYP2D6, 3A4, 1A2	**CYP2D6**		See "Common Features"
Mesoridazine (Serentil)		CYP2D6, 1A2	unknown		See "Common Features"
Molindone (Moban)		CYP2D6 and Phase II	None known		Off US market
Perphenazine (Trilafon)		CYP2D6, 3A4, 1A2, 2C19	**CYP2D6**, 1A2		See "Common Features"

Drug				
Pimozide (Orap)	CYP3A4, 1A2	**CYP2D6**, 3A4	Prolongs QTc	PIs may cause arrhythmias when co-administered with CYP3A4-dependent pimozide and are contraindicated
Thioridazine (Mellaril)	CYP2D6, 1A2, 2C19, FMO3	CYP2D6		
Second-Generation (Atypical) Antipsychotics				
Common Features			Increased risk of metabolic syndrome (additive with PIs)	Most do not interfere with metabolism of other drugs (neither inhibit/induce)
			Risk of:	Combined treatment with ART increases risk of metabolic syndrome due to additive effects
			cognitive/motor impairment	QT prolongation is additive with drugs like saquinavir and lopinavir/ritonavir
			EPS, NMS, TD	
			hyperprolactinemia	
			leukopenia/neutropenia	
			orthostatic hypotension	
			priapism	
			seizures	
			Many are associated with QTc prolongation risk (NOT aripiprazole, lurasidone, olanzapine, cariprazine, brexpiprazole)	
			Increased risk of death in elderly patients with dementia	
Amisulpride	50% excreted in urine unchanged		Not available in the US	
	Minimal CYP metabolism			

(Continued)

Table 10.3 Continued

Antipsychotics	Mechanism of Action	Metabolic Site(s)	Enzymes Inhibited (no inducers)	Clinical Considerations	Potential DDIs with ART
Aripiprazole (Abilify)		CYP2D6, 3A4	None known	Increased risk of akathisia/EPS	Aripiprazole dose reduction 50% with: Potent CYP3A4 inhibitors _e.g.: PIs_ _elvitegravir/cobistat_ Potent CYP2D6 inhibitors; _e.g.: bupropion_ _diphenhydramine_ _paroxetine_ _ritonavir_ Aripiprazole dose reduction 75% with: combined CYP3A4 and 2D6 inhibitors (and combinations of inhibitors of each) _e.g.: ritonavir_ _efavirenz,_ _delavirdine_ Aripiprazole dose increase of up to 100% (2X) with: CYP3A4 inducers _e.g.: "pan-inducers"_ _ritonavir_ _some NNRTIs_
Asenapine (Saphris)		UGT1A4, CYP1A2	CYP2D6	QTc prolongation Not recommended in patients with severe hepatic impairment	Reduce paroxetine (CYP2D6 substrate and inhibitor) dose by 50% when co-administered
Blonanserine		CYP3A4		Not available in the US High risk of EPS	Contraindicated with potent CYP3A4 inhibitors like PIs

Drug	Metabolism	Inhibits	Clinical Notes	Drug Interactions
Brexpiprazole (Rexulti)	CYP2D6, CYP3A4	None known	Increased risk of akathisia	Brexpiprazole dose reduction 50% with: Potent CYP3A4 inhibitors, e.g.: PIs and elvitegravir/cobistat Potent CYP2D6 inhibitors, e.g.: *ritonavir diphenhydramine bupropion paroxetine* Brexpiprazole dose reduction 75% with: *combined* CYP3A4 and 2D6 inhibitors e.g.: *ritonavir efavirenz delavirdine* Brexpiprazole dose increase of up to 100% (2X) with: CYP3A4 inducers e.g.: *"pan-inducers" ritonavir some NNRTIs*
Cariprazine (Vraylar)	CYP3A4	None known	Not approved for dementia-related psychosis Increased risk of akathisia Late-occurring adverse drug reactions (ADRs) due to long half-life; monitor patients for several weeks after starting and each dose change	Potent CYP3A4 inhibitors: reduce cariprazine dosage 50% Co-administration with potent CYP3A4 inducers and "pan-inducers" NOT recommended, may significantly lower serum clozapine levels

(Continued)

Table 10.3 Continued

Antipsychotics	Mechanism of Action	Metabolic Site(s)	Enzymes Inhibited (no inducers)	Clinical Considerations	Potential DDIs with ART
Clozapine (Clozaril)		CYP1A2, 3A4, 2D6, 2C9, 2C19, UGT1A4, 1A3, FMO3	CYP2D6	Risk of agranulocytosis: US mandatory registry, bi-weekly monitoring CBC, ANC x 6 months, monthly thereafter Cardiac risks: bradycardia and syncope QTc prolongation myocarditis/cardiomyopathy orthostatic hypotension seizures Risk of: Anticholinergic toxicity: caution with narrow-angle glaucoma or anticholinergic drugs Eosinophilia Pulmonary embolism	Potent CYP1A2 inhibitors increase clozapine serum levels: must reduce clozapine to 1/3 standard dose Co-administration with potent CYP3A4 inducers and "pan-inducers" NOT recommended, may significantly lower serum clozapine levels Avoid carbamazepine, for adjunctive risk of agranulocytosis. Synergistic bone marrow suppression if co-administered with treatments for cytomegalovirus or *Herpes simplex* virus infections.
Iloperidone (Fanapt)		CYP2D6, 3A4	None known	Significant QTc prolongation; consider alternative if patient has additional risk factors; monitor K^+ and Mg^{2+} Not recommended in patients with severe hepatic impairment	Potent CYP2D6 or CYP3A4 inhibitors: reduce iloperidone dose by 50% Potent CYP3A4 inducers and "pan-inducers" may reduce serum levels of iloperidone Contraindicated: co-administration of iloperidone with drugs that prolong QTc interval

Drug	Metabolism	Enzyme effects	Clinical notes	Drug interactions
Lurasidone (Latuda)	CYP3A4	None known	Not approved for dementia-related psychosis	Contraindicated: co-administration of lurasidone with potent CYP3A4 inhibitors such as PIs or potent CYP3A4 inducers such as rifampin Moderate inhibitors may be used, but lurasidone dosage should be reduced 50%
Olanzapine (Zyprexa)	UGT1A4, CYP1A2, 2D6 (minor), FMO3	None		PAHs in tobacco smoke are inducers of CYP1A2, and may reduce serum levels of olanzapine Potent "pan-inducers" may reduce serum levels of olanzapine Co-administration of fosamprenavir/ritonavir may reduce olanzapine levels
Paliperidone (Invega)	P-glycoproteins CYP (in vitro) 2D6, 3A4 (minimal)	P-glycoproteins (weak)	Major active metabolite of risperidone QTc prolongation GI narrowing Dysphagia	Potent CYP3A4/P-gp inducers (carbamazepine) may reduce serum paliperidone levels and may require increased paliperidone dose Co-administration of divalproex sodium may require increased paliperidone dose, adjust clinically Potent "pan-inducers" may reduce serum levels of paliperidone

(Continued)

Table 10.3 Continued

Antipsychotics	Mechanism of Action	Metabolic Site(s)	Enzymes Inhibited (no inducers)	Clinical Considerations	Potential DDIs with ART
Quetiapine (Seroquel)		CYP3A4 Sulfoxidation Oxidation P-gp substrate	None	Associated with QTc prolongation Elevated blood pressure in children and adolescents Cataracts, routine screening recommended before starting treatment and every six months	Potent CYP3A4 inhibitors: administer 1/6 standard quetiapine dose Significant risk of priapism when co-administered with potent CYP3A4 inhibitors Potent CYP3A4 inducers: increase quetiapine dose up to 5X standard dose with chronic combination treatment Discontinuing potent CYP3A inducer therapy: reduce quetiapine from 5X elevated dose to standard dose over 7–14 days after discontinuation of CYP3A4 inducer
Risperidone (Risperdal)		CYP2D6, 3A4	2D6, 3A4	Not approved for dementia-related psychosis Associated with QTc prolongation	Potent CYP3A4 and /or CYP2D6 inhibitors may increase serum levels of risperidone. Co-administration requires lower initial risperidone dose and maximum dose of 8 mg per day. Potent CYP3A4 inducers and "pan-inducers" may reduce serum levels of risperidone. Increase risperidone dose up to 2X standard dose.

Drug	CYP	Inhibitor/Inducer	Comments	Contraindications/Notes
Sertindole	CYP2D6, 3A4		Significant, dose-related QTc prolongation Not available in the United States	Potent CYP3A4 and /or 2D6 inhibitors may increase serum levels of sertindole, increasing risk of QTc prolongation, and are contraindicated
Ziprasidone (Geodon)	Aldehyde oxidase Minimal CYP 3A4, 1A2	None	Not approved for dementia-related psychosis Associated with significant QTc prolongation, and ziprasidone use should be avoided in patients with bradycardia, hypokalemia, hypomagnesemia, congenital QT prolongation Taken with food increases absorption 2X Severe cutaneous adverse reactions have been reported (DRESS, SJS, SCAR) Intramuscular formulation not recommended in patients with significant renal impairment	May be least effected by CYP inhibitors or inducers Contraindicated with drugs that also affect QTc Contraindicated in patient with recent acute myocardial infarction or with uncompensated heart failure

Bold CYP indicates **potent** inhibitor or inducer of that cytochrome P450 enzyme

CYP = cytochrome; DDIs = drug–drug interactions; EPS = extrapyramidal symptoms; FMO = Flavin monoxygenase (non-CYP450 drug metabolizing enzyme that is considered not readily induceable or inhibited); NMS = neuroleptic malignant syndrome; TD = tardive dyskinesia; UGT = uridine 5ᵉ-diphosphate glucuronosyltransferase; ABCB = ATP binding cassette B transporter (p-glycoprotein transporter)

[a] Pan-inducers: drugs that induce many if not all CYP450 enzymes and include barbiturates, carbamazepine, ethanol, phenytoin, and rifamycins

metabolism. Combined treatment with ART and atypical antipsychotics is associated with significantly higher mean triglycerides, increased risk of developing diabetes, elevated mean arterial pressures, and marginally higher body mass index (Hammerness et al. 2002). Metformin has been identified in two separated meta-analyses as efficacious for weight loss independent of lifestyle modifications in context of continued antipsychotic use (Lavery et al. 2001, Samartzis et al. 2013, Karkow et al. 2017). Additionally et al. critically evaluated two randomized, placebo-controlled trials to investigate the effect of metformin on antipsychotic-associated dyslipidemia. These researchers found significant improvements in antipsychotic-associated dyslipidemia but also improved insulin resistance and weight loss (Ferrarra et al. 2014). Mizuno et al. (2014; Generali and Cada 2013) performed a meta-analysis to evaluate a wide variety of pharmacological interventions utilized across specialties to combat antipsychotic-associated metabolic side effects. They concluded that, of all interventions, the literature supported metformin as first-line for antipsychotic-associated metabolic side effects such as weight gain and dyslipidemias.

A significant number of atypical antipsychotics are associated with a risk of QTc prolongation and require regular cardiac monitoring for patients with additional risk factors for arrhythmias or who are on other medications with similar QTc prolongation profiles, such as saquinavir, macrolide antibiotics, TCAs, venlafaxine, bupropion, or antihistamines (Mizuno et al. 2014, de Silva et al. 2016, Wu et al. 2016). Aripiprazole, brexpiprazole, cariprazine, lurasidone, and olanzapine are not associated with an elevated risk of QTc prolongation (Hill and Lee 2013, Lavery et al. 2013, Maljuric et al. 2015, Otsuka Pharmaceuticals Co Ltd 2016).

Aripiprazole

Aripiprazole has less documented risk of EPS, metabolic syndrome, and QT interval prolongation than other atypical antipsychotics (2015). Aripiprazole is primarily metabolized by CYP2D6 and CYP3A4 and has no effects on P450 activity (2013). Aripiprazole serum concentrations may be vulnerable to co-administration of potent inhibitors of CYP2D6 (e.g., fluoxetine, paroxetine, quinidine, or PIs) and CYP3A4 (e.g., clarithromycin, erythromycin, ketoconazole, or PIs), with the potential of increasing aripiprazole's serum levels. Potent CYP3A4 inducers such as carbamazepine may reduce aripiprazole serum levels, and dose adjustments may be needed to obtain clinical efficacy. The manufacturer suggests using 50% of the standard aripiprazole dose when it is co-administered with potent CYP2D6 inhibitors such as ritonavir or strong CYP3A4 inhibitors such as PIs, ketoconazole, and voriconazole. A 25% standard aripiprazole dose is suggested if co-administering with combined CYP3A4 and 2D6 inhibitors of moderate to severe potency, either as co-administered regimens (e.g., bupropion and PIs), or as single poly-inhibitors like delavirdine, ritonavir, or efavirenz. Aripiprazole doses may need to be doubled (2X) over one to two weeks if co-administered with potent CYP3A4 inducers such as carbamazepine and rifampin to maintain clinical efficacy (Hill and Lee 2013, Maljuric et al. 2015, Otsuka Pharmaceuticals Co Ltd 2016).

Asenapine

Asenapine demonstrates high affinity for adrenergic α1A, α2A, and α2C receptors, resulting in an elevated risk of orthostatic hypotension and syncope (2013, 2016). Asenapine is metabolized via glucuronidation at UGT1A4 and oxidative metabolism at CYP1A2, with minor contributions from CYP2D6 and CYP3A4. It is a weak inhibitor of CYP2D6 (2016). Potent CYP1A2 inhibitors such as fluvoxamine may increase asenapine serum levels, with concern for asenapine toxicity at higher doses (2015; Mandrioli et al. 2015). Potent CYP2D6 inhibitors, including fluoxetine, paroxetine, PIs, ketoconazole, and ritonavir, may increase serum levels of asenapine. Importantly, potent CYP1A2 inducers such as ritonavir and the PAHs in tobacco smoke can reduce asenapine serum concentrations (Cozza and Wynn 2012, Mandrioli et al. 2015). Cessation of smoking in individuals receiving asenapine will lead to gradual increases in asenapine serum concentrations, with resultant side effects or toxicity (2015), and initiation/resumption of smoking tobacco will lead to a gradual reduction of asenapine serum levels and may lead to breakthrough psychosis.

Olanzapine

Olanzapine is commonly associated with significant alterations in weight, glucose dysregulation, and dyslipidemia. Providers need to aggressively monitor for metabolic complications when concurrently prescribing olanzapine. Olanzapine also has affinity for alpha adrenergic receptors, resulting in elevated risk of orthostatic hypotension and syncope, which may be potentiated with co-administration of diazepam and alcohol. Additionally, olanzapine potentiates the efficacy of anti-hypertensive agents when co-administered (Penzak et al. 2002, Eli Lilli and Co. 2015). Olanzapine is primarily metabolized by CYP1A2 and uridine diphosphate glucuronosyltransferase (UGT) ritonavir at a dose of 500 mg twice daily reduced the mean area under the concentration curve (AUC) of olanzapine by 53% in healthy volunteers, presumably due to induction of CYP1A2 and/or UGT (Cozza and Wynn 2012). A more recent study conducted on 24 healthy volunteers replicated those results, where co-administration of fosamprenavir/ritonavir appeared to increase olanzapine's metabolism and reduce antipsychotic serum levels. Jacobs et al. (2014) propose a 50% dosage increase of olanzapine when combined with a ritonavir-boosted PI. They also noted a potential risk of increased anti-retroviral non-nucleoside reverse transcriptase inhibitors NNRTI serum levels with concomitant olanzapine administration, although the mechanism is unclear. Potent CYP1A2 inducers such as ritonavir and PAHs in tobacco smoke can reduce olanzapine concentrations (2015) (Penzak et al. 2002). Discontinuation of potent CYP1A2 inducers like ritonavir and cessation of smoking in individuals receiving olanzapine will lead to gradual increases in olanzapine concentrations, with resultant side effects or toxicity. Additionally, starting olanzapine at standard dosing while in a smoke-free environment places patients at risk for a gradual loss of efficacy and relapse if they initiate/resume smoking and increase the metabolism of olanzapine (Jacobs et al. 2014).

Mood Stabilizers for Depression

Mood stabilizers are a heterogeneous class of drugs, which includes lithium, anticonvulsants, and antipsychotics. This section will discuss lithium and the antiepileptic mood stabilizers commonly used to treat depression and the depression associated with bipolar disorder.

Lithium

Lithium's mechanisms of action are complex and not very clear. A full explanation of its known effects can be found elsewhere (Penzak et al. 2002). Growing evidence suggests that lithium has protective effects against a variety of insults, including glutamate-induced excitotoxicity, ischemia-induced neuronal damage, and other neurodegenerative conditions (Cozza and Wynn 2012). Lithium's side effects include sedation, weight gain, cognitive impairment or "fogginess," bilateral hand tremor, polyuria and polydipsia, and acne. The clearance of lithium is exclusively dependent upon renal excretion as a free ion and decreases with aging (Zullino et al. 2002, Malhi et al. 2013). Symptoms of lithium toxicity (serum levels >1.5 mEq/L) include tremor, nausea, vomiting, diarrhea, vertigo, and confusion. Plasma levels greater than 2.5 mEq/L require hemodialysis and may lead to seizures, coma, cardiac dysrhythmia, and permanent neurological impairment (Chiu and Chuang 2010). Lithium use also requires adequate electrolyte balance, which may be difficult for patients with medical co-morbidities like HIV or GI disease who have diarrhea, nausea, vomiting, and general debility. Patients with renal dysfunction, to include HIV-associated nephropathy, may also be poor candidates for lithium treatment due to the potential for reduced lithium clearance (Speirs and Hirsch 1978, Moscovich 1993). Despite these obstacles, lithium has a favorable DDI profile, and for some treatment-resistant depressed and bipolar patients, it is the only mood stabilizer that is effective. Therefore, therapeutic drug monitoring is a necessity.

Antiepileptics

Many mood-stabilizing antiepileptic drugs (AEDs), particularly the older ones (phenobarbital, phenytoin, carbamazepine, topiramate, and valproic acid [VPA]) induce metabolism by increasing the synthesis of multiple metabolic enzymes, which speeds the metabolism of many drugs and endogenous compounds such as antiretrovirals, analgesics, anticoagulants, other antiepileptics, antihypertensives, cytotoxics, glucocorticoids, immunosuppressants, oral contraceptives, psychotropics, statins, hormones, and lipids. The newer, non-pan-inducing AEDs with efficacy for epilepsy, mood stabilization, and pain management should be considered first-line when choosing an AED for mood stabilization or pain, especially in a patient on polypharmacy. For more complete information on AEDs, the reader is referred to the American Academy of Neurology and the International League Against Epilepsy's evidenced-based guidelines (Chen et al. 2004).

Table 10.4, "Mood Stabilizers," presents the metabolic, DDI, and clinical considerations pertinent to the AEDS in common use.

Table 10.4 Mood Stabilizers in the Treatment of Depression

Mood Stabilizer	Metabolic Site(s)	Enzymes Inhibited	Enzymes Induced	Clinical Considerations	Potential DDIs
Lithium	Renal	None	None	Risk for toxicity with dehydration, especially with diuretic use or when administered with renally toxic medications such as NSAIDs	Lithium serum levels may be increased by NSAIDs, diuretics Lithium levels may be reduced by osmotic diuretics (mannitol), sodium bicarbonate, and acetazolamide
Carbamazepine (CBZ, Tegretol)	CYP3A4 (primary) 2C8, 2B6, 2C9, 1A2 UGT2B7 Transporter ABCB1, ABCC2	CYP2C19 (perhaps) **CYP3A4,** 1A2, 2B6, 2C8, 2C9, UGT1A4	**CYP3A4,** 1A2, 2B6, 2C8, 2C9, UGT1A4	Potential for diminished white blood cell count Narrow therapeutic index Risk of Stevens-Johnson syndrome and toxic epidermal necrolysis HLA-B genotyping for patients of Asian descent necessary	CBZ is considered a potent "pan-inducer" and it auto-induces High risk of reduced effectiveness/treatment failure of co-administered drugs dependent upon many CYPs Potent CYP3A4 inhibitors like PIs, clarithromycin, ketoconazole, and grapefruit juice may increase serum levels of CBZ Other "pan-inducers" may reduce serum levels of CBZ
Clobazam[b] (Frisium, Onfi)	CYP3A4, 2C19	CYP2C9, 2C19			Potent CYP3A4 inhibitors like PIs, clarithromycin, ketoconazole, and grapefruit juice may increase serum levels of clobazam; CYP3A4 inducing drugs and St. John's wort may reduce clobazam serum levels
Ethosuximide (Zarontin)	CYP3A4, Phase II	None known			Potent CYP3A4 inhibitors like PIs, clarithromycin, ketoconazole, and grapefruit juice may increase serum levels CYP3A4 inducers may reduce ethosuximide serum levels

(Continued)

Table 10.4 Continued

Mood Stabilizer	Metabolic Site(s)	Enzymes Inhibited	Enzymes Induced	Clinical Considerations	Potential DDIs
Eslicarbazepine acetate (Aptiom)	Non-microsomal hydrolysis (first pass) UGT2B4 and many others	CYP2C19 (moderate)	CYP3A4	Cognitive impairment Dizziness/gait disturbance SIADH Suicidal thoughts and behavior Visual changes	CYP3A4 induction by eslicarbazepine has clinically reduced serum levels of: CBZ OCPs Statins Warfarin
Felbamate (Felbatol)	CYP3A4, 2E1 Transporter ABCB1	CYP2C19	CYP3A4		CYP3A4 induction by felbamate may reduce serum levels of CYP3A4-dependent drugs Potent CYP3A4 inhibitors like PIs, clarithromycin, ketoconazole, and grapefruit juice may increase serum levels of felbamate CYP3A4 inducers may reduce serum felbamate levels
Gabapentin (Neurontin)	Excreted in urine unchanged	None known	None known	May cause dizziness/gait disturbance, blurred vision Needs dose adjustment in patients with renal dysfunction	
Lamotrigine (Lamictal)	UGT1A4 and excreted in urine unchanged	None known	UGT1A4 (mild, with auto-induction)	Must have slow titration to effective dose to avoid potentially lethal rashes	UGT inducers like efavirenz, ritonavir, lopinavir, and nelfinavir, as well as valproic acid and perhaps sertraline may reduce lamotrigine serum levels

Drug	Metabolism		Induction	Clinical notes / interactions
Levitiracetam (Keppra)	1/3 by non-CYP450, Phase I hydrolysis	None known	None known	May cause depression, suicidal thoughts/attempts, and non-psychotic behavioral changes
Methsuximide (Celontin)	CYP3A4, Phase II	None known	None known	Potent CYP3A4 inhibitors like PIs, clarithromycin, ketoconazole, and grapefruit juice may increase serum levels of methsuximide, CYP3A4 inducers may reduce methsuximide serum levels
Oxcarbazepine (Trileptal)	Non-cytochromal Metabolism UGTs	CYP2C19	CYP3A4 (mild) UGTs (moderate)	Oxcarbazepine's induction of CYP3A4 may reduce serum levels of CYP-dependent drugs, especially PIs
Phenobarbital	CYP2C9, 2C19		**CYP3A4, 1A2, 2C9, 2C19, UGTs**	Phenobarbital is considered a "pan-inducer"[a] Risk of phenobarbital failure when co-administered with CYP2C9 and 2C19 inducers such as ritonavir and pan-inducers[a]
Phenytoin	CYP2C9, 2C19		**CYP3A4, 2C9, 2C19, UGTs**	Phenytoin is considered a "pan-inducer" Phenytoin serum levels may be increased to toxicity when co-administered with CYP2Cp/2C19 inhibitors like fluoxetine and fluvoxamine

(Continued)

Table 10.4 Continued

Mood Stabilizer	Metabolic Site(s)	Enzymes Inhibited	Enzymes Induced	Clinical Considerations	Potential DDIs
Tiagabine (Gabitril)	CYP3A4, UGTs	None known			Potent CYP3A4 inhibitors like PIs, clarithromycin, ketoconazole, and grapefruit juice may increase serum levels of tiagabine
Topiramate (Topamax)	70% excreted unchanged in urine Phase I and II UGTs Transporter ABCB1	2C19	3A4 (mild), UGTs	Associated with weight loss, sedation, depression, and mood changes	
Valproic acid (VPA, Depakote, Depakene)	UGT1A6, UGT1A9, UGT2B7, β-oxidation, CYP2C9, 2C19 2A6	Inhibits: UGT1A4, UGT1A9, UGT2B7, UGT2B15, CYP2D6, 2C9, 2C19 Epoxide hydroxylase	Possibly CYP3A4, ABCB1	Hepatotoxicity, especially with CYP inducers like nevirapine, efavirenz, and ritonavir Hepatotoxic metabolite is not measured in standard lab tests	Very complicated and controversial interaction profile pan-inducers[a], may reduce VPA serum levels

Drug	Metabolism	Inhibits	Induces	Adverse Effects	Drug Interactions
Vigabatrin (Sabril)	Excreted in urine unchanged	None known	CYP2C9	Visual changes to include permanent visual field deficits Suicidal thoughts and behavior Peripheral neuropathy	
Zonisamide (Zonegran)	CYP3A4, 3A5 Acetylation, Sulfonation	CYP2C9, 2C19			Potent CYP3A4 inhibitors like PIs, clarithromycin, ketoconazole, and grapefruit juice may increase serum levels of zonisamide Potent CYP3A4 inducers, like St. John's wort, ritonavir, and pan-inhibitors [a], may reduce zonisamide serum levels

---

Bold CYP indicates **potent** inhibitor or inducer of that cytochrome P450 enzyme

CYP = cytochrome, DDIs = drug–drug interactions, UGT = uridine 5'-diphosphate glucuronosyltransferase, ABCB = ATP binding cassette B transporter (p-glycoprotein transporters), OCP = oral contraceptive pills

[a] Pan-inducers: drugs that induce many if not all CYPP450 enzymes, and include barbiturates, carbamazepine, ethanol, phenytoin, and rifamycins

[b] Clobazam is a 1, 5-benzodiazepine1-5 (BZD) that is used as an antiepileptic drug.

Stimulants/Alerting Agents for Depression

Since stimulants are sometimes used to treat asthenia, fatigue, and depression in severe medical illnesses, we have included the drug characteristics in table format here for the reader.

Stimulant/ Alerting Drug	Mechanism of Action	Metabolism Site (s)	Enzyme (s) Inhibited	Enzyme (s) Induced	Clinical Considerations	Potential DDIs with ART
Amphetamine-based:						
Dextroamphetamine (Dexedrine, ProCentra, Zenzedi)		CYP2D6	CYP2D6 (weak)	None known	Myocardial infarction Hypertension QT prolongation Mania	Caution with other serotonergic/ noradrenergic medications due to additive pharmacodynamic effects Pan-inhibitors† and potent CYP2D6 inhibitors such as paroxetine, fluoxetine, and quinidine may increase serum levels of dextroamphetamine
Methylphenidate (Concerta, Metadate, Ritalin, Methylin, Quillivant)		Plasma esterases	None known	None known	Myocardial infarction Hypertension QT prolongation Mania	Alcohol can denature the Concerta capsule and cause an immediate release of medication; e.g.: *tipranavir*
Non-amphetamine based:						
Atomoxetine (Strattera)		CYP2D6	None known	None known	Myocardial infarction Hypertension QT prolongation Mania	Pan-inhibitors and potent CYP2D6 inhibitors such as paroxetine, fluoxetine, and quinidine may increase serum levels of amphetamine
Modafinil (Provigil)/ Armodafinil (Nuvigil)		CYP3A4 glucuronidation ABCB1	CYP2C19, 2C9	CYP3A4		CYP3A4 induction by modafinil and armodafinil may reduce serum levels of drugs dependent upon CYP3A4; e.g.: *cyclosporine*, *PIs*

CYP = cytochrome

†Pan-inducers: drugs that induce many if not all CYPP450 enzymes and include barbiturates, carbamazepine, ethanol, phenytoin, and rifamycins

SUMMARY

Depression in all of its forms is indeed a systemic illness, affecting patients in every clinic and hospital setting. Many in primary care will be first-line evaluators and prescribers, requiring a broad and facile understanding of the mechanisms of action, side effects, possible toxicities, and potential drug interactions of these medications. Clinicians in all medical fields will encounter patients in the midst of treatment for their depressive symptoms, plus all of the myriad symptoms that are addressed with antidepressants and mood stabilizers, such as pain, anxiety, and sleep disturbances. Understanding these medications . . . and knowing where to learn more . . . is critical to safe and effective care.

REFERENCES

Abdallah, C., et al. (2014). "Glutamate metabolism in major depressive disorder." *Am J Psychiatry* **171** (12): 1320–1327.

Albert, P. R. et al. (2014). "Serotonin-prefrontal cortical circuitry in anxiety and depression phenotypes: pivotal role of pre-and post-synaptic 5-HT1A receptor expression." *Front Behav Neurosci* **8**: 199.

Alderman, J., et al. (1997). "Desipramine pharmacokinetics when coadministered with paroxetine or sertraline in extensive metabolizers." *J Clin Psychopharmacol* **17** (4): 284–291.

Alderman, C. P., et al. (2001). "Possible interaction of zopiclone and nefazodone." *Ann Pharmacother* **35** (11): 1378–1380.

Alpert, J., et al. (2008). "Difference in treatment outcome in outpatients with anxious versus nonanxious depression: a STAR*D report." *Am J Psychiatry* **165** (3): 342–351.

Anderson, G. (2008). "Gender Differences in pharmacological response." *Int Rev Neurobiol* **83**: 1–10.

Andrade, C., et al. (2010). "Serotonin reuptake inhibitor antidepressants and abnormal bleeding: a review for clinicians and a reconsideration of mechanisma." *J Clin Psychiatry* **71** (12): 1565–1575.

Andrews, P., et al. (2015). "Is serotonin an upper or a downer? The evolution of the serotonergic system and its role in depression and the antidepressant response." *Neurosci Biobehav Rev* **51** (1): 164–188.

Anglin, R., et al. (2014). "Risk of upper gastrointestinal bleeding with selective serotonin reuptake inhibitors with or without concurrent nonsteroidal anti-inflammatory use: a systematic review and meta-analysis." *Am J Gastroenterol* **109** (6): 811–819.

Anttila, A. K., et al. (2001). "Fluvoxamine augmentation increases serum mirtazapine concentrations three- to fourfold." *Ann Pharmacother* **35** (10): 1221–1223.

Arinzon, Z. H., et al. (2002). "Delayed recurrent SIADH associated with SSRIs." *Ann Pharmacother* **36** (7–8): 1175–1177.

Armstrong, S. C. and S. M. Schweitzer (1997). "Delirium associated with paroxetine and benztropine combination." *Am J Psychiatry* **154** (4): 581–582.

Arnold, L., et al. (2004). "A double-blind, multicenter trial comparing duloxetine with placebo in the treatment of fibromyalgia patients with or without major depressive disorder." *Arthritis Rheumatology* **50** (9): 2974–2984.

Baird, P. (2003). "The interactive metabolism effect of oxcarbazepine coadministered with tricyclic antidepressant therapy for OCD symptoms." *J Clin Psychopharmacol* **23** (4): 419–420.

Ball, S. E., et al. (1997). "Venlafaxine: in vitro inhibition of CYP2D6 dependent imipramine and desipramine metabolism; comparative studies with selected SSRIs, and effects on human hepatic CYP3A4, CYP2C9 and CYP1A2." *Br J Clin Pharmacol* **43** (6): 619–626.

Begre, S., et al. (2002). "Paroxetine increases steady-state concentrations of (R)-methadone in CYP2D6 extensive but not poor metabolizers." *J Clin Psychopharmacol* **22** (2): 211–215.

Bell, I. R. and J. O. Cole (1988). "Fluoxetine induces elevation of desipramine level and exacerbation of geriatric nonpsychotic depression." *J Clin Psychopharmacol* **8** (6): 447–448.

Belpaire, F. M., et al. (1998). "The oxidative metabolism of metoprolol in human liver microsomes: inhibition by the selective serotonin reuptake inhibitors." *Eur J Clin Pharmacol* **54** (3): 261–264.

Belzer, K. and F. Schneier (2004). "Comorbidity of anxiety and depressive disorders: issues in conceptualization, assessment, and treatment." *J Psychiatr Pract* **10** (5): 296–306.

Bertelsen, K. M., et al. (2003). "Apparent mechanism-based inhibition of human CYP2D6 in vitro by paroxetine: comparison with fluoxetine and quinidine." *Drug Metab Dispos* **31** (3): 289–293.

Binkhorst, L., et al. (2013). "Unjustified prescribing of CYP2D6 inhibiting SSRIs in women treated with tamoxifen." *Breast Cancer Res Treat* **139** (3): 923–929.

Blier, P. (2013). "Neurotransmitter targeting in the treatment of depression." *J Clinical Psychiatry* **74** (suppl 2): 19–24.

Boinpally, R., et al. (2014). "Influence of CYP3A4 induction/inhibition on the pharmacokinetics of vilazodone in healthy subjects." *Clin Ther* **36** (11): 1638–1649.

Brannan, S., et al. (2005). "Duloxetine 60mg once-daily in the treatment of painful physical symptoms in patients with major depressive disorder." *J Psychiatr Res* **39** (1): 43–53.

Brosen, K. (2004). "Some aspects of genetic polymorphism in the biotransformation of antidepressants." *Therapie* **59** (1): 5–12.

Brosen, K. and C. A. Naranjo (2001). "Review of pharmacokinetic and pharmacodynamic interaction studies with citalopram." *Eur Neuropsychopharmacol* **11** (4): 275–283.

Caccia, S. (2004). "Metabolism of the newest antidepressants: comparisons with related predecessors." *IDrugs* **7** (2): 143–150.

Cardozo, L., et al. (2004). "Pharmacological treatment of women awaiting surgery for stress urinary incontinence." *Obstetrics Gynecology* **104** (3): 511–519.

Carrillo, J. A. and J. Benitez (2000). "Clinically significant pharmacokinetic interactions between dietary caffeine and medications." *Clin Pharmacokinet* **39** (2): 127–153.

Cavanaugh, S. V. (1990). "Drug-drug interactions of fluoxetine with tricyclics." *Psychosomatics* **31** (3): 273–276.

Cavuto, N., et al. (1996). "Pharmacies and prevention of potentially fatal drug interactions." *JAMA* **275** (14): 1086–1087.

Centorrino, F., et al. (1996). "Serum levels of clozapine and norclozapine in patients treated with selective serotonin reuptake inhibitors." *Am J Psychiatry* **153** (6): 820–822.

Chau, N., et al. (2014). "Morphine glucuronidation and glucosidation represent complementary metabolic pathways that are both catalyzed by UDP-glucuronosyltransferase 2B7: kinetic, inhibition, and molecular modeling studies." *J Pharmacol Exp Ther* **349** (1): 126–137.

Chen, K., et al. (2004). "Implication of serum concentration monitoring in patients with lithium intoxication." *Psychiatry Clin Neurosci* **58** (1): 25–29.

Chiu, C. and D. Chuang (2010). "Molecular actions and therapeutic potential of lithium in preclinical and clinical studies of CNS disorders." *Pharmacol Ther* **128** (2): 281–304.

Christensen, M., et al. (2002). "Low daily 10-mg and 20-mg doses of fluvoxamine inhibit the metabolism of both caffeine (cytochrome P4501A2) and omeprazole (cytochrome P4502C19)." *Clin Pharmacol Ther* **71** (3): 141–152.

Court, M. H. (2009). *Metabolism in Depth: Phase II. Clinical Manual of Drug Interaction Principles for Medical Practice.* Washington, DC: American Psychiatric Publishing: 23–41.

Cozza, K., et al. (2003). *Drug Interaction Principles for Medical Practice Cytochrome P450s, UGTs and P-glycoproteins.* Washington, DC: APPI, Inc.

Cozza, K. L. and G. H. Wynn (2012). "Pharmacology updates for psychosomatic medicine: smoking and metabolism; asenapine; irreversible MAOIs." *Psychosomatics* **53** (5): 499–502.

Dalton, S., et al. (2003). "Use of selective serotonin reuptake inhibitors and risk of upper gastrointestinal tract bleeding: a population-based cohort study." *Arch Intern Med* **163** (1): 59–64.

Davies, S., et al. (2004). "Potential for drug interactions involving cytochromes P450 2D6 and 3A4 on general adult psychiatric and functional elderly psychiatric wards." *Br J Clin Pharmacol* **57** (4): 464–472.

Davis, A., et al. (2011). "Carbamazepine coadminstration with an oral contraceptive: effects on steriod pharmacokinetics, ovulation, and bleeding." *Epilepsia* **52** (2): 243–247.

de Silva, V. A., et al. (2016). "Metformin in prevention and treatment of antipsychotic induced weight gain: a systematic review and meta-analysis." *BMC Psychiatry* **16**: 341.

DePriest, A., et al. (2015). "Metabolism and disposition of prescription opioids: a review." *Forensic Sci Rev* **27** (2): 115–145.

DeSilva, K. E., et al. (2001). "Serotonin syndrome in HIV-infected individuals receiving antiretroviral therapy and fluoxetine." *Aids* **15** (10): 1281–1285.

DeVane, C. L., et al. (2004). "Comparative CYP3A4 inhibitory effects of venlafaxine, fluoxetine, sertraline, and nefazodone in healthy volunteers." *J Clin Psychopharmacol* **24** (1): 4–10.

DiMatteo, M. R., et al. (2000). "Depression is a risk factor for noncompliance with medical treatment: meta-analysis of the effects of anxiety and depression on patient adherence." *Arch Intern Med* **160** (14): 2101–2107.

Duman, R. S. (2014). "Pathophysiology of depression and innovative treatments: remodeling glutamatergic synaptic connections." *Dialogues Clin Neurosci* **16** (1): 11–27.

Egberts, A. C., et al. (1997). "Serotonin syndrome attributed to tramadol addition to paroxetine therapy." *Int Clin Psychopharmacol* **12** (3): 181–182.

ElMansari, M., et al. (2010). "Relevance of norepinephrine–dopamine interactions in the treatment of major depressive disorder." *CNS Neurosci Ther* **16** (3): e1–17.

Ferrarra, M., et al. (2014). "The concomitant use of second-generation antipsychotics and long-term antiretroviral therapy may be associated with increased cardiovascular risk." *Psychiatry Res* **218** (1): 201–208.

Fiedorowicz, J. G. and K. L. Swartz (2004). "The role of monoamine oxidase inhibitors in current psychiatric practice." *J Psychiatr Pract* **10** (4): 239–248.

Fijal, B., et al. (2015). "CYP2D6 predicted metabolizer status and safety in adult patients with attention deficit hyperactivity disorder participating in a large placebo-controlled atomoxetine maintenance of response clinical trial." *J Clin Pharmacol* **55** (10): 1167–1174.

Fogelman, S. M., et al. (1999). "O- and N-demethylation of venlafaxine in vitro by human liver microsomes and by microsomes from cDNA-transfected cells: effect of metabolic inhibitors and SSRI antidepressants." *Neuropsychopharmacology* **20** (5): 480–490.

Food and Drug Administration (FDA) (2012). *FDA Drug Safety Communication: Revised Recommendations for Celexa (Citalopram Hydrobromide) Related to a Potential Risk of Abnormal Heart Rhythms with High Doses*. Silver Spring, MD: U. S. Food and Drug Administration.

Ford, N., et al. (2015). "Benzodiazepines may reduce the effectiveness of ketamine in the treatment of depression." *Aust N Z J Psychiatry* **49** (12): 1227.

Fried, E. and R. Nesse (2015). "Depression sum-scores don't add up: why analyzing specific depression symptoms is essential." *BMC Med* **13** (1): 1.

Gaedigk, A. (2013). "Complexities of CYP2D6 gene analysis and interpretation." *Int Rev Psychiatry* **25** (5): 534–553.

Galetin, A., et al. (2010). "Contributions of intestinal cytochrome p450-mediated metabolism to drug-drug inhibition and induction interactions." *Drug Metab Pharmacokinet* **25** (1): 28–47.

Gareri, P., et al. (2008). "Venlafaxine-propafenone interaction resulting in hallucinations and psychomotor agitation." *Ann Pharmacother* **42** (3): 434–438.

Generali, J. A. and D. J. Cada (2013). "Metformin: Prevention and Treatment of Antipsychotic-Induced Weight Gain." *Hosp Pharm* **48** (9): 734–735, 777.

Ghassemi, M., et al. (2014). "Leveraging a critical care database: selective serotonin reuptake inhibitor use prior to ICU admission is associated with increased hospital mortality." *Chest* **145** (4): 745–752.

Gillman, P. K. (2007). "Tricyclic antidepressant pharmacology and therapeutic drug interactions updated." *Br J Pharmacol* **151** (6): 737–748.

Gonzalez, J. S., et al. (2011). "Depression and HIV/AIDS treatment nonadherence: a review and meta-analysis." *J Acquir Immune Defic Syndr* **58** (2): 181–187.

Grandjean, E. and J. M. Aubry (2009). "Lithium: updated human knowledge using and evidence-based approach. Part II: Clinical Pharmacology and Therapeutic Monitoring." *CNS Drugs* **23** (4): 331–349.

Granfors, M. T., et al. (2004). "Fluvoxamine drastically increases concentrations and effects of tizanidine: a potentially hazardous interaction." *Clin Pharmacol Ther* **75** (4): 331–341.

Grasmader, K., et al. (2004). "Impact of polymorphisms of cytochrome-P450 isoenzymes 2C9, 2C19, and 2D6 on plasma concentrations and clinical effects of antidepressants in a naturalistic clincal setting." *Eur J Clin Pharmacol* **60** (5): 329–336.

Greenblatt, D. J., et al. (2003). "Short-term exposure to low-dose ritonavir impairs clearance and enhances adverse effects of trazodone." *J Clin Pharmacol* **43** (4): 414–422.

Greene, D. S. and R. H. Barbhaiya (1997). "Clinical Pharmacokinetics of Nefazodone." *Clin Pharmacokinet* **33** (4): 260–275.

Guzey, C., et al. (2002). "Change from the CYP2D6 extensive metabolizer to the poor metabolizer phenotype during treatment with bupropion." *Ther Drug Monit* **24** (3): 436–437.

Hall, J., et al. (2003). "Pharmacokinetic and pharmacodynamic evaluation of the inhibition of alprazolam by citalopram and fluoxetine." *J Clin Psychopharmacol* **23** (4): 349–357.

Hammerness, P., et al. (2002). "Linezolid: MAOI activity and potential drug interactions." *Psychosomatics* **43** (3): 248–249.

Hamon, M. and P. Blier (2013). "Monoamine neurocircuitry in depression and strategies for new treatments." *Prog Neuropsychopharmacol Biol Psychiatry* **45**: 54–63.

Hansen, R., et al. (2005). "Efficacy and safety of second-generation antidepressants in the treatment of major depressive disorder." *Ann Intern Med* **143** (6): 415–426.

Harrison, J. E., et al. (2016). "Which cognitive domains are improved by treatment with vortioxetine?" *Int J Neuropsychopharmacol* pii: pyw054.

Hemeryck, A., et al. (2001). "Metoprolol-paroxetine interaction in human liver microsomes: stereoselective aspects and prediction of the in vivo interaction." *Drug Metab Dispos* **29** (5): 656–663.

Herbild, L., et al. (2013). "Does pharmacogenetic testing for CYP450 2D6 and 2C19 among patients with diagnoses within the schizophrenic spectrum reduce treatment costs?" *Basic Clin Pharmacol Toxicol* **113** (4): 266–272.

Hesse, L. M., et al. (2000). "CYP2B6 mediates the in vitro hydroxylation of bupropion: potential drug interactions with other antidepressants." *Drug Metab Dispos* **28** (10): 1176–1183.

Hesse, L. M., et al. (2001). "Ritonavir, efavirenz, and nelfinavir inhibit CYP2B6 activity in vitro: potential drug interactions with bupropion." *Drug Metab Dispos* **29** (2): 100–102.

Hill, L. and K. C. Lee (2013). "Pharmacotherapy considerations in patients with HIV and psychiatric disorders: focus on antidepressants and antipsychotics." *Ann Pharmacother* **47** (1): 75–89.

Himei, A. and T. Okamura (2006). "Discontinuation syndrome associated with paroxetine in depressed patients: a retrospective analysis of factors involved in the occurrence of the syndrome." *CNS Drugs* **20** (8): 665–672.

Hori, H., et al. (2003). "Grapefruit juice-fluvoxamine interaction—is it risky or not?" *J Clin Psychopharmacol* **23** (4): 422–424.

Imbs, J., et al. (1997). "Mechanism of drug interactions with renal elimination of lithium." *Bull Acad Natl Med* **181** (4): 695–697.

Jacobs, B. S., et al. (2014). "Effect of fosamprenavir/ritonavir on the pharmacokinetics of single-dose olanzapine in healthy volunteers." *Int J Antimicrob Agents* **44** (2): 173–177.

Jiang, H., et al. (2015). "Use of selective serotonin reuptake inhibitors and risk of upper gastrointestinal bleeding: a systematic review and meta-analysis." *Clin Gastroenterol Hepatol* **13** (1): 42–50.e43.

Joos, A. A., et al. (1997). "Dose-dependent pharmacokinetic interaction of clozapine and paroxetine in an extensive metabolizer." *Pharmacopsychiatry* **30** (6): 266–270.

Kalgutkar, A. S., et al. (2005). "Bioactivation of the nontricyclic antidepressant nefazodone to a reactive quinone-imine species in human liver microsomes and recombinant cytochrome P450 3A4." *Drug Metab Dispos* **33** (2): 243–253.

Karkow, D. C., Kauer, J. F., Ernst, E. J. (2017). "Incidence of serotonin syndrome with combined use of linezolid and serotonin reuptake inhibitors compared with linezolid monotherapy." *J Clin Psychopharmacol* **37**(5): 518–523. doi:10.1097/JCP.0000000000000751.

Kaufman, K. R. and R. Gerner (1998). "Lamotrigine toxicity secondary to sertraline." *Seizure* **7** (2): 163–165.

Kennedy, S. H., et al. (2002). "Combining bupropion SR with venlafaxine, paroxetine, or fluoxetine: a preliminary report on pharmacokinetic, therapeutic, and sexual dysfunction effects." *J Clin Psychiatry* **63** (3): 181–186.

Khairul, M. F., et al. (2006). "Fluoxetine potentiates chloroquine and mefloquine effect on multidrug-resistant Plasmodium falciparum in vitro." *Jpn J Infect Dis* **59** (5): 329–331.

Khan, A. Y. and S. H. Preskorn (2001). "Increase in plasma levels of clozapine and norclozapine after administration of nefazodone." *J Clin Psychiatry* **62** (5): 375–376.

Kobayashi, T., et al. (2010). "Inhibition of G-protein-activated inwardly rectifying K+ channels by the selective norepinephrine reuptake inhibitors atomoxetine and reboxetine." *Neuropsychopharmacology* **35** (7): 1560–1569.

Köhler, S., et al. (2016). "The serotonergic system in the neurobiology of depression: Relevance for novel antidepressants." *J Psychopharmacol* 30 (1): 13–22.

Kotlyar, M., et al. (2003). "Nefazodone inhibits methylprednisolone disposition and enhances its adrenal-suppressant effect." *J Clin Psychopharmacol* 23 (6): 652–656.

Kurdyak, P. A., et al. (2012). "Antidepressants, metoprolol and the risk of bradycardia." *Ther Adv Psychopharmacol* 2 (2): 43–49. doi: 10.1177/2045125311433580.

Lam, Y. W., et al. (2003). "Pharmacokinetic and harmacodynamics interactions of oral midazolam with ketoconazole, fluoxetine, fluvoxamine, and nefazodone." *J Clin Pharmacol* 43 (11): 1274–1282.

Lance, S. and I. Ternouth (2015). "Fluoxetine-induced phenytoin toxicity: a clinical reminder about the perils of polypharmacy." *NZ Med J* 128 (1422): 78–79.

Lantz, M. S., et al. (1998). "Serotonin syndrome following the administration of tramadol with paroxetine." *Int J Geriatr Psychiatry* 13 (5): 343–345.

Lantz, R., et al. (2003). "Metabolism, excretion, and pharmacokinetics of duloxetine in healthy human subjects." *Drug Metabolism Dispos* 31 (9): 1142–1150.

Laroudie, C., et al. (2000). "Carbamazepine-nefazodone interaction in healthy subjects." *J Clin Psychopharmacol* 20 (1): 46–53.

Larsen, F., et al. (2001). "Lack of citalopram effect on oral digoxin pharmacokinetics." *J Clin Pharmacol* 41 (3): 340–346.

Laugesen, S., et al. (2005). "Paroxetine, a cytochrome P450 2D6 inhibitor, diminishes the stereoselective O-desmethylation and reduces the hypoalgesic effect of tramadol." *Clin Pharmacol Ther* 77 (4): 312–323.

Lavery, S., Ravi, H., McDaniel, W. W., Pushkin, Y. R. (2001). "Linezolid and Serotonin Syndrome." *Psychosomatics* 42 (5): 432–434.

Lee, E. and E. Emanuel (2013). "Shared decision making to improve care and reduce costs." *NEJM* 368 (1): 6–8.

Leo, R. J. (1996). "Movement disorders associated with the serotonin selective reuptake inhibitors." *J Clin Psychiatry* 57 (10): 449–454.

Lessard, E., et al. (2001). "Diphenhydramine alters the disposition of venlafaxine through inhibition of CYP2D6 activity in humans." *J Clin Psychopharmacol* 21 (2): 175–184.

Leucht, S., et al. (2000). "Effect of adjunctive paroxetine on serum levels and side-effects of tricyclic antidepressants in depressive inpatients." *Psychopharmacology (Berl)* 147 (4): 378–383.

Leucht, S., et al. (2013). "Comparative efficacy and tolerability of 15 antipsychotic drugs in schizophrenia: a multiple-treatments meta-analysis." *Lancet* 382 (9896): 951–962.

Levin, G., et al. (2001). "A pharmacokinetic drug-drug interaction study of venlafaxine and indinavir. Psychopharm Bull." *Psychopharm Bull* 35 (2): 62–71.

Lindh, J. D., et al. (2003). "Effect of ketoconazole on venlafaxine plasma concentrations in extensive and poor metabolisers of debrisoquine." *Eur J Clin Pharmacol* 59 (5–6): 401–406.

Liston, H. L., et al. (2001). "Lack of citalopram effect on the pharmacokinetics of cyclosporine." *Psychosomatics* 42 (4): 370–372.

Liston, H. L., et al. (2002). "Differential time course of cytochrome P450 2D6 enzyme inhibition by fluoxetine, sertraline, and paroxetine in healthy volunteers." *J Clin Psychopharmacol* 22 (2): 169–173.

Lobo, E. D., et al. (2008). "In vitro and in vivo evaluations of cytochrome P450 1A2 interactions with duloxetine." *Clin Pharmacokinet* 47 (3): 191–202.

Loga, S., et al. (1981). "Interaction of chlorpromazine and nortriptyline in patients with schizophrenia." *Clin Pharmacokinet* 6 (6): 454–462.

Lusetti, M., et al. (2015). "Cardiac toxicity in selective serotonin reuptake inhibitor use." *Am J Forensic Med Pathol* **35** (4): 293–297.

Maes, M., et al. (1997). "Effects of trazodone and fluoxetine in the treatment of major depression: therapeutic pharmacokinetic and pharmacodynamic interactions through formation of meta-chlorophenylpiperazine." *J Clin Psychopharmacol* **17** (5): 358–364.

Malhi, G., et al. (2013). "Potential mechanisms of action of lithium in bipolar disorder. Current understanding." *CNS Drugs* **27** (2): 135–153.

Maljuric, N., et al. (2015). "Heart rate corrected QT interval in a real-life setting: the population-based Rotterdam Study." *British J of Clin Psychopharmacology* **80** (4): 698–705.

Mandrioli, R., et al. (2006). "Fluoxetine metabolism and pharmacological interactions: the role of cytochrome p450." *Curr Drug Metab* **7** (2): 127–133.

Mandrioli, R., et al. (2015). "Novel Atypical Antipsychotics: Metabolism and Therapeutic Drug Monitoring (TDM)." *Curr Drug Metab* **16** (2): 141–151.

Mark, T. L., et al. (2009). "Datapoints: Psychotropic Drug Prescriptions by Medical Specialty." *Psychiatr Serv* **60** (9): 1167.

McAlpine, D. E., et al. (2007). "Cytochrome P450 2D6 genotype variation and venlafaxine dosage." *Mayo Clin Proc* **82** (9): 1065–1068.

McCollum, D. L., et al. (2004). "Severe sinus bradycardia after initiation of bupropion therapy: a probable drug-drug interaction with metoprolol." *Cardiovasc Drugs Ther* **18** (4): 329–330.

McIntyre, R., et al. (2016). "The effects of vortioxetine on cognitive function in patients with major depressive disorder: a meta-analysis of three randomized controlled trials." *Int J Neuropsychopharmacol* **pii**: pyw055.

Miceli, J. J., et al. (2007). "The effect of food on the absorption of oral ziprasidone." *Psychopharmacol Bull* **40** (3): 58–68.

Mihara, K., et al. (1997). "Increases in plasma concentration of m-chlorophenylpiperazine, but not trazodone, with low-dose haloperidol." *Ther Drug Monit* **19** (1): 43–45.

Miller, O., et al. (2016). "Two cellular hypotheses explaining the initiation of ketamine's antidepressant actions: direct inhibition and disinhibition." *Neuropharmacology* **100**: 17–26.

Mizuno, Y., et al. (2014). "Pharmacological strategies to counteract antipsychotic-induced weight gain and metabolic adverse effects in schizophrenia: a systematic review and meta-analysis." *Schizophr Bull* **40** (6): 1385–1403.

Moller, S. E., et al. (2001). "Lack of effect of citalopram on the steady-state pharmacokinetics of carbamazepine in healthy male subjects." *J Clin Psychopharmacol* **21** (5): 493–499.

Moscovich, D. G. (1993). "Lithium neurotoxicity at normal therapeutic levels." *Br J Psychiatry* **163**: 410–412.

Munhoz, R. P. (2004). "Serotonin syndrome induced by a combination of bupropion and SSRIs." *Clin Neuropharmacol* **27** (5): 219–222.

Nakimuli-Mpungu, E., et al. (2013). "Lifetime depressive disorders and adherence to anti-retroviral therapy in HIV-infected Ugandan adults: a case-control study." *J Affect Discord* **145** (2): 221–226.

Nel, A. and A. Kagee (2013). "The relationship between depression, anxiety and medication adherence among patients receiving antiretroviral treatment in South Africa." *AIDS Care* **25** (8): 948–955.

Newport, D., et al. (2015). "Ketamine and other NMDA antagonists: early clinical trials and possible mechanisms in depression." *Am J Psychiatry* **172** (10): 950–966.

Ninan, P. T. (2001). "Pharmacokinetically induced benzodiazepine withdrawal." *Psychopharmacol Bull* **35** (4): 94–100.

O'Brien, F. E., et al. (2012). "Interactions between antidepressants and P-glycoprotein at the blood0brain barrier: clinical significance of invitro and in vivo findings." *Br J Pharmacol* **165** (2): 289–312.

Oesterheld, J. (2009). "Transporters." In G. Wynn, J. Oesterheld, K. Cozza and S (eds.), *Clinical Manual of Drug Interactions for Medical Practice* (pp. 43–72). Armstrong. Washington, DC: American Psychiatric Press.

Ohno, Y., et al. (2007). "General framework for the quantitative prediction of CYP3A4-mediated oral drug interactions based on the AUC increase by coadministration of standard drugs." *Clin Pharmacokinet* **46** (8): 681–696.

Olyaei, A. J., et al. (1998). "Interaction between tacrolimus and nefazodone in a stable renal transplant recipient." *Pharmacotherapy* **18** (6): 1356–1359.

Orsolini, L., et al. (2016). "Current and future perspectives on the Major Depressive Disorder: Focus on the new multimodal antidepressant Vortioxetine." *CNS Neurol Disord Drug Targets* 16 (1): 65–92.

Otani, K., et al. (1996). "Effects of carbamazepine coadministration on plasma concentrations of trazodone and its active metabolite, m-chlorophenylpiperazine." *Ther Drug Monit* **18** (2): 164–167.

Otton, S. V., et al. (1996). "Venlafaxine oxidation in vitro is catalysed by CYP2D6." *Br J Clin Pharmacol* **41** (2): 149–156.

Outhred, T., et al. (2013). "Acute neural effects of selective serotonin reuptake inhibitors versus noradrenaline reuptake inhibitors on emotion processing: implications for differential treatment efficacy." *Neurosci Biobehav Rev* 37 (8): 1786–1800.

Ozdemir, V., et al. (1997). "Paroxetine potentiates the central nervous system side effects of perphenazine: contribution of cytochrome P4502D6 inhibition in vivo." *Clin Pharmacol Ther* **62** (3): 334–347.

Paris, B., et al. (2009). "In Vitro Inhibition and Induction of Human Liver Cytochrome P450 Enzymes by Milnacipran." *Drug Metab Dispos* 37 (10): 2045–2054.

Park, J., et al. (2010). "Dose-related reduction in bupropion plasma concentrations by ritonavir." *J Clin Pharmacol* **50** (10): 1180–1187.

Park-Wyllie, L. and T. Antoniou (2003). "Concurrent use of bupropion with CYP2B6 inhibitors, nelfinavir, ritonavir and efavirenz: a case series." *Aids* **17** (4): 638–640.

Penzak, S., et al. (2002). "Influence of ritonavir on olanzapine pharmacokinetics in healthy volunteers." *J Clin Psychopharmacol* **22** (4): 366–370.

Perahia, D., et al. (2005). "Symptoms following abrupt discontinuation of duloxetine treatment in patients with major depressive disorder." *J Affect Disord* **89** (1–3): 270–212.

Perahia, D., et al. (2013). "The risk of bleeding with duloxetine treatment in patients who use nonsteroidal anti-inflammatory drugs (NSAIDs): analysis of placebo-controlled trials and post-marketing adverse event reports." *Drug Healthc Patient Saf* **5**: 211–219.

Pihlsgard, M. and E. Eliasson (2002). "Significant reduction of sertraline plasma levels by carbamazepine and phenytoin." *Eur J Clin Pharmacol* **57** (12): 915–916.

Pogliani, L., et al. (2010). "Paroxetine and neonatal withdrawal syndrome." *BMJ Case Rep* **2010**: bcr12.2009.2528.

Prapotnik, M., et al. (2004). "Therapeutic drug monitoring of trazodone: are there pharmacokinetic interactions involving citalopram and fluoxetine?" *Int J Clin Pharmacol Ther* **42** (2): 120–124.

Preskorn, S. H., et al. (1994). "Pharmacokinetics of desipramine coadministered with sertraline or fluoxetine." *J Clin Psychopharmacol* **14**: 90–98.

Quinn, D. K. and T. A. Stern (2009). "Linezolid and Serotonin Syndrome." *Primary Care Companion to The Journal of Clinical Psychiatry* **11** (6): 353–356.

Radominska-Pandya, A., et al. (2002). "Nuclear UDP-glucuronosyltransferases: identification of UGT2B7 and UGT1A6 in human liver nuclear membranes." *Arch Biochem Biophys* **399** (1): 37–48.

Rao, N. (2007). "The clinical pharmacokinetics of escitalopram." *Clin Pharmacokinet* **46** (4): 281–290.

Rasheed, A., et al. (1994). "Interaction of chlorpromazine with tricyclic anti-depressants in schizophrenic patients." *J Pak Med Assoc* **44** (10): 233–234.

Richter, T., et al. (2004). "Potent mechanism-based inhibition of human CYP2B6 by clopidogrel and ticlopidine." *J Pharmacol Exp Ther* **308** (1): 189–197.

Ring, B. J., et al. (2001). "Identification of the human cytochromes P450 responsible for in vitro formation of R- and S-norfluoxetine." *J Pharmacol Exp Ther* **297** (3): 1044–1050.

Robertson, S. M., et al. (2008). "Efavirenz induces CYP2B6-mediated hydroxylation of bupropion in healthy subjects." *J Acquir Immune Defic Syndr* **49** (5): 513–519.

Roerig, P. (2016) Zoloft Package Insert. *labeling.pfizer.com*

Rotzinger, S., et al. (1999). "Metabolism of some 'second'- and 'fourth'-generation antidepressants: iprindole, viloxazine, bupropion, mianserin, maprotiline, trazodone, nefazodone, and venlafaxine." *Cell Mol Neurobiol* **19** (4): 427–442.

Rotzinger, S., et al. (1998). "Trazodone is metabolized to m-chlorophenylpiperazine by CYP3A4 from human sources." *Drug Metab Dispos* **26** (6): 572–575.

Rutherford, B., et al. (2016) "Patient Expectancy as a Mediator of Placebo Effects in Antidepressant Clinical Trials." HYPERLINK "https://www.ncbi.nlm.nih.gov/pubmed/27609242" \o "The American journal of psychiatry." *Am J Psychiatry* **174** (2): 135–142.

Sagud, M., et al. (2009). "Smoking and schizophrenia." *Psychiatr Danub* **21** (3): 371–375.

Samartzis, L., et al. (2013). "Linezolid is associated with serotonin syndrome in a patient receiving amitriptyline, and fentanyl: a case report and review of the literature." *Case Reports in Psychiatry* **2013**: 617251.

Sanchez, C., et al. (2004). "Escitalopram versus citalopram: the surprising role of the R-enantiomer." *Psychopharmocology (Berl)* **174** (2): 163–176.

Schatzberg, A. and C. Nemeroff (2011). *The American Psychiatric Publishing Textbook of Psychopharmacology.* Washington, DC: American Psychiatric Publishing.

Schillevoort, I., et al. (2002). "Extrapyramidal syndromes associated with selective serotonin reuptake inhibitors: a case-control study using spontaneous reports." *Int Clin Psychopharmacol* **17** (2): 75–79.

Shi, S., et al. (2010). "Comparative Bioavailability and tolerability of a single 20-mg dose of two fluoxetine hydrochloride dispersible tablet formulations in fasting, health, Chinese male volunteers: an open-label, randomized-sequence, two-period crossover study." *Clin Ther* **32** (11): 1977–1986.

Sitsen, J., et al. (2001). "Drug-drug interaction studies with mirtazapine and carbamazepine in healthy male subjects." *Eur J Drug Metab Pharmacokinet* **26** (1–2): 109–121.

Sitsen, J. M., et al. (2000). "Concomitant use of mirtazapine and cimetidine: a drug-drug interaction study in healthy male subjects." *Eur J Clin Pharmacol* **56** (5): 389–394.

Skinner, M. H., et al. (2003). "Duloxetine is both an inhibitor and a substrate of cytochrome P4502D6 in healthy volunteers." *Clin Pharmacol Ther* **73** (3): 170–177.

Skrabal, M. Z., et al. (2003). "Rhabdomyolysis associated with simvastatin-nefazodone therapy." *South Med J* **96** (10): 1034–1035.

Speirs, J. and S. R. Hirsch (1978). "Severe lithium toxicity with 'normal' serum concentrations." *Br Med J* **1** (6116): 815–816.

Spina, E., et al. (2001). "Plasma concentrations of risperidone and 9-hydroxyrisperidone during combined treatment with paroxetine." *Ther Drug Monit* **23** (3): 223–227.

Spina E, A. A., et al. (2002). "Inhibition of risperidone metabolism by fluoxetine in patients with schizophrenia: a clinically relevant pharmacokinetic drug interaction." *J Clin Psychopharmacol* **22** (4): 419–423.

Spina, E., et al. (2003). "Metabolic drug interactions with new psychotropic agents." *Fundam Clin Pharmacol* **17** (5): 517–538.

Spina, E., et al. (2012). "Clinically significant drug interactions with newer antidepressants." *CNS Drugs* **26** (1): 39–67.

Stahl, S., et al. (2004). "A review of the neuropharmacology of bupropion, a dual norepinephrine and dopamine reuptake inhibitor." *Prim Care Companion J Clin Psychiatry* **6** (4): 159–166.

Stahl, S. (2013). *Stahl's Essential Psychopharmacology: Neuroscientific Basis and Practical Applications*. New York, NY: Cambridge University Press.

Stevens, D. L., et al. (2004). "A review of linezolid: the first oxazolidinone antibiotic." *Expert Rev Anti Infect Ther* **2** (1): 51–59.

Stewart, D. E. (2002). "Hepatic adverse reactions associated with nefazodone." *Can J Psychiatry* **47** (4): 375–377.

Störmer, E., et al. (2000). "Metabolism of the antidepressant mirtazapine in vitro: contribution of cytochromes P-450 1A2, 2D6, and 3A4." *Drug Metab Dispos* **28** (10): 1168–1175.

Strain, J., et al. (2004). "Psychotropic drug versus psychotropic drug-update." *Gen Hosp Psychiatry* **26**: 87–105.

Strolin Benedetti, M., et al. (2007). "Factors affecting the relative importance of amine oxidase and monooxygenases in the in vivo metabolism of xenobiotic amines in humans." *J Neural Transm (Vienna)* **114** (6): 787–791.

Taylor, D. (1995). "Selective serotonin reuptake inhibitors and tricyclic antidepressants in combination. Interactions and therapeutic uses." *Br J Psychiatry* **167** (5): 575–580.

Terada, T. and D. Hira (2015). "Intestinal and hepatic drug transporters: pharmacokinetic, pathophysiological, and pharmacogenetic roles." *J Gastroenterol* **50** (5): 508–519.

Timmer, C. J., et al. (2000). "Clinical pharmacokinetics of mirtazapine." *Clin Pharmacokinet* **38** (6): 461–474.

Tirkkonen, T. and K. Laine (2004). "Drug interactions with the potential to prevent prodrug activation as a common source of irrational prescribing in hospital inpatients." *Clin Pharmacol Ther* **76** (6): 639–647.

Troy, S. M., et al. (1998). "The influence of cimetidine on the disposition kinetics of the antidepressant venlafaxine." *J Clin Pharmacol* **38** (5): 467–474.

Uchaipichat, V., et al. (2011). "Effects of ketamine on human UDP-glucuronosyltransferases in vitro predict potential drug-drug interactions arising from ketamine inhibition of codeine and morphine." *Drug Metab Dispos* **39** (8): 1324–1328.

Vande Griend, J. P. and S. L. Anderson (2012). "Histamine-1 receptor antagonism for treatment of insomnia." *J Am Pharm Assoc (2003)* **52** (6): e210–219.

Vandenberghe, F., et al. (2015). "Genetics-based population pharmacokinetics and pharmacodynamics of risperidone in a psychiatric cohort." *Clin Pharmacokinet* **54** (12): 1259–1272.

Vaughan, D. (1988). "Interactions of fluoxetine with tricyclic antidepressants." *Am J Psychiatry* **145** (1): 1478.

Von Ammon Cavanaugh, S. (1990). "Drug-drug interactions of fluoxetine with tricyclics." *Psychosomatics* **31** (3): 273–276.

von Moltke, L. L., et al. (1997). "Venlafaxine and metabolites are very weak inhibitors of human cytochrome P450-3A isoforms." *Biol Psychiatry* **41** (3): 377–380.

von Moltke, L. L., et al. (1999). "Nefazodone, meta-chlorophenylpiperazine, and their metabolites in vitro: cytochromes mediating transformation, and P450-3A4 inhibitory actions." *Psychopharmacology (Berl)* **145** (1): 113–122.

von Moltke, L. L., et al. (2001). "Escitalopram (S-citalopram) and its metabolites in vitro: cytochromes mediating biotransformation, inhibitory effects, and comparison to R-citalopram." *Drug Metab Dispos* **29** (8): 1102–1109.

von Wincklemann, S., et al. (2008). "Therapeutic drug monitoring of phenytoin in critically ill patients." *Pharmacotherapy* **28** (11): 1391–1400.

Waring, W., et al. (2010). "Evaluation of a QT nomogram for risk assessment after antidepressant overdose." *Br J Clin Psychopharmacol* **70** (6): 881–885.

Wienkers, L. C., et al. (1999). "Cytochrome P-450-mediated metabolism of the individual enantiomers of the antidepressant agent reboxetine in human liver microsomes." *Drug Metab Dispos* **27** (11): 1334–1340.

Wiseman, C. (2012). "Does bupropion exacerbate anxiety?." Curr Psychiatr **11** (6): E3–4.

Wright, D. H., et al. (1999). "Nefazodone and cyclosporine drug-drug interaction." *J Heart Lung Transplant* **18** (9): 913–915.

Wu, R., et al. (2016). "Metformin treatment of antipsychotic-induced dyslipidemia: an analysis of two randomized, placebo-controlled trials." *Molecular Psychiatry* **21**: 1537–1544.

Wynn, G., et al. (2009). *Clinical Manual of Drug Interaction Principles for Medical Practice.* Washington, DC: American Psychiatric Publishing.

Zalma, A., et al. (2000). "In vitro metabolism of trazodone by CYP3A: inhibition by ketoconazole and human immunodeficiency viral protease inhibitors." *Biol Psychiatry* **47** (7): 655–661.

Zorina, O., et al. (2013). "Comparative performance of two drug interaction screening programmes analysing a cross-sectional prescription dataset of 84,625 psychiatric inpatients." *Drug Saf* **36** (4): 247–258.

Zullino, D., et al. (2002). "Tobacco and cannabis smoking cessation can lead to intoxication with clozapine or olanzapine." *Int Clin Psychopharmacol* **17** (3): 141–143.

Celexa. (2014). CELEXA-citalopram hydrobromide tablet, film coated. New York, Forest Laboratories, Inc. https://medlibrary.org/lib/rx/meds/celexa-3/. Accessed November 18, 2017.

Cymbalta. (2016). CYMBALTA (duloxetine delayed-release capsules) for oral use. Indianapolis, Eli Lilly and Company. http://pi.lilly.com/us/cymbalta-pi.pdf. Accessed November 19, 2017.

Otsuks. (2016). Abilify, manufacturere's website: https://www.otsuka-us.com/media/static/Abilify-PI.pdf?_ga=2.251074753.631697756.1515971908-192168919.1515971908. Accessed January 14, 2018.

Serzone. (2004). SERZONE® (nefazodone hydrochloride). New York, Bristol-Meyers-Squibb. https://www.fda.gov/ohrms/dockets/ac/04/briefing/2004-4065b1-25-tab11F-Serzone-SLR034.pdf. Accessed November 19, 2017.

(2013)   Latuda package insert.

(2014)   Med Library.

(2015)   Rexulti (brexpiprazole) Prescribing Information.

(2015)   Saphris (asenapine) Package insert. St. Louis, Missouri.

(2015)   Zyprexa-Eli Lilly and Company.

(2015)   Zyprexa Prescribing Information.

(2016)   Abilify Prescribing Information.

(2016)   Wellbutrin.

11

Diagnostic Dilemmas

James J. Strain, Patricia Casey, and Peter Tyrer

Diagnosis is obviously an essential component of treatment. To date, the diagnosis of depression is subjective, phenomenologically driven, and has no universal biological or genetic markers. This makes it difficult at times to distinguish normality from pathology. Phenomenological definitions may be reliable but are not necessarily valid. A new conceptual framework for the diagnosis of depression is mandatory for clinicians to move forward and especially if the diagnosis and treatment of depression—a systemic disease—is to migrate more intensively toward primary care medicine and other non-psychiatric service delivery personnel. These seminal issues will be elaborated upon in this chapter.

NORMALITY VERSUS PATHOLOGY IN PSYCHIATRIC DISORDERS

As Casey has described there is a need to distinguish between normal adaptive responses from recognized disorders.[1] For decades, the distinction between psychiatric disorders—distinct from each other—and from normality has exercised the most important philosophical and psychiatric minds.[2-4] The thinking is that discrete categorical disorders should possess natural boundaries from each other and from normal distress, a perspective that is deeply rooted in the disease entity assumption.

The cleavage that separates various diagnostic categories from each other and from normality is called a *zone of rarity*. Using this concept, there should be a clear demarcation between those who were ill and those who were not, with few, if any, in the intermediate zone. This is the approach used in general medicine, where various diseases are recognized and distinguished from others by their symptoms, etiology, pathophysiology, course and prognosis, and their response to treatment. The process involved in each of these domains is termed *validation*. For example, sickle cell anemia is either present or absent (with only a small cohort where there is uncertainty); this model does not apply to all medical conditions. Similar to most common mental illnesses, obesity and hypertension are examples of conditions that exist on a continuum.

It was envisaged by the architects of the *Diagnostic and Statistical Manual of Mental Disorders III* (DSM-III; APA 1980)[5] that, over time, the descriptive approach to classification would allow the validation of the various diagnoses. These would be the foundations for research by relating them to genetics, psychobiology, treatment, and so on. This has not been realized. Some have suggested that DSM-5 should have defined as mental disorders the syndromal categories that have been validated[6,7] based on key measures such as prognostic significance, evidence of psychobiological disruption, or prediction of response to treatment. (Unfortunately, only one biological marker is listed in this most recent taxonomy—for narcolepsy—and DSM-5 therefore remains a phenomenologically driven classification of disorders).

One of the problems is that in psychopathology, "zones of rarity" do not exist between various psychiatric conditions, especially the common mental disorders such as major depression, adjustment disorder, post-traumatic stress disorder (PTSD), and generalized anxiety, etc. The symptoms of one condition are also often found in others, calling into question the validity of many of the syndromes conventionally regarded as discrete psychiatric disorders.[4] The impact of the failure to find "zones of rarity" is that definitive diagnosis has become difficult. So diagnostic categories are heterogenous, and symptoms of one condition are present in others.

Major depression, for example, is not a single entity as is commonly believed, but can have different manifestations and responses to treatment. Symptoms of abnormal grief overlap with those of major depression; adjustment disorder overlaps with major depression,[8] and PTSD symptoms such as intrusive memories may be found in major depression.[9] This tendency to falsely diagnose a psychiatric disorder when there is none is referred to as the *false-positive dilemma*.

The consequences of false diagnoses in those who are not mentally ill are well recognized. These include the medicalization of ordinary suffering; the use of interventions (pharmacological or psychological) for emotional responses where none are needed, since most of those reactions are self-limiting; the possible stigmatization of those so diagnosed; the implications for those newly seeking health insurance coverage who have been so diagnosed; and the change in self-perspective that a person experiences when diagnosed with a psychiatric disorder. Finally, identifying an illness when there is none may inflate prevalence data in epidemiological studies, and in those experiencing continuing sadness, may increase beliefs about chronicity.

In response to the false-positive challenge, DSM-5 has adopted a particular approach to minimize this. Judging what constitutes a normal or expectable response, as against a pathological one, in a particular context requires wisdom in the absence of any assistance from science. This is important, as the reach of psychiatry increasingly extends into the management of common mental disorders, with a concomitant danger of pathologizing normal responses. Clearly, the incorporation of clinical significance is helpful in reducing the false-positive rate.

THE DISTRESS-IMPAIRMENT CRITERION

In attempting to define what a psychiatric disorder is, stimulated by a discussion regarding homosexuality, Robert Spitzer proposed that psychiatric illness in its manifestations should be associated with clinically significant distress or impairment in social, occupational, or other important areas of functioning.

Critics of the DSM system point out that the clinical significance criterion is tautological,[10] since it is merely saying that symptoms are clinically significant if they are judged to be clinically significant by doctors treating them! No further operationalization of this is provided. But what if *both* distress due to symptoms and functional impairment were required rather than one or the other? This might further strengthen the boundary between normal responses to problems of living and recognized mental disorders. The superior power of functional impairment as a predictor of outcome compared to symptom severity has been demonstrated,[11] suggesting that it warrants serious attention in the assessment of symptoms.

This heterogeneity stems from the fact that not all the specified symptoms are required to make the diagnosis, and all are regarded as equally important. This is known as the *polythetic* approach and is the one used by the DSM. So individuals with the same diagnosis present with diverse clinical pictures. One way to address this would be to require that certain symptoms might be essential to making the diagnosis of PTSD; e.g., flashbacks, re-experiencing the trauma. (It is clear that PTSD criterion A requires a traumatic stressor, but even this single requirement can be questioned—when is a stressor traumatic?) This would represent the *monothetic* approach in which each category is associated with specific criteria, all of which are considered essential to that category's definition (also called *classical categorization*). A mixed approach would include symptoms that were weighted more heavily than others in contributing to a particular diagnosis.

Thresholds: One must ask if the threshold cut-offs have been derived scientifically or pragmatically. The decision on a cut-off for the threshold is often an arbitrary one, since there are no natural boundaries. If the symptom threshold is not met, or the distress/impairment criteria are not met, then the diagnosis cannot be made. Arguably, this should lead to the assumption that no disorder is present.

THE DIMENSIONAL APPROACH

In light of the absence of zones of rarity between different psychiatric disorders and between normality and mental illness, some have proposed the use of dimensional measures instead of categorical labels,[4,12] or, alternatively, a combination of both to augment each other. The dimensions might range from biological measures, to symptom severity scores or measures of social functioning, although little work has been done on these. Yet for all the problems with the categorical approach, there is no agreement on what dimensions should be measured or to which diagnostic groups they should apply. Importantly, a dimensional approach would not assist in deciding on the boundary between what a normal reaction to stress is and what is pathological, unless the cut-off point was defined by research evidence.

In an attempt to capture the continuum from normality to pathology that is the hallmark of mental illness, DSM-5 (APA 2013)[6] has incorporated a dimensional as well as categorical approach. In this way, the gradient in domains that are obscured by a simple categorical approach can be captured. The process involves three stages—the first measures 12 core domains (anger, depression, psychosis, personality functioning, and so on) using 23 self-rated questions in adults. This is known as the "Level 1 Cross Cutting Measure." A score of 2 (mild) out of 5 on any item requires the application of a level 2 Cross

Cutting Symptom Measure to provide more detailed information on the level of symptoms within that domain. For example: those scoring in the level 1 depression domain would be administered the Patient Reported Outcome Measurement Information System Emotional Distress-Depression–Short Form at level 2, and this could be used to establish the severity of symptoms and track them over time. The third stage would involve a clinical assessment to make a diagnosis. DSM-5 also includes the World Health Organization (WHO) Disability Assessment Schedule, which can be used to track changes in overall functioning as clinically indicated.

Notwithstanding the attempts to introduce dimensional measures into DSM-5, it is questionable if these will be used, since the dimensional measures that were incorporated in DSM-IV, such as measures of severity and the 100-point Global Assessment of Functioning (GAF) were seldom employed either in practice or in research,[12] possibly because they were regarded as burdensome. One skeptic comments that dimensions are "appealing ideas whose time has not yet arrived."[12] It is also unclear if the combined use of dimensions and categories will assist in separating normal from pathological responses to stress.

CLINICAL JUDGMENT

The original idea behind DSM-III (APA 1980)[5] was to improve the reliability of psychiatric diagnosis, a source of great difficulty before that, which relied heavily on the vagaries of clinical judgment. In deciding where to draw the line between reactions that are normal and those that are pathological, DSM has attempted to deal with this using the clinical significance (symptoms or impairment) and threshold criteria, since there are no zones of rarity as discussed before. Yet many commentators are agreed that this approach is unsatisfactory.[13]

Clinical judgment, it seems, cannot be operationalized, and the problem of overdiagnosis based on the approach of DSM continues to be a concern. There are those who believe that, despite the value set by DSM-III (1980)[5] and DSM-IV (1994)[14] and restated by DSM-5 (APA 2013)[6] on clinical judgment alongside the application of specific criteria, diagnosis has become largely a cursory exercise, divorced from the thorough clinical assessment and reflective approach recommended by these manuals.[15] They argue that the bottom-up approach in which detailed information is gleamed from the patient, third parties, and an evaluation of the person's life history has been replaced by one that is top-down in which diagnosis is based on symptom checklists. A WHO survey of psychiatrists internationally found that the majority wanted diagnostic manuals to contain flexible guidance so that clinical judgment could be factored into diagnostic decision-making rather than having fixed diagnostic criteria.[16] Others have called for clinicians to make the decision as to whether a response to a stressor was proportionate or excessive,[13] while some saw this as "more a step backward than forward for our field," pointing to the subjectivity of deciding on "understandability."[17]

It requires clinical training to recognize when the combination of predisposing, precipitating, perpetuating, and protective factors has resulted in a psychopathological condition in which physical signs and symptoms exceed "normal ranges." The DSM-5 manual places much emphasis on clinical judgment. The fact is that if judgment plays such a major role in determining what is normal and what is excessive in response to psychosocial stressors, it places a huge onus on the clinician. In the absence of biological markers to demarcate the boundaries between various disorders, we are only left with our clinical judgment.

PHENOMENOLOGY, DSM, AND RELIABILITY

It is a matter of argument whether phenomenology is a science. Science depends on measurement and independent validation, and the phenomenology of mental illness constitutes a formal description of the subjective experiences of psychiatric patients without any independent confirmation that they are true. The subjective experiences of a patient with delirium associated with physical illness and those of schizophrenia can be remarkably similar, but the causes are very different. But this does not make phenomenology valueless. If there is no good way of communicating the experiences of patients to others, every single psychiatric phenomenon becomes a unique event that will never again be experienced in the same way. The advantage of phenomenology is that it groups the common elements of psychiatric disorders in a meaningful way. The meaning may not be necessarily a manifestation of truth, but it represents a practical way of communicating between professionals and also aids to some extent in diagnosis.

Psychiatric classifications rely on a mix of hard objective data (e.g., a magnetic resonance imaging [MRI] scan), softer objective data (e.g., neuropsychological testing), and careful clinical observation (observed behavior, symptoms and phenomenology). Before DSM-III was published in 1980, these classifications were in disarray as, although consistency of diagnosis could be achieved within an individual over the course of time, there was tremendous inconsistency between psychiatrists in their interpretations of mental manifestations of illness.[5]

As recently as the early 1970s, there was a considerable divergence of opinion between American and British psychiatrists in the diagnosis of schizophrenia. This culminated in the U.S./U.K. Diagnostic Project[18,19] in which clinicians in both settings assessed vignettes of psychiatric patients and came to a set of poor agreement levels that was worst for the diagnosis of schizophrenia. The Washington school, under the far-seeing Samuel Guze, was also a major influence, helping to remove the notion that somatic symptoms were equivalent to conversion symptoms,[20] defining the importance of follow-up studies,[21,22] and setting forth the notion that diagnosis might be best made by clearly defined operational criteria.[23]

When we move on 40 years, the self-confidence of these pioneers has been replaced with a heavy aura of doubt. Successive DSM revisions have come in for greater criticism than their predecessors, and the absence of any independent validation has troubled those responsible for reforming classification systems. Thus David Kupfer, the chair of the DSM-5 Task Force, wrote gloomily at the beginning of their deliberations that it was disturbing that "not one laboratory marker has been found to be specific in identifying any of the DSM-defined syndromes." (One diagnosis, of narcolepsy, does have a biological marker). Epidemiological and clinical studies have shown extremely high rates of comorbidity among the disorders, undermining the hypothesis that the syndromes represent distinct etiologies. Furthermore, epidemiological studies have shown a high degree of short-term diagnostic instability for many disorders. With regard to treatment, lack of treatment specificity is the rule rather than the exception.[24]

There are now many people who are getting disillusioned with the DSM classification, as it gives a spurious impression of solidity in diagnostic practice that is lacking for so many disorders.[25] The considered view that diagnosis is still developing but is overall going forward is expressed by Craddock and Mynors-Wallis[26]: They write that the future is likely to require a willingness to use both categorical and dimensional approaches. It will also be necessary to ensure consistency between the diagnoses used in all aspects of medicine that relate to brain and behavioral disorders. Further, like all medical classifications, it is likely to involve a pragmatic mix of approaches that reflect the differing levels of understanding of each diagnostic entity.

Few would disagree that some form of classification is essential to communicate effectively with colleagues and with the general public, and if every problem is considered unique, there is little to be gained from previous knowledge. The success of DSM-III was largely grounded on the evidence that it was possible for psychiatrists to agree on diagnostic categories at a sufficiently acceptable level. There was no need to write reams of qualifying information to communicate the essential nature of the conditions, so it was a great step forward.

What has been realized in the ensuing years is that good reliability is not enough to make a good diagnosis. Trained assessors can always achieve good reliability, but a highly reliable diagnosis can still be completely invalid. As a consequence, the emphasis on operational criteria as the gold standard of diagnosis has suffered a serious knock, and subsequent editions of DSM, despite accommodating this concern, have been viewed much more circumspectly and often critically, especially when they seem to expand to include what many would consider as normal variation that is not pathological.[27]

THE IMPACT OF RESEARCH DOMAIN CRITERIA (RDOC) ON DIAGNOSIS

The National Institute of Mental Health (NIMH) in the United States is at the forefront of research development. So, when it makes pungent criticisms of both DSM and the *International Classification of Diseases 11th Ed.* (ICD-11) and formulates a radically different model of classification of mental disorders, it is bound to lead to a great deal of debate and rethinking. The Research Domain Criteria (RDoC) model proposed by Thomas Insel of NIMH and his colleagues uses, probably correctly, the overused phrase "paradigm shift" in reviewing the classification of mental disorders.[28] It does not accept the traditional view of mental disorders as symptom complexes that can be identified through clinical description. Instead, it examines the primary behavioral functions of the brain and the neural systems that are responsible for implementing this behavior.

UNDERSTANDING THE RESEARCH DOMAIN CRITERIA FORMAT (RDOC)

In an attempt to "speed the translation of new knowledge to classifying mental disorders based on dimensions of observable behavior and neurobiological measures," the NIMH under its former director Tom Insel promoted a strategy named the RDoC Project (http://www.nimh.nih.gov//index.shtml). It is important to note this was not initially proposed for the clinical setting, but was focused on research investigation offering a guide to the classification of patients for research studies, not as an immediately useful clinical tool.

The goal is to build a sufficient research foundation that can best inform the best approaches for clinical diagnosis and treatment. It is hoped that by creating a framework that interfaces directly with genomics, neuroscience, and behavioral science, progress in explicating etiology and suggesting new treatments will be markedly facilitated. It does, however, offer a template for reconceptualizing diagnoses in the psychiatric setting.

The RDoC concept is organized around basic neural circuits, their genetic and molecular/cellular building blocks and the dimensions of function that they implement. The intent of the RDoC matrix will enhance the study of both developmental aspects and interactions with the environment by promoting a systematic focus on their relationship to specific circuits and functions (http://www.nimh.nih.gov//index.shtml).

Cuthbert and Insel[29] recently reformulated the Seven Pillars of RDoC (Table 11.1). The word "domain" is an appropriate one here because it describes the territory of disorder. Rather than walling off specific areas for diagnostic purposes, it asks the clinician to look at the whole area covered by the symptoms or behavior. The same general principle has been used in the ICD-11's revised classification of personality disorder.[30] Understandably, the link between neural mechanisms and behavior in most psychiatric disorders is a long way off.

Another overall schema of the essential elements embodied in the RDoC conceptual framework is presented (Table 11.2).[31] It is apparent that there are *five domains*— constructs: (1) negative valence systems, (2) positive valence systems, (3) cognitive

Table 11.1 The Seven Pillars of RDoC

The Seven Pillars of RDoC	*Central Elements of Pillar*
Translational research perspective	Basic science is the driving force behind the classification
Dimensional approach to Classification	Need to accommodate the full range of normality and pathology
Reliable and valid measures of diagnosis	Need for measures that are not artificially diagnosis-specific and that cover the range of all pathology
Broader design of research studies	Need to acknowledge that treatments are effective across a range of disorders and the important variables are rarely diagnostic ones
Integration of behavior and neural science	Neural science determines behavior, and this should never be forgotten
Concentration on core concepts	Acceptance that a large number of disorders in DSM and ICD have limited validity and sustainability
Flexibility in accommodating new concepts	Currently too much attention is being paid to a range of specific DSM disorders that interfere with the evaluation of new ideas that may be of much greater heuristic value

Table 11.2 The RDoC Levels of Information

Domins			Levels of information					
		Genes	Molecules	cells	Circuits	Physiology	Behavior	Self-Report
Negative Valence Systems	Acute threat		GABA		Autonomic NS	HR, BP, Resp	Avoidance	"Fear"
	Potential threat		Cortisol			Startle reflex	Worry	"Anxiety"
	Sustained threat		ACTH		Vigilance Network	HPA	Avoidance	"Fatigue"
	Loss	5-HTTLPR	Glucocorticoid		Reward Circuit	HPA	Depression	"Sadness"
	Frustrative nonreward	5HTR	Serotonin		Amygdala-ACC		Withdrawal/ Aggression	"Helpless"
Positive Valence Systems	Approach Motivation		Dopamine		Basal ganglia	HR	Conditioning	"Craving"
	Initial Responsiveness to Reward		Endocannabinoids		Lateral hypothalamus		Appetite	"Hunger"
	Sustained Responsiveness to Reward		hypocretin		VM hypothalmus		Satiety	"Binge eating"
	Reward Learning		Dopamine		Striatum		Addiction	"Urges"
	Habit		Serotonin		Basal ganglia		Compulsions "	"Obsessions"
Cognitive Systems	Attention		Acetylcholine		Attention networks	EEG	Delirium	Attentional testing
	Perception		NMDA	Pyramidal	Various		Psychosis	Hallucinations
	Declarative Memory				hippocampal circuits		Poor recall	memory problems

Domain / Construct	Molecules	Circuits	Physiology	Behavior	Self-Report
Language		Various		Aphasia	language problems
Cognitive contro		DLPFC		Impulsivity D	Disorganized
Working memory	Glutamate	DLPFC		ADHD	Poor concentration
Social Processes — Affiliation and Attachment			immune response	Attachment	anxiety
Social Communication				Verbal/Non-Verbal	loneliness
Perception and Understaning of Self				Delusions	Paranoia
Perception and Understanding of Others				Empathy	Love
Arousal and Regulatory — Arousal	Hypocretin	hypothalamic	Autonomic	waking	"not restful sleep"
Circadian Rhythms	Melatonin	Suprachiasmatic nucleus		sleep-wake	"insomnia"
Sleep and Wakefulness	GABA	Mesopontine nuclei	EEG	Parasomnias	"night terror"

Elements of the current RdoC Matrix November 2016. Examples which are clinically used are highlighted green with examples.

symptoms, (4) social processes, (5) arousal and regulatory systems. This is companioned by *seven levels of information*: (1) genes, (2) molecules, (3) cells, (4) circuits, (5) physiology, (6) behavior, and (7) self-reports. Table 11.2 shows where certain information is currently available; e.g., molecules, circuits, behavior, self-reports; but also where there are major omissions of knowledge; e.g., minimal information regarding genes and cells.

The RDoC Matrix (Table 11.2) reveals that psychiatrists regularly utilize molecular and circuit models to understand and treat patients with deficits in various domains (threat, loss, reward learning, habit, cognitive systems, and rousal/regulatory systems). For example, "acute threat" is a well-understood phenomenon with measurable physiological phenomena—e.g., blood pressure, heart rate—while bio-markers for molecular and cellular targets are still lacking. Working-memory problems attentional disabilities that cross various neuropsychiatric disorders are correlated with slowing on the EEG, but full understanding of their impact on cellular dysfunction is lacking. Arousal, sleep, and wakefulness have powerful molecular targets, including hypocretin deficiency, along with objective measures beyond behavior and self-report; yet genetic testing and targets are only current goals.

The neurobiology of psychiatric disorders is complex and multidimensional. This tabular representation of what is known and what is needed is essential to the development of a new taxonomy. Genetic assessments from "big data" integrated with other levels of information will also advance diagnosis and treatment.

In summary: the intention of the RDoC concept is to accelerate new discoveries by fostering research that translates findings from basic science into new treatments addressing fundamental mechanisms that cut across current diagnostic categories. It is important to note that the conceptual framework for RDoC is "explicitly agnostic."

The importance of this framework for the message of this volume of *Depression as a Systemic Illness* is that, as a clinical syndrome, depression is related to abnormal activity in the prefrontal cortex, amygdala, anterior cingulate cortex, nucleus accumbens, and multiple monoamine systems, and undoubtedly to other central nervous system components. Clearly, the physiological correlates with those adumbrated in other chapters—e.g., relationship to glucose metabolism, platelet activation, cytokine activity, and alterations in cortisone—all underscore the fact that depression is not just a mental disorder, but a *systemic disorder* that could and should be in the hands of PCPs—especially uncomplicated depressions that are responsive to first-line treatment.

Markowitz has recently written that the emphasis on neuroscience—and as an example the RDoC model—may be an important research tool, but it overlooks the importance, benefits, and evidence base of the current psychological tools we already do have for the depressed patient: cognitive behavioral therapy (CBT), interpersonal therapy, and other talking therapies (NY Times John Markowitz, There's Such a Thing as Too Much Neuroscience October 15, 2016 p A21). He says: We could wait for decades before tantalizing neural findings translated to useful human treatments. And what do we do for patients in the meantime? He pleads for a balance between neuroscience and clinical research. Nevertheless, medicine as a specialty gave up symptom diagnosis years ago and went to the understanding of mechanisms causing symptoms.[33]

GENETICS AND THE DIAGNOSIS
OF DEPRESSION

Flint knew that genetic studies of 9,000 persons with depression did not yield a genetic linkage, nor did a follow-up study of 17,000 individuals. However, in *Nature* (2015),[34] from a DNA analysis of 5,303 Chinese women with depression and 5, 337 controls, Flint, Kendler, and the Converge Consortium reported using sparse whole-gene sequencing and observing two genetic markers—two genetic sequences reproducibly linked to major depressive disorder.[34] The researchers examined persons with a major depressive disorder and who were from the same Han Chinese ethnicity. The researchers identified, and subsequently replicated in an independent sample, two loci contributing to risk of major depressive disorder on chromosome 10: one near the *SIRT1* gene, the other in an intron of the *LHPP* gene. Kendler and Flint, studying the genome of 5,000 members of the Han tribe in China, found three groups of depressed cohorts, genetically distinct from each other, and not in concordance with the diagnostic classifications found in the DSM-5, the ICD-10, or the ICD-11.[34,35]

As Ledford wrote: "The hope is that as more genetic links are found, they will flag up groups of proteins known to work together to affect certain cellular functions.[36] These pathways could be investigated as drug targets and for their potential to make the diagnosis of depression more definitive" (www.nature.com/news). (This underscores the category of "*levels of information*" in the RDoC schema of genes [Table 11.2).

BIOLOGICAL MARKERS

Mossner, Mikova, Koutsilier, et al., in their important report "Consensus Paper of the World Federation of Societies of Biological Psychiatry (WFSBP) Task Force on Biological Markers: Biological Markers in Depression," identify a series of entities regarded as potential biomarkers for major depressive disorders.[37] They include: neurotrophic factors, serotonergic markers, biochemical markers, immunological markers, neuroimaging, neurophysiological findings, and neuropsychological markers. They also include decreased platelet imipramine binding, decreased 5-HT1A receptor expression, increase of soluble interleukin-2 receptor and interleukin-6 in serum, decreased brain-derived neurotrophic factor in serum, hypocholesterolemia, low blood folate levels, and impaired suppression of the dexamethasone suppression test. However, they state in regard to the DSM-5 and ICD-11: "no biological markers for major depression are sufficiently specific to be included in the diagnostic lexicons." Lopresti, Maker, Hood, and Drummond, after reviewing the potential of inflammatory and oxidative stress biomarkers, also conclude that much more research is needed before biomarkers can be employed for the assessment of depression.[38]

The Annals of the New York Academy of Sciences highlighted "Translational Neuroscience in Psychiatry: Light at the End of the Tunnel" and emphasized the need to "find translatable biomarkers that can be used to predict the efficacy of a psychiatric drug, before commencing costly phase III studies" (www.nyas.org/annals). In addition to predicting efficacy, there is a need for translational biomarkers that can inform researchers about the unmistakable presence of a drug in the brain and its time course, using noninvasive and inexpensive approaches. One approach may be "qualitative electroencephalography," which records electrical activity in the brain that arises from electrochemical communication between brain cells, and different frequencies of activity are strongly related to aspects of cognition.

The findings that Flint, Kendler, and collaborators report are extremely important in assisting the identification of patients at risk for depressive disorders, providing a genetic model, and eventually establishing the genetic biological markers for easy and ready identification of probands for depressive illness. Such an addition to the diagnostic tools available will help the PCPs identify patients who might otherwise not be observed as depressed, and with treatment protocols based on genetic algorithms yet to be developed. This would be reminiscent of the glycated hemoglobin A1C for the detection of diabetes, and prostate-specific antigen (PSA) for early identification of prostate cancer. Such important work and findings also underscore the proposal that depression is a *systemic disease* involving genes, molecules, cell circuits, and physiological correlates affecting bodily processes. Although biological markers are currently unavailable, it is clear that the future holds great promise for them to be discovered and allow the demarcation and identification of disorders of the brain that heretofore have been most commonly identified phenomenologically and often based on clinical judgment.

REFERENCES

1. Casey P. Borderline between normal and pathological responses. In: Casey P, Strain JJ, eds. *Trauma and stressor-related disorders: handbook for clinicians.* Washington, DC: American Psychiatric Association Publishing; 2016:1–19.
2. Cooper R. Avoiding false positives: zones of rarity, the threshold problem and the DSM clinical significance criterion. *Can J Psychiatry.* 2013;58(11):606–611.
3. Wakefield J. Diagnosing DSM-IV part 1: DSM-IV and the concept of disorder. *Behav Res Ther.* 1997;35(7):633–649.
4. Kendell R, Jablensky A. Distinguishing between the validity and utility of psychiatric diagnosis. *Am J Psychiatry.* 2003;160(1):4–12.
5. American Psychiatric Association. *Diagnostic and Statistical Manual of Mental Disorders,* 3rd ed. Washington, DC: American Psychiatric Association; 1980.
6. American Psychiatric Association. *Diagnostic and Statistical Manual of Mental Disorders,* 5th ed. Washington, DC: American Psychiatric Association; 2013.
7. Stein DJ, Phillips KA, Bolton D, et al. What is a mental/psychiatric disorder? From DSM-IV to DSM-5. *Psychol Med.* 2010;40(11):1759–1765.
8. Casey P, Marcy M, Kelly BD, et al. Can adjustment disorder and depressive episode be distinguished? Results from ODIN. *J Affect Disord.* 2006;92(2–3):291–297.
9. Reynolds M, Brewin CR. Intrusive memories in depression and posttraumatic stress disorder. *Behav Res Ther.* 1999;37(3):201–215.
10. Frances A. Problems in defining clinical significance in epidemiological studies. *Arch Gen Psychiatry.* 1998;55(2):119.
11. Casey P, Birbeck G, McDonagh C, et al. Personality disorder, depression and functioning: results from the ODIN study. *J Affect Disord.* 2004;82(2)277–283.
12. Frances A. Whither DSM-V? *Br J Psychiatry.* 2009;195(5):391–392.

13. Horowitz M, Wakefield JC. *The loss of sadness. How psychiatry transformed normal sorrow into depressive disorder.* Oxford, UK: Oxford University Press; 2007.

14. American Psychiatric Association: *Diagnostic and Statistical Manual of Mental Disorders,* 4th ed. Washington, DC: American Psychiatric Association; 1994.

15. McHugh PR, Slavney PR. Mental illness—comprehensive evaluation or checklist? *NEJM.* 2012;366(20):1853–1855.

16. Reed GM, Mendonca, Correia J, et al. The WPA-WHO global survey of psychiatrists' attitudes toward mental disorders classification. *World Psychiatry.* 2011;10(2): 118–131.

17. Kendler K. Book review: *The loss of sadness: how psychiatry transformed normal sorrow into depressive disorder,* by Horwitz AV and Wakefield JC. *Psychol Med.* 2008;38:148–150.

18. Cooper JE, Kendell RE, Gurland BJ, Sharpe L, Copeland JRM, Simon R. *Psychiatric diagnosis in New York and London.* London: Oxford University Press; 1972.

19. Sharpe L, Gurland BJ, Fleiss JL, Kendell RE, Cooper JE, Copeland JR. Comparisons of American, Canadian and British psychiatrists in their diagnostic concepts. *Can Psychiatr Assoc J.* 1974;19:235–245.

20. Guze SB, Woodruff RA, Clayton PJ. A study of conversion symptoms in psychiatric outpatients. *Am J Psychiatry.* 1971;128:643–646.

21. Guze SB. The role of follow-up studies: their contribution to diagnostic classification as applied to hysteria. *Semin Psychiatry.* 1970;2:392–402.

22. Guze SB, Cloninger CR, Martin RL, Clayton PJ. A follow-up and family study of Briquet's syndrome. *Br J Psychiatry.* 1986;149:17–23.

23. Feighner JP, Robins E, Guze SB. Diagnostic criteria for use in psychiatric research. *Arch Gen Psychiatry.* 1972;26:57–63.

24. Kupfer DJ, First MB, Regier D, eds. *A research agenda for DSM-V.* Washington, DC: American Psychiatric Press, 2002:xv–xxiii.

25. Paris J. *The intelligent clinician's guide to the DSM-5.* Oxford: Oxford University Press; 2013.

26. Craddock N, Mynors-Wallis L. Psychiatric diagnosis: impersonal, imperfect and important. *Br J Psychiatry.* 2014;204:93–95.

27. Frances A. *Saving normal: an insider's revolt against out-of-control psychiatric diagnosis, DSM-5, Big Pharma, and the medicalization of ordinary life.* New York: William Morrow; 2013.

28. Insel TR. The NIMH Research Domain Criteria (RDoC) Project: precision medicine for psychiatry. *Am J Psychiatry.* 2014;171:395–397. Available at http://www.nimh.hih.gov//index.shtml. Accessed August 8, 2016.

29. Cuthbert BN, Insel TR. Toward the future of psychiatric diagnosis: the seven pillars of RDoC. *BMC Med,* 2013;11:126.

30. Tyrer P, Reed GM, Crawford MJ. Classification, assessment, prevalence and effect of personality disorder. *Lancet.* 2015;385:717–726.

31. Strain JJ, Shenoy A. The dimensions of the RDoc: their applications to psychosomatic medicine. Abstract Academy of Psychosomatic Medicine Annual Meeting, Austin, TX, November 10, 2016.

32. Cai N, Li Y, Chang S, et al. Genetic control over mtDNA and its relationship to major depressive disorder. *Curr Biol.* 2015;25(24):3170–3177.

33. McHugh P, Slavney PR. Diagnostic and classificatory dilemmas. In: Blumenfeld M, Strain JJ, eds. *Psychosomatic medicine.* Baltimore, MD: Lippincott, Williams & Wilkins; 2007:39–46.

34. CONVERGE Consortium. Sparse whole-genome sequencing identifies two loci for major depressive disorder. *Nature.* 2015;523:588–591.

35. Geschwind DH, Flint J. Genetics and genomics of psychiatric disease. *Science.* 2015;349:1489–1493.

36. Ledford H. First robust links to depression emerge. Available at www.nature.com/news. Accessed August 10, 2016.

37. Mossner R, Mikova O, Koutsilier E, et al. Consensus paper of the WFSBP Task Force on Biological Markers: biological markers in depression. *World J Biol Psychiatry.* 2007;8(3):141–174.

38. Lopresti AL, Maker GL, Hood SD, Drummond PD. A review of peripheral biomarkers in major depression: the potential of inflammatory and oxidative stress biomarkers. *Prog Neuro-Psychopharmacol Biol Psychiatry.* 2014;48:102–111.

12

Models of Mental Health Training for Non-Psychiatric Physicians

Beyond Collaborative Care

James J. Strain

INTRODUCTION

This chapter will review the evolution of psychiatry's involvement with teaching mental health issues to other medical disciplines over the last 60 years in order to support the thesis that depression is a systemic disease and its initial diagnosis and management should be incorporated into the primary care treatment setting. The characterization of the pedagogical models of mental health training for primary care physicians (PCP) that have evolved over the years to share knowledge and skills that need to be incorporated into the PCP's skill set will be presented. The rationale for moving standard assessment and treatment for depression to the PCP will be explored. Finally, the need to advance beyond the collaborative care model—the current *headwind* as a primary and integrative teaching of psychiatry to non-psychiatrists—not only in the international setting, but also in the industrialized and developed countries of the world as well—will be described.

HISTORICAL BACKGROUND

There has been a remarkable evolution of mental health inpatient care from the asylum in the country, to the asylum in town, to a psychiatric unit in a general hospital, to psychiatry-medicine units (or medical-psychiatric units), or to a "scatter bed"—a medical psychiatric bed—on a general medical ward, and to the ambulatory setting. There has been an innovative evolution as well in the development of teaching models to improve mental health care delivered by the non-psychiatric physician in the inpatient and the ambulatory settings. This will be described in detail later.

But there are several issues driving this need to enhance the PCPs' capacity to deal with depression in their patients. PCPs are the most common gateway into the health care system for patients with depression.[1-3] The Centers for Disease Control and Prevention (CDC) estimates that 6.8–8.7% of the U.S. population suffers from depression.[4,5] Eight million ambulatory care visits for depression diagnosis and management occur each year, costing more than $12 billion.[6] The CDC estimates that depression results in the loss of 200 million workdays annually, costing employers $17–$44 billion each year.[7] Patients with chronic diseases and depressive disorders results in increased risk of morbidity and mortality.[8–10] Of the eight million ambulatory annual visits for depression in the U.S. more than half are to a PCP.[5,6]

It is unclear whether PCPs are well equipped to manage depression as a chronic illness by utilizing proactive population-based care and having patients play an active role in their health care.[11–13] However, the PCPs in the United States are already prescribing 70% of the antidepressant medication utilized.[14] In addition, they are prescribing 90% of the anxiolytics given to the U.S. population.[14] Non-psychiatric medical physicians are expert in knowing how to assess for drug reactions and drug–drug interactions, and they have access to several vehicles—e.g., computer programs, daily fact sheets, hospital drug officers, and pharmaceutical companies themselves. Of the 15% of the population with *Diagnostic and Statistical Manual–5* (DSM-5) diagnosable disorders, 54% are seen exclusively by the PCP or other health professionals.[1] Stigma keeps many patients from seeing mental health specialists or even discussing their mental condition with their PCP. It is estimated that only half of the patients with depression in the United States confer with a physician or mental health specialist about their condition or even seek out a physician.

Another important finding is from the Star-D Study of patient responses to antidepressant drug therapy for their depressive states.[16] From this National Institute of Mental Health (NIMH) observational study of depressed patients, 50% responded to the first family of antidepressants they were prescribed. Of the remaining 50% unimproved, only 5% responded to a second family of antidepressant medication. And, finally, of the 45% unimproved residual group, again only 5% responded to a third family of antidepressants. Clearly, 40% did not improve and needed more specialized treatment; e.g., more than one drug, selective monoamine oxidase inhibitors (MAOIs) (that do not require dietary restrictions), or evaluation for electro-convulsive treatment (ECT). Finally, deep-brain stimulation (DBS) is an experimental therapeutic option for those with refractory depression.[17] Ketamine, which affects the glutamatergic system (rather than the norepinephrine system), is an important investigative drug with a new target.[18–22] It would be important for PCPs to be trained to diagnose and offer the first line of treatment for "uncomplicated depression" (the cohort that responds to the first family of antidepressants prescribed) similar to their caring for uncomplicated asthma, hypertension, congestive heart failure, diabetes, etc. When these illnesses are uncomplicated and not made more refractory by other medical comorbidities, they can usually be cared for by the PCP, and if necessary, referred for specialty care at the time they are unresponsive to first-line therapeutics, or complications arise. Should this therapeutic approach also be applied for uncomplicated depressive disorders? There is no question that the 50% who do not respond to the first-line antidepressant medication approach could, and in many cases should, be referred to a mental health specialist who can engage in more complex treatment modes and professional psychotherapies.

Bishop and co-workers have also studied PCP practices and observed that care-management processes are used less for depression than for other chronic conditions; e.g., asthma, diabetes, and congestive heart failure.[1] Care management processes include disease registries, nurse care managers, feedback of quality data to physicians, reminders to patients, and non-physician staff for patient education. Using national survey data from 2006–2013, these five care management processes were examined for their application in the PCP practices. The study revealed that on average, less than one care management process was utilized for depression. Where larger PCP practices may have a team approach for diabetes that could include a nutritionist, case manager, regulated follow-up, ongoing assessment of important biological markers, such as hemoglobin glycolate A1C, careful monitoring of compliance, meaningful outcomes, and patient and physician education, such teams are rare to nonexistent for depression. Therefore, PCP education and practice management procedures need to be provided for an improvement in identification, initial treatment, assessment of outcome, and/or referral to a mental health specialist for the depressed patient when indicated. Bishop et al.[1] stress that physician education, financial incentives, government guidelines, and regulations may enhance the development of management processes for the identification, treatment, and management of depression in PCP.

MODELS OF MENTAL HEALTH TRAINING FOR PRIMARY CARE

To understand how PCPs are prepared for addressing some of the mental health needs of their patients, three studies were funded by the National Institute of Mental Health (NIMH) to develop a taxonomy of mental health training models for PCP.[23] Six pedagogical models were identified to help the PCP with knowledge and skills to treat behavioral disorders, including depression.[23] (These models may have been superseded by other specific approaches to teaching for various general medicine programs and for family medicine training).

Psychiatric Consultation Model

The consultation model is practiced in most hospitals and especially in teaching hospitals throughout the country.

> The teaching is almost exclusively done around psychiatric consultation requests on specific patients. The amount of exposure is minimal (3 hours/year), the modality is formal and informal consultation, and permeability (exposure to a variety of mental conditions) is minimal. There is little use of educational technology (evaluation of trainee's competence) and no specification of a pedagogical curriculum. The content of the teaching is derived from the case method and depends on which cases are presented to the consultant. Some residents may present *no* psychiatric consultation requests during their entire residency. Both the administration and implementation of this model are almost uniformly delegated to the psychiatric service (p. 99).[23]

This is the model commonly employed in teaching hospitals and in particular in community hospitals; it is not a *liaison* model unless it uses structured formal teaching for the modal resident. It is the universal teaching model in most medical residency programs and, unfortunately, the weakest one.

Liaison Psychiatry Model

Liaison psychiatry utilizes the psychiatric consultation process, but it also provides regular ongoing educational efforts that contain both formal and informal aspects; e.g., regular patient-care liaison conferences, the presence of the psychiatric consultant on ward rounds, and an ongoing relationship with the ward or unit staff, participation in medical surgical grand rounds, seminars, and colloquia. In addition, there is an attempt to create *Islands of Excellence* with carefully appointed medical, surgical, and obstetrical-gynecological physicians assigned to be co-teachers—the *Ombudsman*—who teach with the psychiatrist for extended periods of time, often months or years.[24] This weekly Ombudsman conference on medical/surgical services allows the systematic coverage of diverse topics: depressive disorders, psychopharmacology, anxiety, loss of body parts and function, the dying, the non-compliant, the difficult, the seductive patient, referral techniques, among others. The administration and implementation of this program is generally delegated to psychiatry, although medicine must allocate some of its teaching time for its residents, sometimes assists with funding of the psychiatrist teacher, and provides an important attending in the specific specialty who in effect co-teaches with the psychiatrist. This model allows for 10–20 hours of mental health teaching per year in the medical setting and is an important pedagogical advance above consultation.

Bridge Model

In the bridge model—usually employed in an outpatient setting—there is a more extensive formal pedagogical structure to the program, more total teaching time, and a greater variety of teaching methods devoted to psychiatric issues. The modalities frequently include mechanisms for teaching in an ambulatory setting where patients with chronic illnesses can be followed over time; direct-observation precepting is available as opposed to the abbreviated contacts of acute inpatient medicine. There is greater involvement of the primary care faculty in the teaching of mental health issues. The increase intensity of the training experience and the use of the ambulatory setting allows a greater emphasis on interviewing skills, behavioral risk issues; e.g., noncompliance, and life cycle concerns. Primary care often pays for the psychiatric teaching in the bridge model, more commonly found in general internal medicine and family medicine programs.

Hybrid Model

In this model, a significant amount of time is allotted to mental health teaching, which can be done by psychiatry or other mental health specialists, psychologists, social workers, sociologists, etc. In addition, primary care teachers also emphasize mental health issues, primarily in ambulatory settings. The teacher who is a role model for the trainee not only inquires about mental health issues, but teaches them as well. The majority of primary care attendings discuss cases from a biological as well as a psychosocial perspective, so there is a role model to identify with who assumes responsibility for mental health as well as physical issues; the students observe their teacher working in these two spheres. Primary care retains ultimate administrative control, assumes responsibility for funding of mental health teachers, and often employs this model of mental health teaching in family practice programs.

Autonomous Model

In this model, much of the mental health training occurs by the primary care attendings. For example, most case conferences include a discussion of psychosocial issues. There is less emphasis on formal psychiatric training, and more emphasis on family therapy, behavioral modification, interviewing, or sensitivity training. Administrative control of the mental health teaching component is under the auspices of the family medicine program, and departments of psychiatry may not be involved. Often non-medical behavioral scientists are the teachers in these community-based administered family practice programs.

Postgraduate Specialization Model

This model is a block rotation with considerable formal and informal teaching for graduate physicians who have completed their residencies in disciplines other than psychiatry; e.g., medicine, surgery, and ob-gyn, who want greater expertise in mental health knowledge, skills, and research to add this dimension to their basic medical/surgical skills. They then are equipped to deal with mental health issues in their practices and become teachers of mental health for their specialty students. The program fostered by George Engel at the University of Rochester is the best example of this model, which encompassed a two-year training period after specialty training.[25-27] These graduates could diagnose and treat many of the psychiatric and psychosocial disorders in their patients, but would refer to psychiatry those with serious suicidal thoughts and wishes, new psychosis, refractory disorders not responsive to usual treatment approaches, etc.

Double-Boarded Model

The double-boarded model provided training in a specialty of medicine and, in addition, full training in psychiatry, so that the graduates were fully trained in their desired field of medicine and in psychiatry, having taken dual residencies and often becoming dual-boarded. In a sense, they could refer patients with mental disorders to themselves. This program was costly in time (essentially two residencies) and previously offered at the University of West Virginia and at the University of Virginia. It would be important to know if such trainees cared for psychiatric, medical, or both kinds of patients in their practices, and how many became teachers.

Collaborative Care Model (CoCM)

The *collaborative care model*—the current "***headwind***" for mental health care in non-psychiatric medical settings—is where the psychiatrist becomes part of the treatment team in a physician's office, an ambulatory clinic, or an outpatient setting in which doctors are seeing medical/surgical/obstetrical/pediatric patients. "The CoCM attempts to maximize the effectiveness of current behavioral health treatments by ensuring that patients (Figure 12.1) are identified, treated, and monitored proactively, with clinical guidelines provided by a qualified psychiatric consultant" (letter from Saul Levin to the director of Centers for Medicare and Medicaid Services [CMS]). "In this model PCPs receive

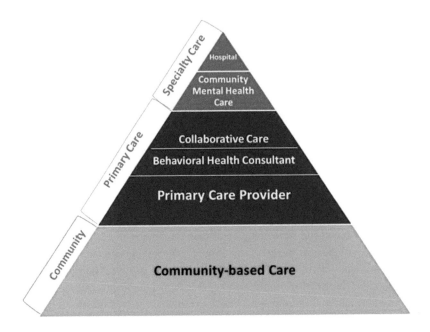

Figure 12.1 With Permission: Jurgen Unutzer, MD, MPH, MA Chair Psychiatry and Behavioral Science Director AIMS Center University of Washington. Don Lipsitt Research Workship, Academy of Psychosomatic Medicine, Austin, Texas. November 2016.

extensive support from a team that includes a trained behavioral health manager and a psychiatric consultant . . . that applies well-established principles of population based behavioral health care and employs specific behavioral health expertise."[28] New codes are available for the PCP to be reimbursed for coverage for collaborative care, i.e., GPP1, GPP2, and GPP3, in 2017. In collaborative care, the psychiatrist is an important participant in the teaching of the medical physicians in an attempt to upgrade their skills in mental health.[29-38] However, there is also collaboration with a team to insure screening, diagnosing, treatment, follow-up, and ongoing assessment of outcome to insure that relapse or failure to respond are quickly identified. The patient is called in if they fail to keep their appointments, if there is noncompliance, or if an educated and informed significant other has concerns for the patient's follow-through of suggested care plans. In this model it is hoped that psychiatric information will be transmitted to non-psychiatric staff so that they may incorporate such knowledge in time into their own, ongoing practices with their patients. Patient and staff education are important components of this model.

Katon and his co-workers originally observed that screening patients and giving the physician this information—e.g., that the patient could be depressed—did not alter the physician's care taking behavior and did not influence the patient's treatment or outcome. Giving the physician screening information and reading material also did not improve care or outcome. Katon and his group, through carefully constructed randomized controlled trials, found that *collaboration* with the non-psychiatric physician and a care team was required to change physician behavior and patient outcomes.[29-38] The nature and content of this collaboration was carefully defined, and when practiced with the intensity required, resulted in improved patient outcomes. In addition, the use of the mental health specialist, namely the psychiatrist, in this way fostered the extension of mental health care through the PCP, where the other models described here (except for the post-graduate and double-boarded), did not measurably change the PCPs' behavior or their patients' outcomes. Therefore, the collaborative care model extended the efforts of the psychiatrist by informing, teaching, and encouraging primary care and care facilities to incorporate behavioral screening, diagnosis, and treatment, and to measure outcomes with rigorous protocols as part of their method of operation. This has extended the reach of psychiatry in an impressive way and allows the treatment of mental problems in the primary care setting.

There is some question of how cohorts of non-psychiatric physicians will align themselves with a psychiatrist; who will pay for the psychiatric teaching (although Medicare now has codes for reimbursing collaborative care); and how long the mental health teacher needs to be involved with the medical caretakers for them to become autonomous in their "medical home." Is autonomy for the PCP with regard to offering mental health care and measuring outcomes the goal?

This model still depends on the availability of psychiatrists, the willingness of non-psychiatric physicians to align themselves collaboratively, establishment of a care team addressing mental health, and funding for this new treatment and pedagogical approach, especially in the non-Medicare setting.

And if one examines not only the developing world but developed countries as well, the shortage of psychiatrists as collaborators is sobering. For example, Rwanda has two psychiatrists, and Tanzania 40 psychiatrists for 44 million persons. Twenty of the psychiatrists in Tanzania are in Dar Es Salaam, of whom 10 are in private practice. There are not enough psychiatrists to engage in collaborative care. In Tanzania, a new model has been employed: training select PCPs for three months/year for four years, so that they may address the majority of mental health issues in their practices. (This training takes place in Losthotol, Tanzania at Sikomo University). The government pay the physicians during training and they are paid an additional 20% of the accustomed salary upon completion of the four years course work.

Even in as developed a nation as Sweden, with 9 million citizens, and with a cohort of 9,000 psychiatrists, most outpatient psychiatry is delivered by non-psychiatrist mental health care workers.[39] In Sweden, all inpatient psychiatric patients are under the care of a psychiatrist. With 30,000 psychiatrists in China—population 1.3 billion; 20,000 psychiatrists in India—population 1.4 billion; collaborative care between psychiatry and non-psychiatric physicians seems unlikely. Even collaborative care in upstate New York seems unlikely, with large sections of the state having no psychiatrist in residence; and 50% of the counties in the United States have no psychiatrist.

Family Practice Model

Family practice has developed a comprehensive model for evaluating and treating mental health issues in its residency programs.[40] This includes attitudes, knowledge, skills, and implementation. It is taught through a comprehensive set of teaching environments throughout the residency. Training in human behavior and mental health should be accomplished in outpatient, in-patient, home-based, nursing home, emergency, and other settings appropriate to the residents' future practice needs. This occurs through a combination of longitudinal experiences, supervision, and didactic teaching. This combination should include experience in diagnostic assessment, psychotherapeutic techniques (e.g., cognitive behavioral therapy, motivational interviewing, self-reflection, narrative medicine, wellness interventions), and psychopharmacological management. Learning tools such as Balint groups, video review of resident interviews with actual or standardized patients, direct observation, feedback, didactics, community-based experiences, and role playing are useful and recommended. Collaborating with multiple mental health professionals and community-based individuals/agencies (e.g., schools, nursing homes/home visits, substance abuse programs, shelters) to work as a team is often essential to providing the most effective, comprehensive, and long-lasting care (p. 2).[40]

With regard to *attitudes,* the Family Practice Training Guidelines state the importance of recognition of the complex bidirectional interaction between family/social factors and individual health. And in regard to *knowledge,* the guidelines emphasize several areas of expected awareness, but three are of particular importance in regard to this volume on depression as a systemic disorder (p. 2):[40]

1. Interrelationships among biological, psychological, and social factors in all patients
2. Differential diagnosis of common mental health disorders
3. Familiarity with *Diagnostic and Statistical Manual of Mental Disorders,* 5th edition (DSM-5) nomenclatures of mental health disorders.

Knowledge and *skills* to be acquired specify the following for depressive disorders in the family practice practitioner's competence, among several others (p. 4–9):[40]

1. Use evaluation tools and interviewing skills to enhance data collection in short periods of time and optimize the physician–patient relationship.
   a. Understand that the nature of questioning influences patient responses (e.g., open ended, nonjudgmental).
   b. Create an environment that allows for honest patient responses.
2. Elicit the context of the visit using BATHE (Background, Affect, Trouble, Handling, Empathy) or other techniques.
3. Perform a mental status examination.
4. Use special procedures in psychiatric disorder diagnoses, including psychological testing, laboratory testing, and brain imaging.
5. Teach patients methods for evaluating and selecting reliable websites for medical information.
6. Screen for depression using the Patient Health Questionnaire (PHQ-9), Beck Depression Inventory, Zung Self-Rating Depression Scale, Hamilton Rating Scale for Depression, and SIG-E-CAPS mnemonic (Sleep, Interest, Guilt, Energy, Concentration, Appetite, Psychomotor, and Suicidal ideation).
7. Refer appropriately to cognitive behavioral therapy and psychiatric consultation.
   a. Understand the central therapeutic role of the primary care provider.
   b. Utilize team-based collaborative care, such as the IMPACT model of evidence-based depression care.
8. Apply techniques to enhance compliance with medical treatment regimens.

9. Initiate management of psychiatric emergencies (e.g., the suicidal patient, the acutely psychotic patient).
10. Properly use psychopharmacological agents, taking into consideration the following:
    a. Diagnostic indications and contraindications.
    b. Dosage; length of use; monitoring of response, side effects, and compliance.
    c. Drug interactions.

Medical Model

Because of the paucity of psychiatrists and the impediments to establishing a mental health care team, not only in the developing world, but in the United States as well, another more far-reaching model that may provide wider mental health care, even beyond collaborative care, is needed—the *medical* model. It would not need to reach the breadth and depth of the American Academy of Family Physicians Training Guidelines, but key elements from those guidelines should apply to all physicians trained in medical schools, and emphasized in their residency training experience. As said before, in the United States, non-psychiatric physicians prescribe 70% of the antidepressants and 90% of the anxiolytics.[14] The CDC estimates that 6.8–8.7% of the U.S. adult population suffers from depression at any given time.[4,5] PCPs are already caring for half of the 8 million patients with depression. As also said before, from the Star D Study, 50% of depressed patients respond positively to the first family of antidepressant medication that they are prescribed.[16] Therefore, as the PCP routinely cares for the uncomplicated diabetic, asthmatic, hypertensive, and congestive heart failure patient, before sending the refractory patients on to sub-specialty care professionals, could they not be trained to provide basic care for the "uncomplicated" depressive disorder? Furthermore, Bishop et al.[1] have shown that PCPs have equipped their practices to care for asthma, congestive heart failure, and diabetes with the use of at least five case management processes mentioned herein, but they have not done so for the depressive disorders they encounter.[1]

Therefore, as medical students are provided training for skills and knowledge to care for these other acute and chronic diseases, and they are expected to have competencies for their patients' care and have further training during their residency years, why cannot medical schools and residencies equip their internal medicine graduates to diagnose, manage, and/or refer as necessary the patients with uncomplicated depression? It is understood if a patient is suicidal or has a paranoid psychosis, that patient should be referred for urgent specialist care. Similarly, cases of depression refractory to ordinary care should also be referred to a trained specialist in mental health management. The importance of experience with depressive disorders in residency training necessitates that they be a part of the residency teaching program. Currently, many internal medicine residency programs do not insure exposure for depressed patients, but rely on in-house psychiatric consultation teams to address these patients. In contrast to medicine, surgery, and ob-gyn residency training programs, pediatric residencies do include behavioral pediatrics and psychological assessments as part of their pedagogic effort. This would mean that the MD PCP cadre of the world could screen, diagnose, treat, and/or refer refractory depressive patients for more advanced mental health care if it were needed and available. This would also mean that, as they have for other illnesses, the PCP could organize care-management processes for their depressed patients: access to social workers, psychologists, case managers (for compliance, keeping appointments), as they do nutritionists, physical therapy, exercise, medication review for their diabetics and patients with congestive heart failure.

The *medical* model would:

1. Improve on collaborative care;
2. Overcome the handicap of the shortage of psychiatrists and even psychologists in so many parts of the world to be collaborators;
3. Avoid the patient stigma of seeing a psychiatrist or mental health care worker;
4. Have important assessments readily available for other medical comorbidities that maybe present; e.g., the Electronic Health Record (EHR) (see Chapter 13); and
5. Have caretakers cognizant of drug side effects and psychiatric drug–medical drug interactions (see Chapter 10).

The PCP would not be expected to do psychotherapy, but that could be made available as one of the care management processes, via a nurse physician assistant, social worker, psychologist, registered nurse, etc. A nurse physician assistant can write her/his own prescriptions, work side by side with the MD or independently, and offer care to depressed patients under their own banner. She/he can also bill for the services rendered.

In addition, a carefully conceived EHR (see Chapter 13), would assist the PCP with prompts and algorithms regarding screening, diagnostic possibilities, treatment options, meaningful outcome, and necessary follow-up. The EHR would be his/her ally—a *collaborating agent*—in providing up-to-date evidence-based care for the depressed patients in their practices. The EHR could, with its database from the patient's contacts and medical history, assist in identifying patients at risk for depression and those that need more thorough evaluation and have important medical comorbidities. The EHR would also highlight medications prescribed, laboratory test results, follow-up studies, etc. Also the technology would suggest diagnostic measures that would identify the biological correlates of depression that could affect the patient's physiological state and other medical comorbidities—the "allostatic load," e.g., the hyperactivation of the HPA-axis, activation of platelets, effects on cytokines, etc. Finally, the EHR could offer alerts for adverse drug side effects and psychiatric drug–medical drug adverse reactions. Meaningful outcome of treatment interventions would be spontaneously generated from algorithms that incorporate objective measures of salutary changes for the patient and might influence physician reimbursement.

In summary, psychiatry cannot care for all of those with depressive disorders; others need to be in the caretaker cohort. Avenues are currently available to move to the *medical model,* which enhances and promulgates better care for depression in the PCP setting, a most important venue already taking care of millions of patients with depression. This would help overcome the handicap of too few psychiatrists, especially in the developing world, to collaborate with PCPs for this enormous global need. With the institution of care management processes, effective care of the depressed patient may take place within the province of the PCP and his/her assistants; e.g., the nurse physician assistant, social worker, psychologist, or case manager.[41] Such a medical model mitigates the shortcomings of current methods of teaching, provides another cohort of essential metal health practitioners, and enhances opportunities for more optimal care for this important segment of our patient population.

REFERENCES

1. Bishop TF, Ramsay PP, Casalino LP, Bao Y, Pincus HA, Shortell SM. Care management processes used less often for depression than for other chronic conditions in US primary care practices. *Health Aff (Millwood)*. 2016;35(3):394–400.

2. Boyd JS, Linsenmeyer A, Woolhandler S, Himmelstein DU, Nardin R. The crisis in mental health care: a preliminary study of access to psychiatric care in Boston. *Ann Emerg Med*. 2011;58(2):218–219.

3. Rhodes KV, Vieth TL, Kushner H, Levy H, Asplin BR. Referral without access: for psychiatric services wait and beep. *Ann Emerg Med*. 2009;54(2):272–278.

4. Centers for Disease Control and Prevention. FastStats: depression [internet]. Atlanta (GA): CDC [Last updated Jul 17, 2015; cited Jan 4, 2016]. Available from: http://www.cec.gov/nchs/faststats/depression.htm.

5. Reeves WC, Strine TW, Pratt LA, et al. Mental illness surveillance among adults in the United States. *MMWR Surveill Summ*. 2011;60(Suppl 3):1–29.

6. Marcus SC, Olfson M. National trends in the treatment for depression from 1998 to 2007. *Arch Gen Psychiatry*. 2010;67(12):1265–1273.

7. Centers for Disease Control and Prevention. Workplace health promotion: depression [Internet]. Atlanta (GA). [Last updated Oct. 23, 2013; cited Jan. 4, 2016.] Available from http://www.cdc.gov/workplacepromotion/implementation/topics/depression.html

8. Katon WJ. Clinical and health services relationships between major depression, depressive symptoms, and general medical illness. *Biol Psychiatry*. 2003;54(3):216–226.

9. Ciechanowski PS, Katon WJ, Russo JE. Depression and diabetes: impact of depressive symptoms on adherence, function, and costs. *Arch Intern Med*. 2000;160(21):3278–3285.

10. Kessler RC, Berglund P, Demler O, et al. The epidemiology of major depressive disorder: results from the National Comorbidity Survey Replications (NCS-R). *JAMA*. 2003;289(23):3095–3105.

11. Wagner EH, Austin BT, Von Korff M. Organizing care for patients with chronic illness. *Milbank Q*. 1996;74(4):511–514.

12. Coleman K, Austin BTG, Brach C, Wagner EH. Evidence on the chronic care model in the new millennium. *Health Aff (Millwood)*. 2009;28(1):75–85.

13. Wagner EH, Groves T. Care for chronic diseases. *BMH*. 2002;325(7370):913–914.

14. Barkil-Oteo A. Collaborative care for depression in primary care: how psychiatry could "trouble shoot" current treatments and practices. *Yale J Biol Med*. 2013;86(2):139–146.

15. Weisberg RB, Dyck I, Culpepper L, Keller MB. Psychiatric treatment in primary care patients with anxiety disorders: a comparison of care received from primary care providers and psychiatrists. *Am J Psychiatry*. 2007;164(2):276.

16. Rush AJ. STAR*D What have we learned? *Am J Psychiatry*. 2007;164(2):201–204.

17. Deeb W, Giordano JJ, Rossi PJ, et al. Proceedings of the Fourth Annual Deep Brain Stimulation Think Tank: a review of emerging issues and technologies. *Front Integr Neurosci*. Nov 22 2016;10:38.

18. Abdallah CG, Averill LA, Collins KA, et al. Ketamine treatment and global brain connectivity in major depression. *Neuropsychopharmacology*. 2017;42:1210–1219.

19. Murrough JW, Collins KA, Fields J, et al. Regulation of neural responses to emotion perception by ketamine in individuals with treatment-resistant major depressive disorder. *Transl Psychiatry*. 2015;5:e509.

20. Murrough JW, Burdick KE, Levitch CF, et al. Neurocognitive effects of ketamine and association with antidepressant response in individuals with treatment-resistant depression: a randomized controlled trial. *Neuropsychopharmacology*. 2015;40(5):1084–1090.

21. Wan LB, Levitch CF, Perez AM, et al. Ketamine safety and tolerability in clinical trials for treatment-resistant depression. *J Clin Psychiatry*. 2015;76(3):247–252.
22. Lapidus KA, Levitch CF, Perez AM, et al. A randomized controlled trial of intranasal ketamine in major depressive disorder. *Biol Psychiatry*. 2014;76(12):970–976.
23. Strain JJ, Pincus HA, Haupt J, Gise L, Taintor Z. Models of mental health training for primary care physicians. *Psychosom Med*. 1985;47(2):95–110.
24. Strain JJ, Hamerman D. Ombudsmen (medical-psychiatric) rounds. An approach to meeting patient-staff needs. *Ann Intern Med*. 1978;88:550–555.
25. Engel GL. The need for a new medical model: a challenge for biomedicine. *Science*. 1977;196(3):129–136.
26. Engel GL. Personal letter to James J. Strain, "The need for a tertiary messenger to teach the biopsychosocial model to non-psychiatric physicians" (1980).
27. Engel GL. The need for a new medical model: a challenge for biomedicine. *Psychodyn Psychiatry*. 2012;40(3):377–396.
28. Levin S. Collaborative care model. *Psychiatric News*. 2016;51:19.
29. Chwastiak L, Vanderlip E, Katon W. Treating complexity: collaborative care for multiple chronic conditions. *Int Rev Psychiatry*. 2014;26:638–647.
30. Huffman JC, Niazi SK, Rundell JR, Sharpe M, Katon WJ. Essential articles on collaborative care models for the treatment of psychiatric disorders in medical settings: a publication by the Academy of Psychosomatic Medicine research and evidence-based practice committee. *Psychosomatics*. 2014;55(2):109–122.
31. Katon W. Collaborative depression care models: from development to dissemination. *Am J Prev Med*. 2012;45:550–552.
32. Katon W, Unutzer J, Wells K, Jones L. Collaborative depression care: history, evolution and ways to enhance dissemination and sustainability. *Gen Hosp Psychiatry*. 2010;32(5):456–464.
33. Katon W. Collaborative care: evidence-based models that improve primary care depressive outcomes. *CNS Spectr*. 2009;14(12 Suppl 14):10–13.
34. Katon WJ, Seelig M. Population-based care of depression: team care approaches to improving outcomes. *J Occup Environ Med*. 2008;50(4):459–467.
35. Davidson WK, Kupfer DJ, Califf RM, et al. Assessment and treatment of depression in patients with cardiovascular disease: National Heart, Lung and Blood Institute working group report. *Psychosom Med*. 2006;68(5):645–650.
36. Davidson WK, Kupfer DJ, Califf RM, et al. Assessment and treatment of depression in patients with cardiovascular disease. National Heart, Lung and Blood Institute working group report. *Ann Behav Med*. 2006;32(2):121–126.
37. Unutzer J, Schoenbaum M, Druss BG, Katon WJ. Transforming mental health care at the interface with general medicine: report for the President's Commission. *Psychiatr Serv*. 2006;57(1):37–47.
38. Katon W, Gonzales J. Primary care and treatment of depression: a response to the NIMH "White Papers." *Gen Hosp Psychiatry*. 2002;24(4):194–196.
39. Sundquist K, Sundquist J. Personal communication, May 23, 2016. Special Mount Sinai grand rounds: Departments of Population Health Science and Policy and Family Medicine and Community Health grand rounds, New York, New York, 10029.
40. Recommended Curriculum Guidelines for Family Practice Residents: AAFP Reprint 270. http://www.aafp.org/dam/aafp/documents/medical_education_residency/program_directors/reprint270_mental.pdf
41. Luthra S. Doctors often fail to treat depression like a chronic illness. Kaiser Health News (NPR). March 7, 2016.

13

An Updated Electronic Health Record (EHR) for Depression Management

Jay J. Strain, Akhil Shenoy, and James J. Strain

INTRODUCTION

Depression is an omnipresent medical illness that recently evolved in the first leading cause of burden of health world wide as proclaimed by the WHO in March of 2017.[1] Depression affects more than 15 million American adults, or about 6.7% of the U.S. population age 18 or older.[2] Certain populations, such as individuals who have experienced acute trauma, may have depression as a co-factor up to 30% of the time, and appropriate involvement of a psychiatrist or mental health care worker would lead to an increase of 78% in the identification and treatment of psychopathology.[3,4] The prevalence of depression is clearly higher in the medical setting and has been shown to increase with the comorbidity of medical illness. Primary care physicians (PCPs) are already identifying and managing 4 million cases of clinical depression out of 8 million patients seen annually in the United States, but still many patients are not identified, and, for the most part, this disease remains under-treated.[5]

This chapter will focus on a new model to manage this ubiquitous illness—depression—which may be acute or chronic. Every physician should be considering depression as free-standing or a possible comorbidity with medical illness, and as such, a potential complicating factor that can affect medical treatment. The question remains how our newest trends in electronic health records (EHRs) and innovative technology can be utilized and mobilized to improve identification, treatment, measurable outcome, and follow-up of this most common illness, and especially in the setting of the PCP. Depression is a systemic illness, and it needs to be approached with an innovative model like other systemic illnesses—e.g., delirium, sepsis, pain, decubitus ulcers, asthma, hypertension, congestive heart failure—within the venue of the PCP. An enhanced and intelligent EHR and innovative technical applications can be important tools to advance the management of depression by the PCP.

The brain is body as much as mind, and its routine assessment is integral to the primary care model, as has occurred in the specialty of family practice. Depression, regarded as a mental disease, is relegated to the background in primary care priorities. Katon and co-workers have shown that simply informing the PCP that a patient has depression does

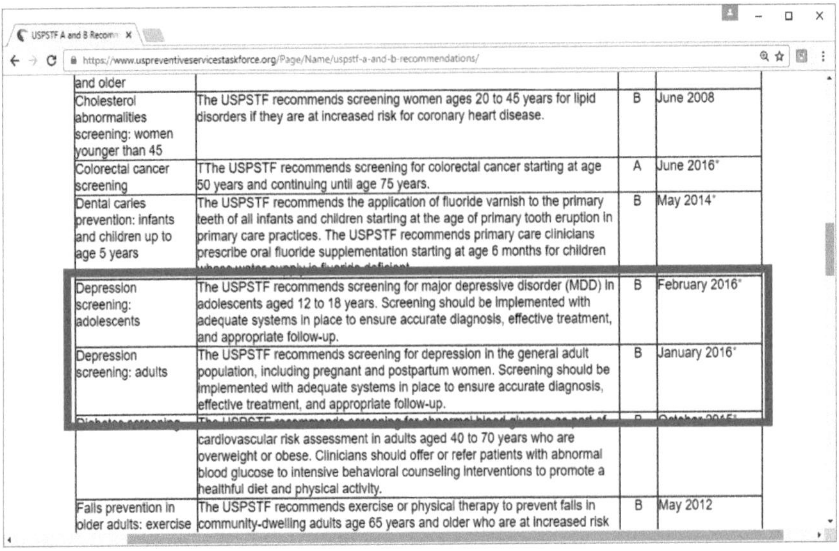

and older			
Cholesterol abnormalities screening: women younger than 45	The USPSTF recommends screening women ages 20 to 45 years for lipid disorders if they are at increased risk for coronary heart disease.	B	June 2008
Colorectal cancer screening	TThe USPSTF recommends screening for colorectal cancer starting at age 50 years and continuing until age 75 years.	A	June 2016*
Dental caries prevention: infants and children up to age 5 years	The USPSTF recommends the application of fluoride varnish to the primary teeth of all infants and children starting at the age of primary tooth eruption in primary care practices. The USPSTF recommends primary care clinicians prescribe oral fluoride supplementation starting at age 6 months for children	B	May 2014*
Depression screening: adolescents	The USPSTF recommends screening for major depressive disorder (MDD) in adolescents aged 12 to 18 years. Screening should be implemented with adequate systems in place to ensure accurate diagnosis, effective treatment, and appropriate follow-up.	B	February 2016*
Depression screening: adults	The USPSTF recommends screening for depression in the general adult population, including pregnant and postpartum women. Screening should be implemented with adequate systems in place to ensure accurate diagnosis, effective treatment, and appropriate follow-up.	B	January 2016*
	cardiovascular risk assessment in adults aged 40 to 70 years who are overweight or obese. Clinicians should offer or refer patients with abnormal blood glucose to intensive behavioral counseling interventions to promote a healthful diet and physical activity.		
Falls prevention in older adults: exercise	The USPSTF recommends exercise or physical therapy to prevent falls in community-dwelling adults age 65 years and older who are at increased risk	B	May 2012

Figure 13.1 US Dept. of Health and Human Services, selected standards for Depression.[5]

not change their management or the outcome with this disease.[6,7] As has been shown with many illnesses, a guided approach using an electronic system can be helpful. Over 50 categories of interventions are recommended, including adolescent and adult depression screening (Figure 13.1).[8] Guidelines exist on the best practices to screen and treat most major illnesses, but the recommendations are often massive and difficult to implement. Many of the easier-to-implement guidelines for physical illnesses are targeted; e.g., where a simple laboratory study can be checked or a procedure like colonoscopy can be suggested. Protocols, guidelines, alerts, and event tracking can all be automated in the background to support the physician. Depression recommendations and guidelines exist, but they are not incorporated as part of most EHRs.

Many medical illnesses are managed more effectively and with improved results by addressing both biological and behavioral components simultaneously. For instance, hypertension treated only with medications will have minimal long-term impact if dietary and behavioral interventions are ignored. A multi-factorial treatment regimen is complicated, time-consuming, and often requires integrated care by multiple providers (e.g., PCP, cardiologist, nutritionist, and physical therapist in the case of hypertension, etc.), and it can be significantly streamlined by the guidance provided with an EHR. Most successful EHR packages now link central data collection with integration and data sharing among providers. Patient data are stored with both "current state" information (e.g., patient's blood pressure and weight at last visit, etc.) and recommendations for actions that need to be completed in the future. Disease screening is often a component of "Health Maintenance" in larger commercial EHRs, which anticipate certain medical diseases, making them simpler to identify and easier to coordinate for treatment (e.g., diabetes mellitus, hyperlipidemia, etc.) (Figure 13.2).[9]

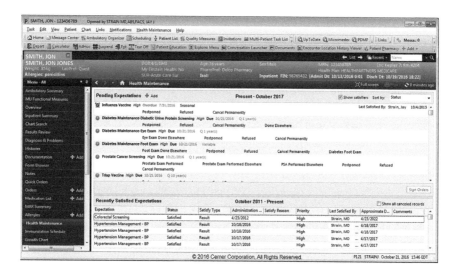

Figure 13.2 Health Maintenance © 2016 Cerner Corporation, All Rights Reserved.[7]

Potentially, depression, like other major health concerns, could be more effectively diagnosed, treated, and monitored using newer tools and techniques not yet incorporated into most advanced EHRs. This chapter will highlight enhanced and creative approaches to capturing depression data for the EHR. Furthermore, methods to elucidate how PCPs can better capture the physiological and behavioral correlates of depressive disorders using EHR systems will be discussed. Several paradigms that allow easier identification of patients, and support more effective cooperation between first-line providers and their psychiatry professionals, are presented. Finally, new research into physiological parameters that might be tracked by the EHR that are secondary to depression and might influence physical illnesses are delineated.

A detailed examination of previously successful algorithmic or computer approaches to handling complex medical illnesses is presented to highlight how the next-generation EHR can be made more effective for depressed-patient care. While genetics may eventually play a significant role in the recognition and management of depression, this bioscience, discussed in earlier chapters, is still on the horizon and not yet appropriate for the EHR.

THE CURRENT EHRS AND A PATH
FOR PROGRESS

In 2012 as part of the Affordable Care Act (ACA, "Obamacare"), hospitals were encouraged and incentivized to convert to EHRs to improve healthcare management. As said earlier, the EHR's potential clinical benefits to improve overall documentation, communication among caregivers, reduce mistakes, and synthesize patient data cannot be overstated. One important example is the use of "electronic prescribing" to avoid pharmaceutical errors. As part of the ACA mandate, the Centers for Medicare and Medicaid

Services (CMS) implemented "meaningful use" measures to improve provider behavior (e.g., updating problem lists, checking allergies and other medications for potential adverse reactions prior to prescribing new medications, and reviewing medications during a transfer of care).

Early implementation of EHRs in large academic centers reported an "increase in the delivery of guideline-adherent care, improvement of quality of care through clinical monitoring, and reduction of medical errors."[7] In parallel, however, there were significant concerns that the ambulatory care quality of medical delivery was not improved with the current EHR methodology.[8] However, improvements to ambulatory systems (e.g., using EHRs customized by the provider, targeting specialized patient care scenarios, etc.) demonstrated that the EHRs could be constructed to benefit outpatients as well. In addition to the reduction in errors and improved safety, 94% of providers employing these improved EHRs reported having medical records available at the point of care, better completion of records, improved alerts about medication conflicts, better risk management, and adherence to best evidence-based practices.[10] Moreover, it was rapidly shown that quality-of-care screenings across a range of common illnesses and improved patient care services were additional benefits.[11] The majority of hospitals have received large government incentives (up to $44,000 per provider) to switch to EHR technologies; it also appears that EHR use enhances and improves financial reimbursement for those who bill Medicare and private insurance carriers.[12,13]

There continues to be physician concern about disruptions and increased distraction in patient care workflow when using an EHR. Many physicians complain about the physical presence of the EHR terminal or laptop between the physician and patient.[14] Multi-step data-capture activities by the intake clerks, office nurses, and physicians are needed to populate the EHR at each patient visit; this can be massively time-consuming and staff-intensive. EHRs with both "boilerplate" and non-adaptable templates make documentation extremely impersonal and often difficult to decipher, because every note appears the same. Additionally, there is a lack of EHR integration among different hospitals (which often use their own proprietary systems), and even among adjacent medical divisions in the same institution.[15]

Mental health care in particular could benefit from many features of the EHR. Electronic security provides a level of access protection that is unequaled in paper-based systems. Levels of access by different caregivers can be regulated to reflect changing needs for those who should have access to a system, while simultaneously protecting privacy.[15] In some EHR implementations, specialized measures were developed to "nest" private psychiatric records and require anyone but the caring psychiatrist to "break the glass" to secure mental health data. For example, emergency room physicians can obtain temporary privileges to unlock key psychiatric records in the case of a patient arriving who has made a suicide attempt. Mental health specifically benefits from having access to *all* previously documented medical information that does not have to be re-entered into the psychiatric note. Trends of laboratory studies can be graphically displayed to show progression of disease markers, electrolyte alteration, lithium or other drug levels, etc., across multiple axes and over time. Minute-by-minute vital signs can be analyzed for data trends. A well-constructed EHR permits the user to move from simple patient data-acquisition to focusing on the medical, laboratory, and psychiatric data elements to assist in the development of a biopsycho-social formulation of the psychiatric patient.

Effective depression identification and management in the PCP setting will demand changes to the existing EHR. Prior customized psychiatry database systems such as MICROCARES™ created a standardized database for psychiatric consultations in the medical setting.[16] This model was designed to capture an extensive 300+-item database uniquely suited for treatment and follow-up of psychiatric patients, but it was a stand-alone system and did not benefit from integration into other hospital services. Each patient's data were recaptured on each visit with secondary completion of customized questionnaires based on the type of psychiatric illness. Data from various sites, even various countries, could be shared due to its unique flexible Standardized Query Language (SQL) data structure (see Figure 13.3).[16]

Newer systems, such as Cerner™ or Epic™, large-scale providers of patient care EHRs, are completely integrated into all aspects of patient encounters—scheduling, order entry, laboratory data collection, nursing and physician documentation, physician support with alerts, and financial management. Immensely powerful, these all-encompassing patient care systems are able to capture enormous amounts of information but require a significant effort by the provider to enter or pull down relevant data. These larger programs, being proprietary, do not readily engage with new software, and they are not open to being self-managed, such as was designed into MICRO-CARES™. In primary care clinics, the addition of "HealthCare Maintenance" templates that prompt the doctor to input elements for depression management has helped, but it does not go far enough.

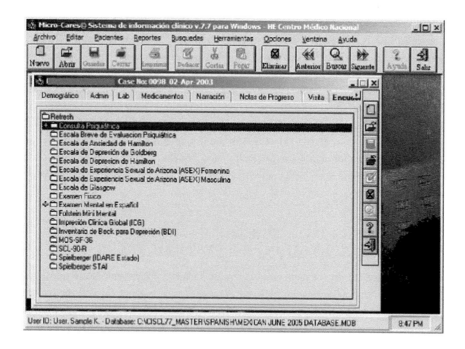

Figure 13.3 Structure, shareable psychiatric data collected into MICRO-CARES™ in Spanish.

Depression, one of the dozens of mandatory components addressed, remains at the bottom of the agenda and a distant target in patient care, only after all other parameters have been fulfilled.[17]

There is no question that the PCP is overwhelmed by requests to review tests, provide preoperative screening, complete enrollment physical exams, address emergency changes in health status, and countless other issues. Secondary to the vast array of care tasks, the PCPs often believe that they are practicing outside their specialty. Fred Pelzman laments in his article "Let Primary Care Be Primary Care" that his specialty is overwhelmed.[14] On asking the PCP to complete the detailed patient evaluation for other specialties (such as psychiatry), he states:

> How are we, as primary care providers, with our 15-to-20-minute visits, going to be able to check all the boxes, do all the things we are supposed to do, and spend enough time to really evaluate and assess all of the multiple symptoms and issues our patients bring to us—especially when we are asked to do someone else's work?[18]

The all-encompassing demands of the PCP environment and acknowledged limitations of the healthcare system today indicate that a new approach to the EHR and evaluating depression is mandatory: it must be an assistant to the physician. Patients and their loved ones may need new ways to report a patient's various depressive symptoms (mood, enjoyment, concentration, energy, pain, sleep, appetite, exercise, and sexual function-libido). The integration of disparate information sources will be required to help all clinicians identify and effectively manage depression. Data from various hospitals, clinics, offices, and even personal observations by family and the patient should be collected, converted into usable patient data, and analyzed into a readily interpretable summary for diagnosis of the disease by any physician. More complex is how to handle incomplete patient data sets: items that are missing for a valid determination of depression must be completed where possible, and unobtainable data must be accounted for in the analysis. Methods of acknowledging that the evaluation is "limited" or "biased" must be described so that the PCP can continue with these known limitations to determine the degree of depression that maybe present. How the PCP is able to intervene has to be streamlined so that early treatment for depression can be initiated, hopefully with the support of a team approach. Then those with refractory illness can be both identified and appropriately referred if necessary.

EHR DATA FOR THE MANAGEMENT OF DEPRESSION AS A SYSTEMIC ILLNESS

Capturing the diagnosis of depression is a multi-factorial process not easily translated into the structured nature of the EHR. All providers must understand that the patient interview provides complex, personal, and narrative data that have always been at the center of making the diagnosis of depression. The human connection is important to the process of diagnosing depression, but it must be supplemented with measureable symptoms and actionable metrics. The nine symptoms according to the *Diagnostic and*

Statistical Manual of Mental Disorders, 5th edition (DSM-5) remain the essential diagnostic keys to the elucidation of both major depression and depressive episodes.[19] Multiple additional biological factors that might simplify diagnosis and treatment are under investigation but are not yet ready for automatic inclusion in the diagnostic algorithm. Several of the techniques and devices that can be implemented or modified to assist in EHR management of depression are presented here.

DIAGNOSIS: POTENTIAL SCREENING TOOLS AND TECHNOLOGY

Ideally, with a valid and simple tool, screening for a depressive disorder can occur in any location—at home, in the PCP's waiting room, in nursing triage, or in any physician's office during a patient visit. Self-screening instruments such as the Patient Health Questionnaire–9 (PHQ9) are particularly useful, since they can be performed by the patient in minutes, consist of only nine questions, are available in multiple languages, and are rapidly scored by any staff or clinical personnel (Figure 13.4).

The PHQ9's validity is confirmed by studies involving eight primary care locations, and has a sensitivity of 88% and a specificity of 88% for major depression.[20] It provides a ranking score for severity of the depressive illness, has built-in treatment recommendations, correlates with other inventories of depressive indicators, and offers a follow-up plan and schedule. The design of this tool can be used to guide both the intensity of care and the level of psychiatric specialist follow-up that is required. Unfortunately, there are significant limitations to the effectiveness of this instrument alone—in the false-positivity rate, and its inability to integrate family history or account for the effects of additional stressors on depression's periodicity.

Additional screening measures for mood, distress, or anxiety, including the *Hamilton Depression Scale,* the *Beck Depression Inventory,* the *Major Depression Inventory,* etc., can also be used to help further identify and document the degree of disease.[21] Continued patient self-monitoring and self-testing are valuable when the diagnosis is already made and ongoing evaluation is necessary, but the collected information must be made available and promulgated back to the primary care provider in addition to the EHR in order to be useful. And, again, as single measures, these instruments can only act as adjuncts to diagnosis when combined with the patient's overall presentation of disease.

To solve these limitations with instruments, it is critical that a communication mechanism be in place to promulgate this information to the care-providing physicians efficiently. Use of electronic mail (email) alone is not sufficient. Lacking HIPAA (Health Insurance Portability and Accountability Act of 1996) compliance, email is difficult to integrate into the EHR, and email lacks the verification necessary to insure that the information has not only been conveyed but also generated an appropriate response and follow-up. An optimized EHR should have a direct link to the tool or instrument utilized in evaluating the patient and should integrate the results into the care record, providing "intelligent alerts" about updated evaluations and continuously reassessing the severity of the disease. However, reporting the results of a questionnaire or survey is not enough. The simplistic solution of having a PHQ9 score of >20 activate an urgent alert to the PCP requesting confirmation of the need for further evaluation and suggesting the use of an

PATIENT HEALTH QUESTIONNAIRE-9 (PHQ-9)

Over the last 2 weeks, how often have you been bothered by any of the following problems? (Use "✔" to indicate your answer)	Not at all	Several days	More than half the days	Nearly every day
1. Little interest or pleasure in doing things	0	1	2	3
2. Feeling down, depressed, or hopeless	0	1	2	3
3. Trouble falling or staying asleep, or sleeping too much	0	1	2	3
4. Feeling tired or having little energy	0	1	2	3
5. Poor appetite or overeating	0	1	2	3
6. Feeling bad about yourself — or that you are a failure or have let yourself or your family down	0	1	2	3
7. Trouble concentrating on things, such as reading the newspaper or watching television	0	1	2	3
8. Moving or speaking so slowly that other people could have noticed? Or the opposite — being so fidgety or restless that you have been moving around a lot more than usual	0	1	2	3
9. Thoughts that you would be better off dead or of hurting yourself in some way	0	1	2	3

FOR OFFICE CODING ___0___ + _____ + _____ + _____

=Total Score: _____

If you checked off any problems, how difficult have these problems made it for you to do your work, take care of things at home, or get along with other people?

Not difficult at all	Somewhat difficult	Very difficult	Extremely difficult
☐	☐	☐	☐

Developed by Drs. Robert L. Spitzer, Janet B.W. Williams, Kurt Kroenke and colleagues, with an educational grant from Pfizer Inc. No permission required to reproduce, translate, display or distribute.

Figure 13.4 Patient Health Questionnaire-9 (PHQ-9).

antidepressant and/or urgent psychotherapy is fraught with peril. The PHQ9 information must be linked to an analysis of patient stressors, family history, and other information to prevent erroneous alerts and false positives.

Once the EHR has detected the potential for a major depressive disorder, the system should begin steps to confirm the diagnosis and protect the patient. If EHR analysis suggests an imminent threat to the patient, remote video communication with an actual provider—a telepresence modality such as Skype™ or Facetime™—could be employed. Video conferencing with on-call therapists would be directly connected to the depressed patient, and a therapist could confirm the severity of the patient's presentation and initiate the patient's appropriate entry into the psychiatric care system.[22] Components of this paradigm exist in modern medicine but are not yet interlinked to provide this level of intervention. Several additional remote-care approaches are in development. The first involves *patient portals*, remote access to dedicated portions of the patient's EHR, which are now becoming standard and part of governmental EHR recommendations.[23] Patient portals are of particular importance because they require no custom software on the part of the patient and can be activated from any remote computer. Smartphone technology, laptops, or even touch-screen kiosks are supported by these remote-access systems. A major advantage is that all on-line portal activities can be unobtrusively monitored by the EHR on the hospital or clinic side. Patient involvement, such as completing a questionnaire, is verifiable. Then, from within the EHR, artificial intelligence or algorithmic alerts are generated; results and recommendations are sent to all appropriate care providers instantly.

The second approach involves custom computer programs—applications or "apps"—which are installed on all types of computing platforms, including desktops, laptops, tablets, and smartphone systems. Whereas patient portals are generic, mobile apps can be personalized to work on a cellphone, remote from access to the EHR. In general, patients have adapted to considerable comfort in using their cells and other mobile devices to communicate, engage in commerce, and manage their daily activities (Figure 13.5).[24,25] They can capture additional details such as location, activity, calls, etc., to assist the patient on a very personal level. As critical information is documented, it can be relayed back to the EHR. Early attempts with self-screening for depression through a mobile app

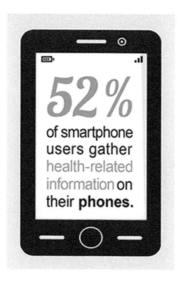

52%
of smartphone users gather health-related information on their phones.

Figure 13.5 Smartphone and HealthCare.[25]

with a direct link to EHR data transfer is promising.[24] The effectiveness of these apps is directly proportional to the tools or instruments they employ. Completing a mobile app is a technology that will be integrated into routine physician office visits in the near future. After-hours nursing, on-call physicians, concerned caregivers at the bedside, and even family members with questions can use these mobile instruments to start a constructive conversation with the PCP or provide support for triggering a direct referral to a mental health clinician.

Dedicated research computer systems can further automate the diagnosis of depression and assist non-psychiatric caregivers. *SimSensi* is a computer software program that utilizes a non-threatening animated "avatar" to communicate with the patient and continues to ask standardized questionnaires until the system has gained sufficient data to support a probable diagnosis of depression or not.[26] *MultiSense* is a separate program that can be run in parallel with SimSensi or other applications.[27] This novel mechanism advances computer evaluation one level further by adding visual sensors and motion-tracking algorithms to capture patterns in body language and facial expressions.[28] A guided-conversation protocol encourages the patient to respond in a predictable physical fashion that can be tracked three-dimensionally, secondarily providing an accurate and repeatable score of the degree of depressive symptoms. Seemingly science fiction, these systems could be placed on computer terminals or robots in the physician's office, allowing patients to perform self-evaluation *prior* to any intervention of the staff or provider. Early trials show promise.

Another approach disassociates early care from the EHR altogether. Recent improvements in providing the general public with access to psychiatric information are seen in the *MindKare* *Kiosk* (Figure 13.6).[29] These stand-alone devices obtain anonymous

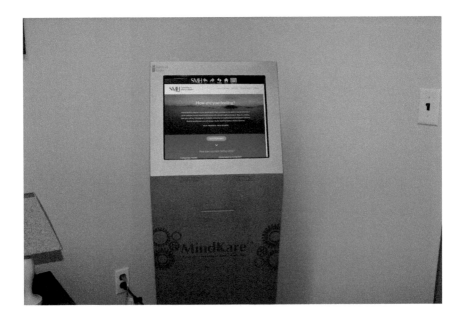

Figure 13.6 The MindKare™ Kiosk. Photo by Sue Thorn, provided to bostonmagazine.com.

information via a touch-screen and examine a range of psychiatric illnesses via question-driven modules on the following disorders: anxiety, depression, post-traumatic stress, bipolar, eating, and alcohol use.[29] As independent kiosks, they reside in a waiting room, in a common area in a mall, or even in a student activity area on college campuses.

In addition to increasing awareness of prevalent psychiatric illnesses, they stimulate dialogue, and provide access to local treatment referrals. While independent of the EHR, this informational approach has the merit of allowing patients and families to begin to address their psychiatric issues outside the confines of the medical system, and gives them guidance towards appropriate psychiatric care. Such methods would be important for the turmoil many persons feel on college campuses and in the military. One can image a next-generation system identifying the patient and transparently linking critical information directly to the patient's personal EHR.

At the forefront of this discussion is that the depressed patient often has difficulty with completing tasks and taking part in the care plan. Fortunately, many of these techniques can be instituted or completed by any associated family member or level of caregiver. A distant family member, student nurse at the bedside, or even a chairperson of a non-psychiatric department can have the tools to begin the diagnosis and treatment process. Further linkage of concerning psychiatric findings into an EHR can then be used to activate the appropriate response by the PCP or psychiatric care provider. Earlier engagement in treatment may move the patient to a higher level of care that will hasten and improve their outcome.

DIAGNOSIS: RISK FACTORS, BIOLOGICAL MARKERS, AND HYBRID METHODS

Known risk factors associated with depression are critical to establishing its diagnosis in some patients (Box 13.1). The EHR is effective at acquiring, in limited detail, some of this information as part of the intake process for creating the patient's visit record. The concept of *allostatic load*—a measure of multiple medical and non-medical factors contributing to a disease—needs a new and flexible approach to be effectively documented in the EHR data. Risk-factor data, when analyzed with experimental evidence using predictive modeling software, can alert a non-psychiatric provider to the possibility of depression in the clinical setting, but it needs useable data to run

---

Box 13.1 Patient-Reported Risk Factors for Depression

Traumatic events, interpersonal stress, financial strain
Childhood trauma
Family history of depression
Other psychiatric illness
Addiction
Other medical illness (diabetes, stroke, cancer, chronic pain, heart disease)
Medications

the analysis.[30] Another similar non-automated depression algorithm using risk factors to increase the predictive value of diagnosis includes demographic, employment, social, past medical history, and family support information, as described by King in 2008.[31] While these allostatic risk factor measures alone are helpful, their combination with additional self-screening tools (previously described) theoretically yields a significantly more robust diagnostic tool. Generating a hybrid score based on this type of predictive modeling approach will augment our identification of at-risk patients.

Patients identified as being at increased risk by this hybrid method would be managed differently by an enhanced EHR. Automated alerts to providers, automated care plans, and even pre-scripted consultation requests to appropriate psychiatric specialists could be instituted. Both major medical-records systems providers—EPIC and Cerner—currently support this automate functionality for care with other disease processes (e.g., venous thromboembolism, cardiac care order sets, etc.). While it is difficult to actually diagnose the presence or degree of depression, it should be within the scope of these systems to appropriately engage the PCP to screen further for a major depressive disorder.

Biological markers to assist in the diagnosis of depression may be ready for clinical use very soon. Potential biomarkers for depression include neurotrophic factors, serotonergic markers, biochemical indicators, and immunological markers.[32] Initial work suggested that no one factor alone is sufficient to allow the direct diagnosis of depression. Acknowledging that a combined panel might be more effective, researchers utilized nine biomarkers to achieve acceptable clinical sensitivity and specificity (92% and 81%, respectively).[33] Further addition of gender and body mass index (BMI) to this combination biomarker model (*MDDScore*) generated one assay for identifying depressed patients for which the validation set accuracy was 91%. Several other biomarker and gene-expression–based tests are under development. While several show promise, and one individual blood transcriptomic biomarker panel was shown to effectively discriminate between depressed patients and non-depressed patients, in general, the sample sizes have been small, and the results have yet to be applied in routine clinical practice.[34] Adaptation of these tests into the decision support of the EHR is a project for the future.

Another multifaceted approach that shows excellent promise is the Research Domain Criteria (*RDoC*).[35] Currently a National Institute of Mental Health (NIMH) research tool, RDoC has the potential of transforming biological, psychological, and social factors into meaningful diagnostic and outcome measures utilizing five cognitive and motivational domains.

Large datasets can be integrated into a searchable knowledge base where a continuum of items from molecular constructs to social/environmental factors can be organized as a starting point for more in-depth research. For example, an RDoC-style methodology was used to join the records of 70,000 individuals with autism and is now identifying common patterns for more accurate diagnosis of the disease.[36] Similarly, in the study of depression, where current research formats use a few major variables, the RDoC can potentially link a wide array of disparate biochemical and biological information into meaningful diagnostic and outcome measures (Box 13.2). Many of these approaches are in their infancy, with statistical methods under development.

Imagine a scenario where the clinical data are captured by the EHR, laboratory studies, mobile apps, and other methods, and are then organized into seven levels of information (genes, molecules, cells, circuits, physiology, behavior, self-reported events). This is then compared to a worldwide RDoC knowledge-base of hundreds of thousands of depressed-patient records. Acquisition of the RDoC elements or "endophenotypes" for our patient then integrates measures of acute threat, motivation, attention, and arousal into the analysis to better define the severity of our patient's depression. A unified and "large-data" method can work with partial information and identify subtle variations in individual patient presentation. Currently, the technical computerized methods for capturing, organizing, accessing, and merging all of these factors do not yet exist for available EHRs. Many of the necessary behavioral variables cannot be seamlessly integrated into the RDoC. Complex disease symptoms such as withdrawal, appetite, and sleep are difficult enough to capture, let alone interpret in conjunction with measureable physiological variables (e.g., heart rate, blood pressure, etc.). Hopefully, the RDoC will evolve into a self-populating template and knowledge base with which to combine these diverse levels of biological, psychological, and motivational information. Hypothetically, genetic and epigenetic depression markers currently under investigation would interface transparently with a RDoC model and could potentially be used to better identify cases of individuals at risk for depression.[36]

CHOOSING TREATMENT

The PCP should benefit from a variety of tools to choose and maintain the best treatment available for their patient. Current EHRs use drug–drug interaction data to alert the provider before a prescription is approved. Medication effects found by evidence-based medicine from Cochrane or other meta-analyses are part of drug–drug interaction databases and analysis engines that optimize medication choice.[37] Already, decision-making software is utilizing massive data analysis and enhanced computational power from multi-institutional resources—"Big Data" and "Predictive Analytics"—to provide continuous pharma-therapeutic feedback on the benefits and side effects of medications.[38] With new, massively high-powered computer "consultants," such as IBM's "Watson" or Google's "Deep Mind," there is now the capacity to provide almost instantaneous decision support on the benefits, side effects, drug–drug interactions, as well as costs and world-wide pharmacy availability.[39] The ability to search global datasets for a patient-specific answer promises to have a profound effect on medical decision-making. Eventually, choosing the appropriate medication and dosage can be simplified and customized to each depressed patient, even perhaps to a molecular level.

Laboratory studies are also becoming more effective at separating components that influence our options in treating patients with depression. For over 20 years, it has been known that drug metabolism can be altered by different isoenzymes that can behave differently on a patient-by-patient basis.[40] One particular target involves profiling the six separate cytochrome p450 enzymes that affect multiple classes of drugs. With the addition of routine isoenzyme identification in the future, it may be possible to better customize the use of pharmacology at a highly individual level.[41] A potentially clinically important example involves testing the variability in the patient's 2D6 gene and characterizing the patient's metabolism of fluoxetine as poor, minimal, intermediate, or ultra-rapid, which would help predict the patient's treatment response or the amount of medication needed. Collecting data about a patient's enzyme profile, current medications, and superimposed drug–drug interactions should provide the type of meta-knowledge highly useful for effective treatment of refractory depression, and anticipate and avoid untoward medication reactions. This is particularly crucial when there is psychiatric and medical comorbidity with drugs employed for both domains. Additional computer decision-support comes in the form of "patient-aware algorithms," which take into account the patient's physiological and psychological ability to successfully complete a course of medication. For example, choosing whether to take apixaban (Eliquist) or warfarin (Coumadin) could be based on a patient's ability to routinely obtain the blood work necessary to check anticoagulation with laboratory measures as is necessary with the second agent.

ASSESSING OUTCOMES

It is well documented that antidepressants are effective in one-third of patients, partially effective in another third, and of no benefit in the remaining patients.[42] Systematically monitoring depressive symptoms with a standardized scale can improve treatment outcomes by providing ongoing assessment of the success of current medication and non-medication therapies.[43] Continuous tracking methods help differentiate where treatments are successful from those where patients are not improving and a different pharmacological and/or psychological approach may be indicated. Monitoring techniques could involve self-reporting, where the patients take the primary responsibility of completing the record on their own, thereby decreasing the time to obtain treatment data by involving the patients at intervals between office visits.

These self-reported tests can also capture more sensitive, personal information than clinician-performed rating scales where the patients feel they are being judged.[44] The self-report Antidepressant Treatment Response Questionnaire (ATRQ; Chandler 2010) is one tool that appears to have good reliability and validity on treatment effect.[45] Physicians have also begun to employ ambulatory monitoring technology that can monitor physiological measures such as skin-conductance response, heart rate variability, and movement.[46] Even vocal characteristics and behavioral measures such as activity context, high-level movements, diurnal sleep patterns, and socialization correlate with improvements in clinical rating scales of depression.[47] Six of the nine major DSM criteria for depression can theoretically be tracked in this fashion. A neuropsychological marker such as documenting a lack of pupillary dilation in reaction to stimuli is also purported to be an effective early sign of relapse and could serve as an outcome-tracking indicator.[28,48]

Consequently, the enhanced EHR has the opportunity to be the important fulcrum for collecting complex outcomes data that mark the patient's progress in a time-independent and continuous format. Signs of depression such as withdrawal and social inactivity can be seamlessly captured through a mobile device, while additional self-monitoring apps track outcome factors such as activity, sleep, and mood. Mobile devices have already been utilized with some success to track behavioral markers for the relapse of depression post-treatment, but it is the integration of this type of technology into the EHR that will allow physicians to truly provide 24-hour care.[49] Patients are already accustomed to consenting to many aspects of the medical care process, including the use of their self-collected data. Now they would have the additional benefit of continuous access to the EHR's analysis of their symptom status, allowing them to become more active participants in their treatment. Continuous monitoring has the potential to identify relapse much earlier than the current practice of intermittent follow-ups.

Ultimately, a simplified depression outcome measure needs to be discovered. Just as the hemoglobin A1C gives guidance for diabetics, and the PSA test aids the assessment of the status of the prostate, a depressive outcomes measure would be ideal to identify the presence or recurrence of depression and/or its response to treatment.[50] A distilled value for depression and relapse may involve a multitude of variables that, when combined, offer a higher positive predictive value, as is seen with the MDDScore biomarker described before. Another robust example of such a measure in another specialty is the Appearance, Pulse, Grimace, Activity, and Respiration scale (APGAR) score for neonates.[51] APGAR has proven to be a great prediction tool for obstetrical teams in correctly identifying babies who need advanced care. It is easily memorized; everyone on the obstetrical team knows the APGAR meaning, and from this score, what their roles are to assist the newborn. In a similar fashion to this well-supported five-point scale, all providers need a specific measure that identifies depression and relapse. The most effective tool for outcome tracking will undoubtedly incorporate a combined effort of self-reporting, and behavioral, physiological, and biological components with the enhanced EHR at its center.

PITFALLS AND PROBLEMS

Non-technical and technical barriers need to be overcome for optimal depression care assisted by a tailored and effective EHR. There is a massive number of depressed patients, estimated to be over 8 million in the United States at any one time. PCPs will on average see or identify 4 million of those patients. Our method and approach with the current

EHR has to evolve to confront this challenge and burden. Physicians need to be stakeholders in these changes, given the dissatisfaction with the work demanded to effectively use the current EHRs:

1. Currently, more physician time is spent on completing the EHR and desk-work than on actually seeing patients;[52]
2. Physicians who use EHRs have decreased satisfaction and a higher risk for professional burnout;[52] and,
3. Patients report lower satisfaction when physicians spend time at the computer performing clerical tasks.[53]

Several design decisions in the EHR could be improved to help with these factors. Customized EHR displays better suited for tablet computers with their lower profile may increase satisfaction. Replacing excessive non-specific alerts with more salient and personalized alarms will unburden the physician from unnecessary, redundant information. A reduction in "click fatigue"—limiting the number of steps to complete a task in the computer record—will also assist the busy professional.

Significant major factors involving the profession of the PCP need to be addressed as well. As witnessed above, the PCP has concerns about becoming a "dumping ground" for all patient care. Multiple excellent analyses say that PCPs see 52% of the patients and receive 5% of the reimbursement.[54] Converting PCPs into our supportive colleagues to manage depression requires creation and implementation of more painless detection methods and automated interlinking to current PCP goals for improved patient health. For instance, if care requirements for smoking and alcohol cessation can be automatically completed as part of their depression management, the PCPs' willingness to assist in psychiatric care will improve. To enhance compliance and support for depression diagnosis and treatment, it is necessary as well to shift the burden of obtaining much of the essential information gathering to the ancillary staff and adjunct providers, such as the physician's assistants.

If patient care portals and mobile applications can energize the patient to provide data entry, this would reduce the burden on the PCPs. Toward this goal, approximately 36% of respondents reported in 2014 that their hospitals provided patients with secure online access to clinical patient information, a significant increase from 12% in 2010.[55] Multimedia tailored to engage the patient, teaching videos to answer patient questions, direct access to after-hours physician support, and continuous access to personal records and information resources can incentivize and assist in increasing patients' portal use.

Intelligent systems and EHR alerts will eventually cooperate in automatically interpreting the patient-input data; hopefully, data sources and studies can be linked into a didactic model that will identify the depression status of a patient. Currently, this is a significant pitfall in that inputting patient data and their subsequent interpretation is an extremely intensive set of individualized assignments. It is essential to convert the diagnosis of depression from an onerous task to an efficient standard of care.

Finally, the EHR systems purchased by hospitals are exorbitant in cost, requiring tremendous resources for both implementation and maintenance. Despite creating common communication standards for computing technologies, individual proprietary database structures have not encouraged local innovation for ready integration or allowed patient records to be shared between institutions with different systems. Complex EHR systems must be restructured to support transparent "bidirectional" data sharing between all medical offices and institutions so that patients may obtain appropriate, data-driven therapies based on the information previously collected in their personal records, regardless of their location or vendor.

APPROACHES TO HANDLING COMPLEX DISEASE— HOW OTHER SPECIALTIES HAVE SUCCEEDED

In terms of EHR diagnosis and treatment recommendations, there is a massive divide between bench research, bedside clinical care, and reality. Depression is in many ways an extremely difficult and complex disease; as evidenced here, it can be identified by a multitude of techniques: from answering questions, observing patients, talking to patient contacts, conducting laboratory studies, and reading facial cues, to tracking performance. Subjective and objective observations vary in importance on a very patient-specific and disease-specific basis. Psychiatrists are laboriously trained in capturing this information in a parallel, simultaneous, and often non-contiguous fashion during their patient evaluations, which are then converted into a DSM Axis diagnosis. Solving this complexity in care is analogous to the difficulties of implementing a "driverless car" where a radical series of new technologies and concepts had to be optimized before it was even conceivable.[56] Accomplishing car transport without a human driver necessitated the creation of both the concept of a "global positioning system" (GPS) and placement into orbit of a minimum of 24 satellites to support continuous access to the GPS information. Traffic data, enhanced and robust car sensors, computer hardware with extremely fast decision-making capacity, and networking and computerized standards all had to be in place before a driverless-car paradigm could be considered. Further modification of state and federal laws, in addition to a willingness by responsible individuals to accept potential catastrophic accidents as an outcome, was a prerequisite before testing could even be considered.[56] Similarly, a modified EHR could assist the PCP in automated depression screening, diagnosis, treatment identification, outcome tracking, and monitoring maintenance, but how is this infrastructure to be realized?

Daunting tasks in the identification and management of complex medical diseases have been successfully breached by unique, multi-specialty approaches. Four models follow that illustrate how kinds of information are obtained and how the algorithms are constructed for identification and action. Success in each of these medical specialties required rethinking the approach to treating the individual disease. In some instances, a "bundle" or guideline was sufficient. In others, empowering someone other than the expert physician was critical to addressing the problem. In most improvements, there was success directly tied to increasing awareness, advertising the importance of attacking the issue, and providing the tools to efficiently fix the disease in a dependable fashion. A novel EHR utilizing these new creative approaches is what we need to bring to our treatment of depression.

One excellent example involves the management of sepsis. Sepsis is a potentially life-threatening complication associated with infection and the body's systemic inflammatory response. Progressive failure leads to severe sepsis, septic shock, and probable death. The source of infection is often unknown, and physicians have struggled for decades to find an approach that works. Fortunately, specialized protocols have changed our approach and success at treating all aspects of this disorder.

The "Surviving Sepsis" campaign has undergone multiple iterations, but is based on a specialty-independent protocol that transparently follows the patient from emergency room to intensive care room or operating room (see Figure 13.7).[57] Sepsis is suspected and therapy begun immediately. Initialization of care has a 30-minute window, is not dependent on a diagnosis or a critical care expert, and does not require availability of specialized equipment; the care progresses even as the specialists are just learning of the patient.

The success of "Surviving Sepsis" has documented a decrease in *mortality* in sepsis patients by 25% or greater.[58] Sepsis protocols—or care "bundles"—allow the expert sepsis specialists to define the goals and guide routine-care providers to take the reins of patient care. All physicians are "kept in the loop," and concrete goals allow the evaluation of every patient for quality of care. The sepsis bundle has become a standard for patient care in all hospitals in the world, and all the algorithms, bundles, and protocols are available free of charge at *Survivingsepsis.org*. Enabling all physicians to initiate the care that experts would routinely provide is remarkably effective.

A similar improvement is seen in targeting decubitus ulcer management in the general hospital setting. Guidelines for pressure-ulcer management have been generated by numerous international coalitions, with varying degrees of success in adoption.[59] It is the hospital-approved *automated nursing* protocols, however, that give bedside providers the power to change care plans instantaneously, based on physical examination findings. Such change is instituted without a physician order and has made the greatest difference in limiting the progression of decubitus disease.[60] The degree of injury is assessed pictographically, the classification and staging are simple and accurate, and the treatment is implemented without delay (Figure 13.8). Protocol instructions on timing, frequency, and methods of documentation are provided.[61] There are multiple benefits to this approach in that the provider closest to the patient—the nurse—is given power to improve care directly, the patient is benefited almost instantaneously, and the entire team is engaged in patient care at all levels of training. Nursing staff are functionally given the decision power that physicians normally wield, with excellent results.

Other modified paradigms have been instrumental in intervening with difficult disease processes. Intensive care unit (ICU) delirium is an extremely difficult problem to treat, with significant long-term worsening of prognosis. New protocol care measures unify Pain, Anxiety, and Delirium care into a single care modality—*P.A.D.*—with assessment, treatment, and prevention as a continuum of care across the spectrum of disease (Figure 13.9). Most major EHRs allow nurses, physicians, and administrators to track where difficulties in the process exist.[62] Again, the structure of the algorithm allows *all* providers to initiate preventative treatment at any time and heightens the awareness of possible pain, anxiety, and delirium. The focus is on prevention and identification by any

Protocol A: Create a protocol and educate users

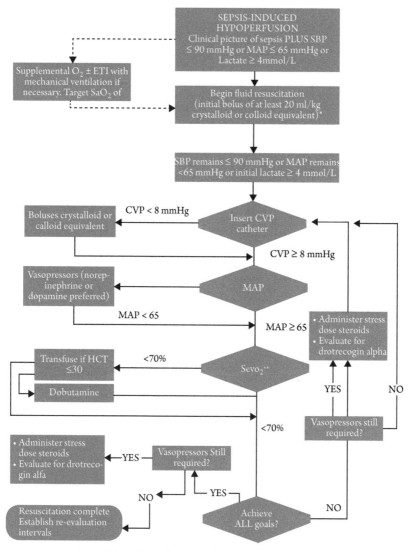

SEPSIS-INDUCED HYPOPERFUSION
Clinical picture of sepsis PLUS SBP ≤ 90 mmHg or MAP ≤ 65 mmHg or Lactate ≥ 4mmol/L

Supplemental O₂ ± ETI with mechanical ventilation if necessary. Target SaO₂ of

Begin fluid resuscitation (initial bolus of at least 20 ml/kg crystalloid or colloid equivalent)*

SBP remains ≤ 90 mmHg or MAP remains <65 mmHg or initial lactate ≥ 4 mmol/L

Boluses crystalloid or colloid equivalent

CVP < 8 mmHg — Insert CVP catheter

CVP ≥ 8 mmHg

Vasopressors (norep-inephrine or dopamine preferred)

MAP

MAP < 65

MAP ≥ 65

• Administer stress dose steroids
• Evaluate for drotrecogin alpha

Transfuse if HCT ≤30

<70%

Sevo₂**

Dobutamine

YES   NO

<70%

Vasopressors still required?

• Administer stress dose steroids
• Evaluate for drotreco-gin alfa

YES — Vasopressors Still required?

NO

YES

Resuscitation complete Establish re-evaluation intervals

Achieve ALL goals?

NO

*In circumstances where MAP is judged to be critically low, vasopressors may be started at any point in this algorithm.

**If pulmonary artery catheter is used, a mixed venous O₂ saturation is an acceptable surrogate and 65% would be the target.

Figure 13.7 Surviving Sepsis Bundle (Dellinger).[58]

nurse or physician provider *before* the disease becomes an extremely difficult management process with a *doubling* of patient morbidity and mortality.[63,64]

Lastly, the National Stroke Campaign has been a global effort with long-lasting impact. Neurological salvage after stroke has a very successful medical therapy involving tissue plasminogen activator (tPA), a systemic anticoagulant, where treatment within three

Category/Stage I: Non-blanchable Erythema Intact skin with non-blanchable redness of a localized area usually over a bony prominence. Darkly pigmented skin may not have visible blanching; its color may differ from the surrounding area. The area may be painful, firm, soft, warmer or cooleras compared to adjacent tissue. Category/Stage I may be difficult to detect in individuals with dark skin tones. May indicate "at risk" individuals (a heralding sign of risk).		
Category/Stage II: Partial Thickness Skin Loss Partial thickness loss of dermis presenting as a shallow open ulcer with a red pink wound bed, without slough. May also present as an intact or open/ruptured serum-filled blister. Presents as a shiny or dry shallow ulcer without slough or bruising.* This Category/Stage should not beused to describe skin tears, tape burns, perineal dermatitis, maceration or excoriation. *Bruising indicates suspected deep tissue injury.*		
Category/Stage III: Full Thickness Skin Loss Full thickness tissue loss. Subcutaneous fat may be visible but bone, tendon or muscle are not exposed. Slough may be present but does not obscure the depth of tissue loss. May include undermining and tunneling. The depth of a Category/Stage III pressure ulcer varies by anatomical location. The bridge of the nose, ear, occiput and malleolus do not have subcutaneous tissue and Category/Stage III ulcers can be shallow. In contrast, areas of significant adiposity can develop extremely deep Category/Stage III pressure ulcers. Bone/tendon is not visible or directly palpable.		
Category/Stage IV: Full Thickness Tissue Loss Full thickness tissue loss with exposed bone, tendon or muscle. Slough or eschar may be present on some parts of the wound bed. Often include undermining and tunneling. The depth of a Category/Stage IV pressure ulcer varies by anatomical location. The bridge of the nose, ear, occiput and malleolus do not have subcutaneous tissue and these ulcers can be shallow. Category/Stage IV ulcers can extend into muscle and/or supporting structures (e.g., fascia, tendon or joint capsule) making osteomyelitis possible. Exposed bone/tendon is visible or directly palpable.		
Unstageable: Depth Unknown Full thickness tissue loss in which the base of the ulcer is covered by slough (yellow, tan, gray, green or brown) and/or eschar (tan, brown or black) in the wound bed. Until enough slough and/or eschar is removed to expose the base of the wound, the true depth, and therefore Category/Stagecannot be determined. Stable (dry, adherent, intact without erythema or fluctuance) eschar on the heels serves as 'the body's natural (biological) cover' and should not be removed.		
Suspected Deep Tissue Injury: Depth Unknown Purple or maroon localized area of discolored intact skin or blood-filled blister due to damage of underlying soft tissue from pressure and/or shear. The area may be preceded by tissue that is painful, firm, mushy, boggy, warmer or cooler as compared to adjacent tissue. Deep tissue injury may be difficult to detect in individuals with dark skin tones. Evolution may include a thin blister over a dark wound bed. The wound may further evolve and become covered by thin eschar. Evolution may be rapid exposing additional layers of tissue even with optimal treatment.		

Figure 13.8 Grading Tool for Decubitus Ulcers (NAPUA).[60]

hours is key to optimizing recovery. Only educating the potential patient and their family can make them arrive at the hospital in time. Recognizing this, the National Stroke Foundation has taken as their task the education of the public. The slogan *"Time Is Brain"* is seen on an endless series of advertisements. The Stroke Associations are quick to observe that 80% of strokes can be prevented, and share their guidelines with the

ICU Pain, Agitation, and Delirium Care Bundle

	PAIN	AGITATION	DELIRIUM
ASSESS	Assess pain ≥ 4x/shift & prn Preferred pain assessment tools: • Patient able to self-report → NRS (0–10) • Unable to self-report → BPS (3–12) or CPOT (0–8) Patient is in significant pain if NRS ≥ 4, BPS > 5, or CPOT ≥ 3	Assess agitation, sedation ≥ 4x/shift & prn Preferred sedation assessment tools: • RASS (−5 to +4) or SAS (1 to 7) • NMB → suggest using brain function monitoring Depth of agitation, sedation defined as: • *agitated* if RASS = +1 to +4, or SAS = 5 to 7 • *awake and calm* if RASS = 0, or SAS = 4 • *lightly sedated* if RASS = −1 to −2, or SAS = 3 • *deeply sedated* if RASS = −3 to −5, or SAS = 1 to 2	Assess delirium Q shift & prn Preferred delirium assessment tools: • CAM-ICU (+ or −) • ICDSC (0 to 8) Delirium present if: • CAM-ICU is positive • ICDSC ≥ 4
TREAT	Treat pain within 30' then reassess: • Non-pharmacologic treatment–relaxation therapy • Pharmacologic treatment: – Non-neuropathic pain → IV opioids +/− non-opioid analgesics – Neuropathic pain → gabapentin or carbamazepine, + IV opioids – S/p AAA repair, rib fractures → thoracic epidural	Targeted sedation or DSI (*Goal: patient purposely follows commands without agitation*): RASS = −2 – 0, SAS = 3–4 • If *under sedated* (RASS > 0, SAS > 4) assess/treat pain → treat w/ sedatives prn (non-benzodiazepines preferred, unless ETOH or benzodiazepine withdrawal is suspected) • If *over sedated* (RASS < −2, SAS < 3) hold sedatives until at target, then restart at 50% of previous dose	• Treat pain as needed • Reorient patients; familiarize surroundings; use patient's eyeglasses, hearing aids if needed • Pharmacologic treatment of delirium: – Avoid benzodiazepines unless ETOH or benzodiazepines withdrawal is suspected – Avoid rivastigmine – Avoid antipsychotics if ↑ risk of Torsades de pointes
PREVENT	• Administer pre-procedural analgesia and/or non-pharmacologic interventions (e.g., relaxation therapy) • Treat pain first, then sedate	• Consider daily SBT, early mobility and exercise when patients are at goal sedation level, unless contraindicated • EEG monitoring if: – at risk for seizures – burst suppression therapy is indicated for ↑ ICP	• Identity delirium risk factors: dementia HTN, ETOH abuse, high severity of illness, coma, benzodiazepine administration • Avoid benzodiazepine use in those at ↑ risk for delirium • Mobilize and exercise patients early • Promote sleep (control light, noise; cluster patient care activities; decrease nocturnal stimuli) • Restart baseline psychiatric meds, if indicated

Figure 13.9 PAD Care Bundle (iculiberation.org).

American Heart Association and other nationally recognized sites.[65] Most importantly, people are learning about stroke. The patient and family have become the diagnosticians, because awareness has been taught and repeatedly emphasized.

FACTORS IN OUR FAVOR

Several recent developments favor implementing a new collaborative paradigm for aggressively targeting depression. Recent years have seen monumental improvements in computing power, mobile technologies, and communications methods and standards. While computers continue to double in power every several years, as had been predicted by Dr. Gordon Moore in 1965, that same progress has led to smartphone technologies capable of accessing secure information sources including EHR data portals.[66] Standards in communication between computers such as hypertext markup language (HTML) and standardized query language (SQL) database design have allowed rapid and safe data sharing across all computers and smartphones. Alternate methods for data collection, including voice recognition and language translation, have also improved exponentially. Computer voice recognition has only recently equaled the 5% error rates seen in routine human-based medical transcription.[67] All of these improvements can support a new collaborative model based on modern technologies built into an enhanced EHR.

Sharing information online via the Internet has become significantly more accepted in our daily lives. As the Internet has become the largest source of medical patient information queries, many more patients are using online learning and social media sites—electronic communication that can create online communities—on a daily basis. With social media sites such as Facebook, Instagram, Twitter, and others becoming the normal mode of communication, sharing information is an everyday occurrence. Mobile approaches are also associated with positive and rewarding feedback. Many physicians' offices supported by their EHRs provide social media access to email, teaching resources, even using social media as a way to reach their patients directly.[68] Previously, a major issue was the lack of staff trained to support a computerized office environment, but this has also significantly improved with revised expectations in staff training and staff comfort with computer usage.[55] Universal adoption of these technologies by patients, providers, and staff makes constructing a robust detection method for depression easier.

Societal norms about discussion of personal medical illness have also changed over the last decade. Television and billboard advertising target diseases and problems that were previously more hidden from view. Stroke, erectile dysfunction, HIV, hepatitis C, constipation, and even psychiatric issues such as suicidal thoughts and antisocial behavior are targeted on a nightly basis in the mainstream media and even on bridges, e.g., the Golden Gate Bridge. Furthermore, patient and families now request new medical therapies and chemotherapies they see advertised on television. Whereas patients would previously defer to their physician's expertise, they now arrive in the office and demand the use of lasers or robots for their surgery[69]—patients in their newfound access to knowledge have begun to drive patient care decisions. Interest in having the most modern therapy as advertised on the media is even redirecting where patients physically decide to pursue their treatment. A greater level of awareness of the patient's wishes and flexibility in our new EHR systems to cater to a patient's technology profile will be necessary to increase the success in the management of depression.

As discussed herein, the use of patient portals continues to expand exponentially. Surprisingly, several studies have examined older patients with chronic illnesses and found they often are the prime portal users, given their desire to minimize exhausting trips to visit the PCP.[70] Proactive strategies to educate potential users about portals are essential to engaging patients into using them and making them ubiquitous.

Portal use is encouraged further with financial and personal incentives, and the technology is now in place to transparently provide rewards to the user. Medical insurance is providing financial rewards to adopters of portal technologies—both patients and physicians.[71] The infrastructure of the Internet now allows for electronic certificates, reward cards, and delivery of gifts to patients who participate in patient portals. This is in addition to the time saved from performing many patient care tasks remotely from the office or hospital.[72] Many employees are encouraged by their companies to use patient portals, with the goal of minimizing office visits and decreasing days lost to disability via preventative care.

PROPOSED PARADIGM FOR AN ENHANCED EHR FOR DEPRESSION RECOGNITION

The future EHR should work on multiple dimensions to aid in identification, management, and treatment of the depressed patient. All levels of care providers and even families need to be encouraged to activate the diagnostic process. Instead of the standard sequential approach with the physician generating an order, which results in studies' being initiated with eventual treatment being prescribed, a parallel process paradigm needs to be developed. In the new collaborative, parallel processing model, any person in contact with the patient can start data collection, minimizing delay to identifying the degree of depression, and effectively bringing the patient "onto the radar" of the health care system as early as possible. The new collaborative care model needs to be expanded to utilize the full technical capabilities of modern society in addition to the current resources of the health care system. The patients are out in the environment, but how do we deliver to them the diagnosis and treatment they need?

There are several design optimizations to the EHR that are crucial to capturing the data. "Health care maintenance" sections of the EHR must include a depression module that requires minimal time to complete, is streamlined to target the disease, and is capable of self-populating with previously entered data points. The goal needs to be generation of an automated system which respects the time limitations of our primary care colleagues. Access to appropriate psychiatric data previously entered into the medical record must happen transparently so the provider knows when depression is appropriately diagnosed. Some depression metrics may even be completely automated and imported from separate devices such as a mobile computing tablet or MindKare‌ Kiosk as described before.[29] In ideal interconnectivity, the PCP would only have to log onto the EHR to acknowledge that depression is a concern; findings from a patient's responses on apps, family observations on Kiosks, events documented in the emergency department, or any other contact made with the EHR would be cataloged and analyzed automatically.

Finally, the care providers' attitude toward depressive illnesses needs to be revised. Critically, they must understand the prevalence and severity of depression to be a first-tier and too common illness. A companion example is the phenomenon of pain and its treatment. Recent preoccupation with the concept of "pain" in patients has led to a revolution in how discomfort is viewed and treated. Patient demands, media coverage, family involvement, legal attitudes, and major physician organizations have promoted pain to the level of a "fifth vital sign" in current medical practice. This has resulted in successful changes in the detection and treatment of pain. Similarly, depression needs to be elevated to a higher level of importance—essentially a "sixth vital sign." While in some ways this may seem an extreme view, the prevalence, disability, and complications associated with depression and adumbrated in the preceding chapters warrant its identification as a preeminent diagnostic consideration.

A new EHR methodology is described in the following discussion: Assumptions include that one's patients have access to a smartphone or home computer and that a patient portal exists to the PCP's office EHR. The communication between the patients and their EHR must include the ability to present new questionnaires and instructions to the patients as needed in a HIPAA-compliant manner. Ideally, backup psychiatric support is available and connected to the EHR used by the PCP. The nature of the decision-making illustrated here is consistent with Federal Drug Administration (FDA) rules for decision support in the EHR setting.

As seen in the section "Approaches to Handling Complex Diseases," the first effort is to educate citizens to the risks of depression and make it a major concern in patients under our care. Warning symptoms should be promoted in office literature and in patient communications. Guidelines of how psychiatrists in a PCP's region would like to have cases of depression referred should be mapped out and subsequently built into our care algorithms to generate backup support for when severe forms of depression are encountered. What medications and formularies are preferred by local psychiatrists need to be implemented in regional guidelines.

Routine patient care office visits should emphasize having access to the enhanced EHR and using it for guidance in care.[73] PCPs have been shown to have the best success when technology is introduced in person; having office staff take patients through access to their own patient portal is critical. Demonstrating the programs on the portal system, including information and social media links to the office, should be encouraged on each patient visit to develop familiarity with the EHR. Providers should educate patients about the simplicity of the portal interface and the amount of time that can be saved by registration at home. Further demonstrations can illustrate access to bills, refill requests, tracking of immunizations, and sharing of records.

With this structured approach, when depression becomes a patient concern, there are many ways to initiate depression care. As shown in Figure 13.10, a patient or their family can navigate to the patient portal and request assistance. A customized mobile app can be initiated, or the patient portal itself can be accessed to begin the data-capture process. Alternately, a patient can schedule a provider visit to discuss depression, or a routine health visit can identify the concern for depression. This "decision for action" phase leads to further evaluation and a search for information to support or rule out the diagnosis.

Once into the evaluation phase, a series of guided tasks is performed:

- *Step One* obtains a PHQ9, which will collect a summary of the past two weeks of symptoms. The PHQ9 can be entered by the patient at home on any device with Internet access, with the assistance of the patient's family online, or via an iPad, tablet, or Kiosk in the medical office.

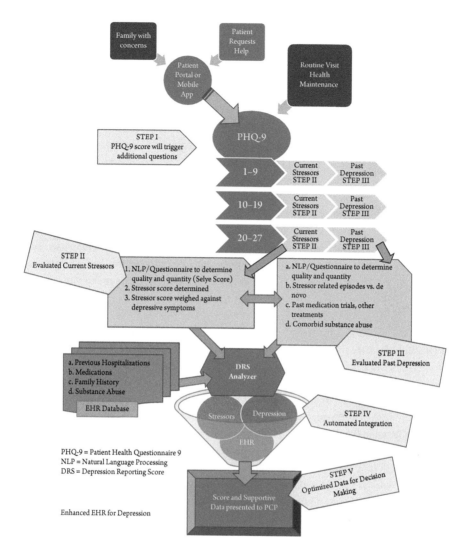

Figure 13.10 Proposed Enhanced EHR for Depression Management.
EHR Database
PHQ-9 = Patient Health Questionnaire 9
NLP = Natural Language Processing
DRS = Depression Reporting Score

- *Step Two* evaluates current *stressors*, along with the premorbid condition and functional status, using written questionnaires or natural language processing to ask questions and complete the documentation. The stressor scores are determined. The stressor scores will be weighed against the depressive symptoms. Sample stem questions to evaluate stressors might include:
  - ✓ "Sounds like you do not have significant depressive symptoms; do you nonetheless have stressors in your life?"
  - ✓ "You seem to have significant depressive symptoms; what stressors could be contributing to this?"

- *Step Three* documents *past depression*, including comorbid substance abuse, quality and quantity of depression, past treatments, and previous medication trials.
- *Step Four* automatically integrates *past medical history* from the EHR with measures of depression, stressors, and EHR records. (Biomedical markers and additional physiological findings would be part of the integration as they become available, valid, and reliable).
- *Step Five*, the *Depression Reporting Score (DRS) Analyzer,* generates a score and supporting data for level and concern for the presence of depression. The algorithm takes data from the previous four Steps and calculates a risk on a scale of 0–5: Zero with no concern for depression, and 5 suggesting the urgent need for professional psychiatric care.
- Information is updated automatically in the background to the medical record "Healthcare Maintenance" section. Both the DRS score and the supporting documentation are presented to the PCP for quick analysis. As additional information, laboratory studies, new substance abuse, or other details of concern (e.g., new questionnaires, outside reports, etc.) become available, the intelligent agent support for the DRS Analyzer would re-process the information to update the DRS Score and the summary of the supporting information.

Of importance, it is only at this final juncture that the PCP becomes a necessary participant in the care process. "Healthcare measures" will be highlighted with the risk of depression, the need for physician evaluation of mental status, and the need for a therapeutic intervention. The patient's severity, physician's comfort with managing the disease, the support that exists to help the patient recover, and multiple other factors will affect the nature of the treatment. Escalation of care is empirically triggered and recommended to the PCP when the current treatment strategy is not successful.

Questions will certainly arise about how the DRS Analyzer will make its decisions. Multiple different methods exist for providing clinical decision support in our model. Certainly, a series of potential scenarios could be entered into a knowledge-base, which is queried by the DRS Analyzer for a match. For example, one simple analytical matrix is shown in Table 13.1. The PHQ9 is separated into <=4 for minimal depression, 5–9 = mild depression, 10–14 = moderate depression, 15–19 = moderately severe depression, and 20–27 as severe depression, consistent with its proven validity as a testing agent. Other key components, including stressors, substance abuse, hospitalizations, gender, and available support, are factored into the decision process.

Table 13.1 emphasizes that a rule-based support algorithm could be tested and implemented. The rule-based system would be verified against expert psychiatric evaluation for specificity and sensitivity. Ideally, each individual category could be given a measure of importance in the decision-making. Bayesian analysis with these weighted values could be employed to generate probability statistics of whether a patient met the criteria of depression.[74] The product of this depression-management module utilized by an enhanced EHR is a pre-processed report of the likelihood that depression is present. The physician's clinical assessment and evaluation remains the "gold standard" for the validation of the diagnosis of depression from the mental status examination, and incorporating all the data generated from the methodology just delineated. The EHR will provide some guidance as to the choices a practitioner can use to treat the patient. The PCP will

Table 13.1 DRS Analyzer—Rule-Based Clinical Decision Support

DRS	PHQ9	Stressors	Depression	Substance Abuse	Hospitalizations	Gender	Support
0	0–4	Minimal	None	None	0	Male	Many close family
1	5–9	Mild	1 episode	Occasionally	1	Female	Many friends
2	10–14	Moderate	2 with occasional med treatment	Weekly	2	Homosexual	Few friends
3	15–19	Severe	3–5 episodes with continued med treatment	Recent escalation to daily	3–5	Transgender	Alternate support available
4	20–27	Extreme	4 intermittent hospitalization, continuous meds	Polysubstance, continuous, years	>5		None
5	3 or more of any category > 3						

be able to walk into the exam room with the patient, review the findings with the patient, perform a mental status exam, and come to a rational and data-supported conclusion as to what the diagnosis is and what the therapeutic intervention should be. Much of the preliminary evaluation is accomplished before the PCP sees the patient. Tracking of a patient's future evaluations will demonstrate progress or lack of success—but most importantly, the patient is identified, assisted, and has a starting point for necessary care and future improvement.

Looking to the future with enhancements to technology, infrastructure, and communication standards, the EHR should include national patient identification, integration of all major vendor EHRs, and transparent collaboration between inpatient and outpatient services. The capacity for integrating "big data" mining and "predictive analytics" should allow a higher level of automated physician support—provision of rapid clinical answers that would benefit all levels of patient care. How these newer approaches will work is yet to be determined, but it is anticipated that predictive modeling, machine learning, text analytics, and ad-hoc statistical analysis will allow systems such as IBM's Watson to provide direct optimization of a patient's care on an extremely efficient, effective, and personal level.[34,75]

CONCLUSIONS

An aging population will continue to increase in its prevalence of psychiatric disease. It is highly likely that the incidence and importance of uncovering depression will continue to rise as well. An enhanced EHR with the capability to provide better diagnosis, continuous tracking, identification of relapse, and personalized optimization of therapy and medications is sorely needed. Who or what provides the initial diagnosis of depression becomes less important than having the efficient tools to identify the patients in need of psychiatric care. Involving the PCP in this process will be necessary to accomplish this monumental task.

There is a great promise for the EHR to aid any clinician in the management of depression as a medical illness. Ideally, the EHR becomes the entity that brings the data together seamlessly from all potential sources and obtains the necessary information quickly and without compromising the quality of the encounter. As with the effective management of diabetes and other chronic medical illnesses, successful depression therapy will require multidisciplinary team-based care—careful, accurate documentation, flexible multi-provider interaction, elegantly tailored medical therapy, and robust outcome measures. Along with these interventions, the EHR will eventually provide automated, evidence-based decision support. The intelligent capabilities of an EHR could help make depression care less cumbersome and more effective. Depression, given its importance as a primary cause of worldwide disability, needs to have easier identification and more aggressive tracking. With the assistance of the EHR, depression may very well take on its role as the next vital sign.

REFERENCES

1. Global Burden of Disease Study 2013 Collaborators. Global, regional, and national incidence, prevalence, and years lived with disability for 301 acute and chronic diseases and injuries in 188 countries, 1990–2013: a systematic analysis for the Global Burden of Disease Study. *Lancet*. 2015;386:743–800.

2. Anxiety and Depression Society of America. Facts & Figures. 2016. https://www.adaa.org/about-adaa/press-room/facts-statistics. Accessed October 11, 2017.

3. Shalev AY, Freeman S, Peri T, et al. Prospective study of posttraumatic stress disorder and depression following trauma. *Am J Psychiatry*. 1998;155:630–637.

4. Findley JK, Sanders KB, Groves JE. The role of psychiatry in the management of acute trauma surgery patients. *J Clin Psychiatry*. 2003;5:195–200.

5. Thornicroft G, Chatterji S, Evans-Lacko S, et al. Undertreatment of people with major depressive disorder in 21 countries. *Br J Psychiatry*. Dec 2016. doi:10.1192/bjp.bp.116.188078.

6. Katon WJ, Lin EH, Von Korff M, et al. Collaborative care for patients with depression and chronic illnesses. *NEJM*. 2010;363(27):2611–2620.

7. Katon, W, Ciechanowski, P. Impact of major depression on chronic medical illness. *J Psychosom Res*. 2002;53:859–863.

8. U.S. Preventive Services Task Force. USPSTF A and B Recommendations. April 2017. https://www.uspreventiveservicestaskforce.org/Page/Name/uspstf-a-and-b-recommendations/. Accessed October 10, 2017

9. Cerner. Hospital & Health Systems. March 2017. http://www.cerner.com/solutions/hospitals_and_health_systems/. Accessed October 10, 2017.

10. Chaudhry B, Wang J, Wu S, et al. Systematic review: impact of health information technology on quality, efficiency, and costs of medical care. *Ann Intern Med*. 2006;144(10):742–752.

11. Linder JA, Ma J, Bates DW, et al. Electronic health record use and the quality of ambulatory care in the United States. *Arch Intern Med*. 2007;167(13):1400–1405.

12. Couch JB. CCHIT certified electronic health records may reduce malpractice risk. 2007. https://www.texmed.org/WorkArea/DownloadAsset.aspx?id=19497. Accessed October 10, 2017.

13. Kern L, Barron Y, Dhopeshwarkar RV, et al. Electronic health records and ambulatory quality of care. J Gen Intern Med. 2013 Apr;28(4):496–503. doi: 10.1007/s11606-012-2237-8.

14. Viederman M. The computer age: beware the loss of the narrative. *Gen Hosp Psychiatry*. 1995;17(3):157–159. https://doi.org/10.1016/0163-8343(95)00020-R

15. HealthIT.gov. Information about the EHR Incentive Program and EHR Incentive Payments. Providers & Professionals. January 15, 2013. https://www.healthit.gov/providers-professionals/ehr-incentive-programs. Accessed October 10, 2017.

16. Hammer JS, Lyons JS, Strain JJ. MICRO-CARES: an information management system for psychosocial services in hospital settings. *Proc Annu Symp Comput Appl Med Care*. 1984 Nov 7:234–237.

17. AMA Wire. Eight top challenges and solutions for making EHRs usable. September 16, 2014. http://www.ama-assn.org/ama/ama-wire/post/8-top-challenges-solutions-making-ehrs-usable. Accessed October 10, 2017.

18. Medpage Today. Let Primary Care be Primary Care. March 31, 2016. http://www.medpagetoday.com/patientcenteredmedicalhome/patientcenteredmedicalhome/57070. Accessed October 10, 2017.

19. DSM-5. 2017. https://www.psychiatry.org/psychiatrists/practice/dsm. Accessed October 10, 2017.

20. Kroenke K, Spitzer R, Williams W. The PHQ-9: validity of a brief depression severity measure. *JGIM*. 2001;16:606–616.

21. US Preventative Services Task Force. Final Recommendations Statement: Depression in Adults Screening. January 2016. https://www.uspreventiveservicestaskforce.org/Page/

Document/RecommendationStatementFinal/depression-in-adults-screening1. Accessed October 10, 2017.

22. Loane M, Wooton R. A review of guidelines and standards for telemedicine. *J Telemed Telecare*. 2002;8:63–71.

23. Centers for Medicare & Medicaid Services. Health Care Reform Insurance Web Portal Requirements. 2010. https://www.cms.gov/CCIIO/Resources/Files/webportal.html. Accessed October 10, 2017.

24. BinDhim NF, Alanazi EM, Aljadhey H, et al. Does a mobile phone depression-screening app motivate mobile phone users with high depressive symptoms to seek a health care professional's help? *J Med Internet Res*. 2016;18(6):e156.

25. Klick Health. 52% of smartphone users look up health information. 2012. https://www.klick.com/health/news/blog/mhealth/52-of-smartphone-users-look-up-health-information/. Accessed October 8, 2017.

26. DeVault D, Artstein ER, Benn G, et al. SimSensei Kiosk: a virtual human interviewer for healthcare decision support. In Proceedings of the 13th International Conference on Autonomous Agents and Multiagent Systems (AAMAS 2014); May 5–9, 2014; International Foundation for Autonomous Agents and Multiagent Systems Richland, Paris, France.

27. Rizzo A, Lucas G, Gratch J, et al. Clinical interviewing by a virtual human agent with automatic behavior analysis. In 2016 Proceedings of the International Conference on Disability, Virtual Reality and Associated Technologies; Sept 20–22, 2016; ICDVRAT and the University of Reading, Los Angelos, California.

28. Siegel GJ, Steinhauer SR, Friedman ES, Thompson WS, Thase ME. Remission prognosis for cognitive therapy for recurrent depression using the pupil: utility and neural correlates. *Biol Psychiatry*. 2011;69(8):726–733.

29. MindCare® Kiosks Program: Screening for Mental Health. 2017. https://mentalhealth-screening.org/programs/mindkare. Accessed October 11, 2017.

30. McEwen B. Protection and damage from acute and chronic stress: allostasis and allostatic overload and relevance to the pathophysiology of psychiatric disorders. *Ann NY Acad Sci*. 2004;1032:1–7.

31. King M, Walker C, Levy G, et al. Development and validation of an international risk prediction algorithm for episodes of major depression in general practice attendees: the PredictD Study. *Arch Gen Psychiatry*. 2008;65(12):1368–1376. doi:10.1001/archpsyc.65.12.1368.

32. Mössner R, Mikova O, Koutsilieri E, et al. Consensus paper of the WFSBP Task Force on biological markers: biological markers in depression. *World J Biol Psychiatry*. 2007;8(3):141–74.

33. Bilello JA, Thurmond LM, Smith KM, et al. MDDScore: confirmation of a blood test to aid in the diagnosis of major depressive disorder. *J Clin Psychiatry*. Feb 2015;76(2):e199–e206. doi:10.4088/JCP.14m09029.

34. Redei E, Andrus B, Kwasny M, et al. Blood transcriptomic biomarkers in adult primary care patients with major depressive disorder undergoing cognitive behavioral therapy. *Transl Psychiatry*. 2014;4:e442. doi:10.1038/tp.2014.66

35. Insel T. The NIMH Research Domain Criteria (RDoC) Project: precision medicine for psychiatry. *Am J Psychol*. 2014;171(4):395–397.

33. Sparse whole-genome sequencing identifies two loci

34. for major depressive disorder

35. Sparse whole-genome sequencing identifies two loci
36. for major depressive disorder
37. Sparse whole-genome sequencing identifies two loci
38. for major depressive disorder

36. Converge Consortium, Kendler K, Flint J, et al. Sparse whole-genome sequencing identifies two loci for major depressive disorder. *Nature*. 2015;523:588–591.

37 Cochrane Drugs and Alcohol. Our Reviews. 2017. http://cda.cochrane.org/our-reviews. Accessed October 11, 2017.

38. Dhar V. Big Data and predictive analytics in health care. *Big Data*. 2014;2(3):113–116.

39. IBM Watson Analytics. 2017. https://www.ibm.com/marketplace/cloud/watson-analytics/us/en-us. Accessed October 11, 2017.

40. Transon C, Leemann T, Dayer P. In vitro comparative inhibition profiles of major human drug metabolising cytochrome P450 isozymes (CYP2C9, CYP2D6 and CYP3A4) by HMG-CoA reductase inhibitors. *Eur J Clin Pharmacol*. 1996;50(3):209–215.

41. Ogu C, Maxa J. Drug interactions due to cytochrome P450. *Proc (Bayl Univ Med Cent)*. 2000 Oct;13(4):421–423.

42. Antonuccio DO, Danton WG. Psychotherapy versus medication for depression: challenging the conventional wisdom with data. Professional Psychology: *Research and Practice*. 1995;26(6):574–585.

43. Wang Y, Gorenstein C. Assessment of depression in medical patients: a systematic review of the utility of the Beck Depression Inventory–II. *Clinics (Sao Paulo)*. 2013 Sep;68(9):1274–1287.

44. Spitzer R, Kroenke K, Williams J. Validation and utility of a self-report version of PRIME-MD: The PHQ Primary Care Study. *JAMA*. 1999;282(18):1737–1744. doi:10.1001/jama.282.18.1737

45. Chandler GM, Iosifescu DV, Pollack MH, et al. RESEARCH: validation of the Massachusetts General Hospital Antidepressant Treatment History Questionnaire (ATRQ). *CNS Neurosci Ther*. 2010 Oct;16(5):322–325. doi:10.1111/j.1755-5949.2009.00102.x

46. Sung M, Marci C, Pentland A. Wearable feedback systems for rehabilitation. *J Neuro Engineer Rehabil*. 2005;2:17. doi:10.1186/1743-0003-2-17

47. Kanter J, Busch A, Weeks C, et al. The nature of clinical depression: symptoms, syndromes, and behavior analysis. *Behav Anal*. 2008;31(1):1–2.

48. Siegel J. REM sleep: a biological and psychological paradox. *Sleep Med Rev*. 2011;15(3):139–142.

49. Saeb S, Zhang M, Karr CJ, et al. Mobile phone sensor correlates of depressive symptom severity in daily-life behavior: an exploratory study. *J Med Internet Res*. 2015;17(7):e175.

50. Sacco W, Bykowski C. Depression and hemoglobin A1c in type 1 and type 2 diabetes: the role of self-efficacy. *Diabetes Res Clin Pract*. 2010;90(2):141–146.

51. ACOG. The Apgar Score. 2017. http://www.acog.org/Resources-And-Publications/Committee-Opinions/Committee-on-Obstetric-Practice/The-Apgar-Score. Accessed October 11, 2017.

52. Shanafelt T, Dyrbye L, Sinsky C, et al. Relationship between clerical burden and characteristics of the electronic environment with physician burnout and professional satisfaction. *Mayo Clin Proc*. 2016;91(7):836–848.

53. Kazley A, Diana M, Ford E, Menachemi N. Is electronic health record use associated with patient satisfaction in hospitals? *Health Care Manag Rev*. 2012;37(1):23–30.

54. Agency for Healthcare Research and Quality. Module 17. Electronic Health Records and Meaningful Use. 2013. http://www.ahrq.gov/professionals/prevention-chronic-care/improve/system/pfhandbook/mod17.html. Accessed October 11, 2017.

55. Incentives to Promote Technology Use in Healthcare Working. 2014. http://www.medscape.com/viewarticle/821053. Accessed October 11, 2017.

56. Anderson JM, Kalra N, Stanley K, et al. Autonomous vehicle technology: a guide for policymakers. RAND Corporation (www.rand.org), 2014. Available at https://www.rand.org/pubs/research_reports/RR443-2.html. Accessed October 11, 2017.

57. Singer M, Deutschman CS, Seymour CW, et al. The Third International Consensus definitions for sepsis and septic shock (Sepsis-3). *JAMA*. 2016;23;315(8):801–810.

58. Dellinger RP, Townsend S, Levy M. The Surviving Sepsis campaign. The Hospitalist. 2005. http://www.the-hospitalist.org/hospitalist/article/123024/surviving-sepsis-campaign. Accessed October 11, 2017.

59. Kruger KA, Pires M, Ngann Y, et al. Comprehensive management of pressure ulcers in spinal cord injury: current concepts and future trends. *J Spinal Cord Med*. 2013 Nov;36(6): 572–585.

60. National Pressure Ulcer Advisory Panel. Quick Reference Guide. 2014. http://www.npuap.org/wp-content/uploads/2014/08/Quick-Reference-Guide-DIGITAL-NPUAP-EPUAP-PPPIA-Jan2016.pdf. Accessed October 11, 2017.

61 Tissue Viability. 2016. http://www.healthcareimprovementscotland.org/our_work/patient_safety/tissue_viability.aspx. Accessed October 11, 2017.

62. Pain, Agitation, Delirium. SCCM. 2013. http://www.sccm.org/Research/Quality/Pages/Pain-Agitation-Delirium.aspx. Accessed October 11, 2017.

63. Barr J, Gilles, LF, Puntillo K, et al. Clinical practice guidelines for the management of pain, agitation, and delirium in adult patients in the intensive care unit. *Crit Care Med*. 2013;41:263–306.

64. Ely EW, Shintani A, Truman B, et al. Delirium as a predictor of mortality in mechanically ventilated patients in the intensive care unit. *JAMA*. 2004;291(1):753–1762.

65. Stay Informed—National Stroke Association. 2016. http://support.stroke.org/site/PageServer?pagename=sem_stayinformed_prev. Accessed October 11, 2017.

66. 50 Years of Moore's Law. 2015. http://www.intel.com/content/www/us/en/silicon-innovations/moores-law-technology.html. Accessed October 11, 2017.

67. The AI Blog. Historic Achievement: Microsoft researchers reach human parity in conversational speech recognition. 2016. http://blogs.microsoft.com/next/2016/10/18/historic-achievement-microsoft-researchers-reach-human-parity-conversational-speech-recognition. Accessed October 11, 2017.

68. Business Insider. 6 Ways Technology is Improving Healthcare. 2010. http://www.businessinsider.com/6-ways-technology-is-improving-healthcare-2010-12?op=1/#the-internet-has-become-a-main-source-of-medical-information-1. Accessed October 11, 2017.

69. da Vinci Surgery. Robot-Assisted Surgery. 2017. http://www.davincisurgery.com/. Accessed October 11, 2017.

70. Krist A, Woolf A, Bello G, et al. Engaging primary care patients to use a patient-centered personal health record. *Ann Fam Med*. 2014;12(5):418–426.

71. The Federal Government Has Put Billions into Promoting Electronic Health Record Use: How Is It Going? 2011. http://www.commonwealthfund.org/publications/newsletters/quality-matters/2011/june-july-2011/in-focus. Accessed October 11, 2017.

72. Baltierra NB, Muessig KE, Pike EC, et al. More than just tracking time: complex measures of user engagement with an internet-based health promotion intervention. *J Biomed Inform*. 2016;28(59):299–307.
73. Ten Ways to Convince Patients to Use the Patient Portal. 2015. http://www.physicianspractice.com/patient-portals/ten-ways-convince-patients-use-patient-portal. Accessed October 11, 2017.
74. Raftery A. Bayesian model selection in social research. *Sociol Methodol*. 1995;25:111–163.
75. Schmidhuber J. Deep learning in neural networks: an overview. *Neural Net*. 2015;61:85–117.

Epilogue

James J. Strain and Michael Blumenfield

Depression will continue to haunt the world for the foreseeable future. No society, no people, no country is immune from its presence and its torment. New ways to identify, diagnose, treat, manage, assess outcome, and prevent recurrence are under development. We need to find these patients and see that they are treated. Our volume examines this ubiquitous illness, from animal studies to allostatic load, to its precipitation and exacerbation of physical disease, to new models of teaching its management—the *medical model*; and the technology to alert, record, and guide the evidence-based management of depressive disorders, an innovative dynamic electronic health record, or EHR. Research currently underway is examining depression's underlying pathophysiological mechanisms. Depression appears to disrupt the neuroimmune axis that interfaces the immune system and central nervous system to effect behavior.[1] These studies attempt to examine the peripheral immune system's effects on the brain, its response to stress and an individual's vulnerability to mood disorder. Inflammation has been suggested as a possible mechanism for depression.[2] This offers new targets for therapeutic agents for the nearly half of depressive patients who will not respond to our current arsenal of antidepressant drugs. Viewing depression as a systemic illness changes our approaches to understanding its mechanisms of causation and its effect on physiological processes including other medical disorders and comorbidity. It also mandates we have changes in the curricula of medical schools and the competencies expected from residency training. It is our hope this volume adumbrates the needs for research, education, and treatment that lie before us.

The major handicap to identification of depression and its adequate care lies in the inability of today's caretakers to find these patients, make an appropriate diagnosis, offer evidenced-based interventions, and refer to a specialist when the basic guidelines for "*garden variety depression*" do not produce acceptable results. And, even in advanced countries, we do not have enough experienced caretakers. To improve the management of stroke, the public was given information on the symptoms and the need for an immediate emergency intervention, and this was promulgated in the public forum. Early intervention initiated by the populace has decreased the morbidity and mortality from cerebral vascular accidents. To decrease the mortality and morbidity of sepsis, protocols were established in hospitals where any member of the caretaking team, most often nurses, could start the necessary procedures immediately if the diagnostic guidelines of the protocol were fulfilled. Decubitus ulcer is now managed with a nursing protocol and begun as soon as the prescribed physical conditions are met. Pain has become a fifth "vital sign." Perhaps depression should become a *sixth* vital sign. It is essential to discover new methods to identify depression, bring these patients to appropriate care, and have health teams sufficiently trained to administer evidenced-based interventions initially. And when that procedure does not show measureable improvement, referrals can be made to specialty physicians for more advanced interventions.

Many models have been tried, and new developments are being enacted to solve this problem: the Chronic Care, the Collaborative Care, and TEAM Care were all summarized and orchestrated in the Care of Mental, Physical And Substance-use Syndromes (COMPASS) initiative implementing a complex integrated-care program.[3-7] This effort was to advance the "Triple Aim" promoted by Berwick: (1) improved health care, (2) better patient experience of care, and (3) lower costs.[8] But all must take into account that depression is a systemic disease, with significant and at times pernicious biological correlates that adversely affect the body and other medical illnesses (comorbidity), and that depression is bidirectional.

First, changes are mandatory in the medical school curricula to have the management of depression be a competency for the primary care physician (PCP)—*the medical model.* Second, changes are needed in residency programs so that PCPs have sufficient experience in the management of depressed patients. Third, physician-assistant nurse practitioners need to be trained to manage this disorder. Fourth, collaborative care models should be installed as designed by Katon and the University of Washington group, TEAMcare, Chronic Care, to enhance the practices of PCPs. Fifth, the PCPs need to be helped to establish care teams specifically for depression, like they have for asthma, diabetes, hypertension, and congestive heart failure; and support funding needs to be arranged for this essential effort.[8] Sixth, in the developing world, we must propose incentives for PCPs, nurses, and village health care workers to have competencies in the screening, diagnosis, and management of this ubiquitous disorder, such as has occurred in Tanzania.

In time, we may have a biological marker that will help immeasurably with the objectification of diagnostic validity. It is time to recognize that depression is a medical illness with critical physiological impacts on the body and other physical diseases, and that it is bidirectional—from mind to body; from body to mind. There are over 600,000 physicians in the United States and hundreds of thousands worldwide. They are a most important resource to cope with this burden of illness—depression. It needs to be approached from as many positions as we can, including enhancing the physicians' and the physician extenders' capacities; the world and our patients are entitled to no less.

REFERENCES

1. Hodes GE, Kana V, Menard C, Merad M, and Russo S. Neuroimmune mechanisms of depression. *Nat Neurosci.* 2015;18:1386–1393.
2. American Psychiatric Association. Diagnostic and Statistical Manual of Mental Disorders. 5th ed. Arlington Virginia: American Psychiatric Association; 2013.
3. Rundell JR, Huffman JC. The Compass Initiative: implementing a complex integrated care program. *Gen Hosp Psychiatry.* 2017;44:67–68.

4. Coleman KJ, Magnan S, Neely C, et al. The COMPASS initiative: description of a nation-wide collaborative approach to the care of patients with depression and diabetes and/or cardiovascular disease. *Gen Hosp Psychiatry.* 2017;44:69–76.
5. Rossom RC, Solberg LI, Magnan S, et al. Impact of a national collaborative care initiative for patients with depression and diabetes or cardiovascular disease. *Gen Hosp Psychiatry.* 2017;44:77–85.
6. Coleman KJ, Hemmila T, Valentia MD, et al. Understanding the experience of care managers and relationship with patient outcomes: the Compass Initiative. *Gen Hosp Psychiatry.* 2017;44:86–90.
7. Whitebird RR, Solberg LI, Crain AL, et al. Clinician burnout and satisfaction with resources in caring for complex patients. *Gen Hosp Psychiatry.* 2017;44:91–95.
8. Bishop TF, Ramsay PP, Casalino LP, Bao Y, Pincus HA, Shortell SM. Care management processes used less often for depression than for other chronic conditions in US primary care practices. *Health Aff (Millwood).* 2016;35(3):394–400.

Index

Page numbers followed by *f, t,* and *b* refer to figures, tables, and boxes, respectively.

Autonomous model, of mental health training for primary care, 247
Axelson, D., 49
Ayerbe, L., 90

Balint groups, in mental health training for primary care, 250
Baltimore Epidemiological Catchment Area Study, 63
Bcl-2 (gene family), 73
BDNF. *See* Brain-derived neurotrophic factor
Beck Depression Inventory (BDI), 65, 74, 131–32, 250, 261
Benztropine, 192
Biological markers
  in diagnosis of depression, 239–40
  and electronic health records, 266
Biphasic actions, of stress, 16
Bipolar disorder
  ADHD vs., 53
  and childhood, 51–52
  and long-term prevention of depression, 41, 45, 46, 47, 48, 49, 51–53
  and neurological disorders, 125
  and wound healing, 159
Bishop, T. F., 245, 251
Black, P. H., 87, 147
Blanzapine, 205*t*
Bleeding, 182
Bleuler, E., 129
Blonanserine, 202*t*
Blood pressure, 62, 74, 76
Blumer, D., 129
Body mass index (BMI), 74, 147
Boyce, Tom, 18
Brain
  and allostatic load, 15–17, 15*f*, 23
  and mood regulation, 5*f*
  responses of, to stress, 4
  as target of stress, 19
Brain-derived neurotrophic factor (BDNF), 9, 91
  and allostatic load, 20
  in hippocampus, 26
  substance abuse, 41

Brazilian Longitudinal Study of Adult Health (ELSA-Brasil), 68
Breast cancer, 100, 106
  and cardiac illness, 75
  progression and stress, 107–9
  and wound healing, 159
Breslau, N., 126, 133
Brexpiprazole (Rexulti), 201*t*, 203*t*, 208
Bridge model, of mental health training for primary care, 246
Brintellix. *See* Vortioxetine
Bupropion (Wellbutin, Zyban), 170, 179*t*, 183*t*, 185*t*, 187*t*, 194–95, 202*t*–203*t*, 208
Burton, Robert, 98
Buspirone, 179*t*

CABG (pre-coronary artery bypass graft), 63
CAD (coronary artery disease), 61–62
Caffeine, 173, 179*t*, 184*t*, 191–92
CAM (complementary and alternative medice), 161
Canada, 124–25
Canadian Nova Scotia Health Survey, 65
Cancer, 91–114
  depression and initiation of, 101–2
  and depression in context of psycho-oncology, 98–100
  effects of stress on, 107–9
  and prevalence of depression, 100–101
  "sickness behavior" of advanced, 103, 105–6
  and social influences on inflammation processes, 111–14
  tumor progression, stress and, 109–11
  and wound healing, 159
Cancer Care for the Whole Patient: Meeting Psychosocial Health Needs (report), 99
Carbamazepine (CBZ, Tegretol), 133, 177, 179*t*, 190, 192, 196, 197, 204*t*, 211*t*
Cardiac arrhythmia, 88
Cardiac illness, 61–77
  and biological mechanisms of depression, 73–74
  and chronic exposure to stressors, 74–75
  and endothelial dysfunction, 72–73
  epidemiology, 62–64

Cognitive behavioral therapy (CBT), 113–14
  and diabetes, 149
  and diagnosis of depression, 238
  and wound healing, 161
Cognitive dysfunction, and long-term
  prevention of depression, 49
Cognitive impairment, and stroke, 89
Cognitive schemas, 74
Cognitive symptoms, of depression, 68
Cohort effect, and long-term prevention of
  depression, 46, 47
Coley's vaccine, 109
Collaborative care model (CoCM), of
  mental health training for primary
  care, 247
Comorbidity, 233
  and allostatic load, 14
  with cancer, 98, 100
  medical, 87
  and negative course of neurological
    disorders, 132–37
  with stroke, 89
  with wound healing, 156–57
Complementary and alternative medice
  (CAM), 161
Computer systems, 264
Concerta. *See* Methylphenidate
Conrad, A., 70
"Consensus Paper of the World Federation
  of Societies of Biological Psychiatry"
  (Mossner, Mikova, and Koutsilier), 239
Conserved transcriptional response to
  adversity (CTRA), 112–13
Converge Consortium, 239
Copenhagen City Heart Study, 67
Copenhagen General Population Study, 67
Cornell Scale for Depression and Dementia
  (CSDD), 131
Coronary artery disease (CAD), 61–62
Corticosteroids, 104*t*
Corticotrophin-releasing hormone (CRH),
  69, 106–7
Cortisol, 69–70
  and cancer, 104*t*, 106, 107–8, 110, 114
  and diabetes, 148
  in RDOC model, 236*t*
Coupland, C., 88

Craddock, N., 234
C-reactive protein (CRP), 64, 65, 75, 147
CRH (corticotrophin-releasing hormone),
  69, 106–7
Cross-sensitization, and long-term
  prevention of depression, 42, 43*f*
CRP. *See* C-reactive protein
CSDD (Cornell Scale for Depression and
  Dementia), 131
CTRA (conserved transcriptional response
  to adversity), 112–13
Cushings disease, 23
Cuthbert, B. N., 235
CVD (cardiovascular disease), 61–62
Cyclobenzaprine, 179*t*
Cyclophosphamide, 179*t*
Cyclosporine, 104*t*, 179*t*, 187*t*, 190
Cymbalta. *See* Duloxetine
Cytochrome P450 enzymes, 179*t*
Cytokine hypothesis, 103, 104*t*
Cytokines
  in allostatic load, 16
  in animal models, 9
  and atherosclerotic plaques, 64
  and cancer, 103, 105, 107, 109, 112, 114
  and cardiac illness, 69
  and diabetes, 147–48
  and strole, 91
Czech Republic, 65

Danese, A., 75
Danish Case Registry, 40
Danish Psychiatric Central Research
  Register, 63
Dar Es Salaam, Tanzania, 249
DDIs. *See* Drug-drug interactions
Decubitus ulcer, 272, 274*f*
Delavirdine, 197, 202*t*–203*t*
Dementia
  and hippocampus, 24–28, 27
  and neurological disorders, 131
  and wound healing, 160–61
  See also Alzheimer's dementia
Demographic considerations, in depression
  and stroke, 86, 89
Denmark, 48, 85
Depakene/Depakote. *See* Valproic acid

Depression
    animal models of, 1–10
    and cancer, 97–114
    cardiac illness and biological mechanisms of, 73–74
    in context of psycho-oncology, 98–100
    diagnostic dilemmas with, 229–40
    and electronic health records, 255–82
    and insulin resistance, 26
    and long-term prevention of depression, 37–54
    monoamine hypothesis in theory of, 169–71
    neurobiology of, 4–9
    and neurological disorders, 123–37
    post-stroke, 90–92
    as risk factor for stroke, 84–88
    and stress response, 106–7
    stroke as risk factor for, 88–91
Depression Reporting Score (DRS) Analyzer, 280, 281*t*
De Ryck, A., 89
Deseryl. *See* Trazodone
Designer receptors activated by designer drugs (DREADD), 5
Desipramine, 182, 189*t*, 192, 198. *See also* Clomipramine
Desvenlafaxine (Pristiq), 185*t*, 193, 194
Dexamethasone-suppression test, 70
Dexedrine. *See* Dextroamphetamine
Dextroamphetamine (Dexedrine, ProCentra, Zenzedi), 216*t*
Diabetes, 87, 144–50
    bidirectional relationship of, with depression, 146
    and cardiac illness, 68, 74
    depression rates in, 145–46
    and HPA axis, 148
    and inflammation, 147–48
    as risk factor for depression, 146
    treatment, 149–50
Diabetes Prevention Program, 145
Diagnosis of depression, 229–40
    biological markers, 239–40
    in cancer patients, 98–99
    clinical judgment in, 232–33
    dimensional approach to, 231–32

distress-impairment criterion in, 230–31
    and DSM classifications, 233–34
    and electronic health records, 261
    genetics and, 239
    and neurological disorders, 128, 131–32
    and normality vs. pathology in psychiatric disorders, 229–30
    and phenomenology of mental illness, 233
    and Research Domain Criteria (RDoC) model, 234–35, 235*t*–237*t*, 238
Diagnostic and Statistical Manual of Mental Disorders (DSM), 124, 128, 130, 145, 230–33, 239, 244, 250, 260–61, 271
Diagnostic and Statistical Manual of Mental Disorders III (DSM-III), 90
Diagnostic and Statistical Manual of Mental Disorders, 5th Edition (DSM-5), 61, 62, 230–32
Dialogue in Diabetes and Depression, 145
Digoxin, 190
Diltiazem, 179*t*
Diphenhydramine, 179*t*, 194, 202*t*–203*t*
Disabilities
    and depression, 155
    as risk factor for depression after stroke, 89
    and stroke recovery, 92
Disability Assessment Schedule, 232
Distress, in cancer patients, 99–100
Distress-impairment criteria, and diagnosis of depression, 230–31
Distress screening, in cancer patients, 99
Diurnal mood variation, 129
Divalproex, 205*t*
DNA methyltransferase3a (DNMT3a), 7
Dome, P., 72–73
Dopamine
    and antidepressants, 193–94, 198
    and cancer, 103, 107, 111
    in RDOC model, 236*t*
Double-boarded model, of mental health training for primary care, 247
Dowlati, Y., 147
Doxepin (Adapin, Sinequan), 189*t*
DREADD (designer receptors activated by designer drugs), 5
DRS Analyzer, 280, 281*t*

Monoaminergic pathways, and stroke, 90
Monocytes, 66
Mood disorders
  intervention in, 54
  and long-term prevention of depression,
    47, 48f, 49–50
  and neurological disorders, 123
Mood regulation, 4, 20
Mood stabilizers, 210, 211t–215t
Moore, Gordon, 275f
Morris, P. L., 90
Mortality
  and cancer, 102
  and cardiac illness, 77
  and chronic illness, 68–70
  and depression scores, 63–64
  and electronic health records, 272
  and mental health training for primary
    care, 241
  post-stroke, 85–87, 89, 90, 92
  and post-traumatic stress disorder, 133
Mortriptyline, 198
Mossner, R., 239
Mostowik, M., 65
Multiple Risk Factor Intervention
  Trail, 86
Multiple sclerosis (MS), 124, 132
MultiSense, 264
Musselman, D. L., 71
Mynors-Wallis, L., 234
Myocardial apoptosis, 64
Myocardial contractility, 64
Myocardial infarction (MI), 61, 88

N-acetylcysteine (NAC), 43, 44b
Nardi. See Phenelzine
Narushima, K., 91
National Academics of Science, 155
National Comorbidity Study, 62
National Comprehensive Cancer Network
  (NCCN), 99
National Health and Nutrition Examination
  Study (NHANES), 63, 64, 86, 147
National Health Examination Follow-up
  Study, 62–63
National Health Insurance Research
  Database, 88

National Institute of Mental Health
  (NIMH), 130, 234, 244, 245, 266
National Institutes of Health, 10
National Stroke Campaign, 273
National Stroke Foundation, 274
NCCN (National Comprehensive Cancer
  Network), 99
NDDI-E (Neurological Disorders
  Depression Inventory for Epilepsy), 131
Nefazodone (Serzone), 179t, 187t, 196
Negative schemas, 74
Nelfinavir, 212t
Nemeroff, C. B., 71
Nervous system, and cancer, 107
Netherlands, 45, 46t, 49f, 51, 127
Neural circuitry, 4–6, 5f
Neural systems, and cardiac illness, 75
Neurodegeneration, and cancer, 103
Neuroendocrine system, 75, 105, 109
Neurological disorders, 123–37
  Alzheimer's dementia, 125, 127–28, 130,
    131, 134
  clinical manifestations of depressive
    disorders in, 128–30
  comorbid depression and negative course
    of, 132–37
  epidemiological data on depressive
    disorders and, 124–26
  epilepsy, 124, 126, 131–33
  migraine, 125–26, 128, 133–34
  mild cognitive impairment, 134
  multiple sclerosis, 124, 132
  Parkinson's disease, 125, 127, 130,
    132, 134
  risk for development of, 126–28
  screening instruments of depression
    in, 131–32
  stroke, 124–25, 127, 129–31, 133
Neurological Disorders Depression
  Inventory for Epilepsy (NDDI-E), 131
Neurontin. See Gabapentin
Neurotransmitter receptor hypothesis, 103
Neurotransmitters, 64, 135–36
Neurotrophic factor hypothesis, 103
Neutrophic hypothesis, 9
Neutrophils, 66
Nevirapine, 214t

Phenelzine (Nardi), 172, 187*t*
Phenobarbital, 104*t*, 184*t*, 213*t*
Phenotypic assays, 3
Phenytoin, 173, 184*t*, 191, 192, 213*t*
PHQ-9. *See* Patient Health Questionnare
Physiological stress, 106–7
Piletz, J. E., 71
Pimozide (Orap), 177, 192, 201*t*
Placebo treatments, 158
Plaque, 70
Plasma, 66, 69
Platelet(s)
  cardiac illness and clotting of, 70–72
  dysfunction of, in drug-drug
    interactions, 182
  dysfunction of, in stroke, 87
Platelet activating factor (PAF), 71
Platelet factor IV (PF4), 71
Plethysmography, arterial, 72
PMs. *See* Poor metabolizers
Polycystic ovary syndrome
  (PCOS), 25, 27
Polymorphisms, genetic, and cardiac
  illness, 76
Polythetic approach, 231
Poor metabolizers (PMs), 181,
  194–96, 199
Positron emission topography (PET), 135
Post, R. M., 39
Postgraduate specialization model, of
  mental health training for primary
  care, 247
Postictal symptoms (epilepsy), 129
Post-stroke depression (PSD), 90–92,
  124, 129
Post-Stroke Depression Scale (PSDS), 131
Post-traumatic stress disorder (PTSD), 1
  diagnosing, 231
  and wound healing, 156
Pre-coronary artery bypass graft
  (CABG), 63
Prefrontal cortex
  and allostatic load, 20
  and mood regulation, 4, 5*f*
  and wound healing, 159
Pre-ictal symptoms, 129
"Prescribing paralysis," 168

Primary care physicians (PCPs)
  and electronic health records, 255–56,
    260, 269–70
  and mental health training, 240–45,
    248–49, 251
PRIME study, 65
Pristiq. *See* Desvenlafaxine
ProCentra. *See* Dextroamphetamine
Prodromal symptoms, and
  long-term prevention of
  depression, 52, 53
Prolixin. *See* Fluphenazine
Propanolol, 104*t*
Prospective Epidemiologic Study of
  Myocardial Infarction (PRIME
  study), 65
Prostate-specific antigen (PSA), 240
Protein-bound drugs, in drug-drug
  interactions, 173
Protriptyline (Vivactil), 189*t*
Provigil. *See* Modafinil
"Provisional Diagnostic Criteria for
  Depression of Alzheimer's Disease"
  (NIMH), 130
Prozac. *See* Fluoxetine
PSA (prostate-specific antigen), 240
PSD. *See* Post-stroke depression
PSDS (Post-Stroke Depression Scale), 131
Psychiatric classifications, and diagnosis of
  depression, 233
Psychiatric comorbidity, in neurological
  disorders, 124, 132
Psychiatric consultation model, 245–46
Psychiatric disorders
  in cancer patients, 98, 106
  and diagnosis of depression, 230
  and electronic health records, 265
  and insulin resistance, 25
Psychiatric treatment, and wound
  healing, 158–59
Psychiatrists, and mental health training for
  primary care, 248–49
Psychological interventions, with
  diabetes, 149
Psychomotor retardation, 129–30
Psychoneuroimmunology, 97, 98, 105, 114
Psycho-oncology, 98–100

sertraline, 192–93
and sexual dysfunction, 27
and stroke, 88, 92
Selegiline (Emsam), 187t, 199
Self-reporting, and electronic health
records, 268
Selye, Hans, 106
Sensitization, and long-term prevention of
depression, 37–38
Sepsis, 272
Septal nuclei, 4
Serentil. *See* Mesoridazine
Seroquel. *See* Quetiapine
Serotonin
and antidepressants, 193
in monoamine hypothesis, 170
and neurological disorders, 135
in RDOC model, 236t
and stroke, 87, 90–91
Serotonin-norepinephrine reuptake
inhibitors (SNRIs), 185t–186t, 193–94
desvenlafaxine, 193
duloxetine, 193–94
levomilnacipran, 194
in monoamine hypothesis, 169–70
venlafaxine, 194
Serotonin syndrome, 172, 182, 191
Sertindole, 207t
Sertraline (Zoloft), 92, 149, 185t,
192–93, 212t
Serzone. *See* Nefazodone
Seven Pillars of RDoC, 235, 235t
Sex differences, and allostatic load, 21–22
Sex hormones, and brain disorders, 22
SHEEP (Stockholm Heart Epidemiology
Program), 63
Shonkoff, J. P., 51–52
SIADH (syndrome of inappropriate
antidiuretic hormone secretion), 182
"Sickness behavior" (advanced cancer),
103, 105–6
Sickness syndrome, 103, 105, 107
SIG-E-CAPS mnemonic, 250
SimSensi, 264
Sinequan. *See* Doxepin
Skype, 263
Slavich, G. M., 40

Sleep disorders, 62
Smartphones, 263f
Smoking, 74. *See also* Cigarette smoke
SNRIs. *See* Serotonin-norepinephrine
reuptake inhibitors
SNS (sympathetic nervous system), 111–13
Social defeat, 3, 6–7
Social engagement, and HRV, 67–68
Social factors, in depression, 97
Social genomics, and cancer, 111
Social phobia, 125
Societal norms, and electronic health
records, 276
Somatic symptoms, of depression, 68, 106
South London Register, 90
Spalletta, G., 91
Spiperone binding, 90
Spirituality, and wound healing, 161
Spitzer, Robert, 230–31
Sprague-Dawley rats, 108
SSRIs. *See* Selective serotonin reuptake
inhibitors
Standardized Query Language (SQL),
259, 276
Star-D Study, 244, 251
Statine, 179t
Stockholm Female Coronary
Risk Study, 63
Stockholm Heart Epidemiology Program
(SHEEP), 63
Strattera. *See* Atomoxetine
Stress
and allostatic load, 17
in animal models, 1–3, 6
and cancer, 98, 101–2, 105–10, 113
and cardiac illness, 69, 73–75
and diabetes, 147
in long-term prevention of depression, 39
sensitization to, and long-term prevention
of depression, 38–41, 43f
and wound healing, 157, 160
Stroke, 84–93, 124–25, 129–31, 133
demographic considerations in
depression and, 86, 89
depression and post-stroke morbidity/
mortality, 86–87
depression as risk factor for, 84–88

Stroke (*cont.*)
  mechanisms underlying association
      between depression and, 87–88
  as neurological disorder, 127
  post-stroke depression, 90–92
  as risk factor for depression, 88–91
  treatment and prevention
      considerations, 88
Stroke Aphasic Depression Questionnaire
      (SADQ), 131
Stroke lesions, 90–91
Strolin Benedetti, M., 175
Stromal signals, in tumor progression, 109
Stroud, C. B., 40
Su, S., 68
Substance abuse, and long-term prevention
      of depression, 41–42
Suicide, 126
Suomi, S. J., 18
Surmontil. *See* Trimipramine
"Surviving Sepsis," 272, 273*f*
Sweden, 86, 249
Sympathetic nervous system (SNS), 111–13
Symptoms
  of depression in cancer, 97
  of depression in neurological
      disorders, 128–30
  and electronic health records, 267
  extrapyramidal, in drug-drug
      interactions, 182
  withdrawal, with paroxetine, 192
Syndrome of inappropriate antidiuretic
      hormone secretion (SIADH), 182
Systemic hormones, and allostatic load, 23

Taiwan, 88
Tamoxifen, 104*t*, 176–77, 184*t*–187*t*, 192
Tang, W. K., 91
Task Force on Biological Markers: Biological
      Markers in Depression, 239
TAU. *See* Treatment as usual
TCAs. *See* Tricyclic antidepressants
TDM (therapeutic drug monitoring), 176
Tegretol. *See* Carbamazepine
Telomere shortening, and long-term
      prevention of depression, 52
Temazepam, 175

Thalamus, 4
Theophylline, 173, 190
Therapeutic drug monitoring (TDM), 176
Thioridazine (Mellari), 201*t*
Thorazine. *See* Chlorpromazine
Thresholds, in diagnosis of depression, 231
Thrombin, 65
Thrombus formation, in cardiac
      illness, 70–71
TIA (transient ischemic attack), 88
Tiagabine (Gabitril), 214*t*
Tizanidine, 191
TNF (tumor necrosis factor), 64
Tofranil. *See* Imipramine
Tomfohr, L. M., 72
Topiramate (Topamax), 128, 179*t*, 214*t*
Toxicity, drug, 177
Toxic stress
  in children and long-term prevention of
      depression, 51
  and long-term prevention of
      depression, 52
Tramadol, 174, 179*t*, 184*t*–187*t*, 192, 194
Transcriptomics, 6–8, 8*f*
Transient ischemic attack (TIA), 88
"Translational Neuroscience in
      Psychiatry: Light at the End of the
      Tunnel" (article), 239
Transporters, in drug-drug interactions, 176
Tranylcypromine (Parnate), 187*t*
Trauma, and cardiac illness, 74–75
Trazodone (Deseryl), 188*t*, 190, 191, 197
Treadway, M. T., 40
Treatment(s)
  of depression, in diabetes, 149
  and electronic health records, 256, 267
  placebo, 158
  for stroke, 84, 88
  and wound healing, 156, 161
Treatment as usual (TAU)
  in bipolar disorder, 48
  for children with depression, 50
Triazolobenzodiazepines
      (triazoloBZDs), 179*t*
Tricyclic antidepressants (TCAs), 88,
      179*t*, 184*t*, 185*t*, 188*t*–189*t*, 190–92,
      198–99, 208

Trilafon. *See* Perphenazine
Trileptal. *See* Oxcarbazepine
Trimipramine (Surmontil), 189*t*
Troponin, 70
Tumerigenesis, 109
Tumor(s)
    growth of, 107
    microenvironment of, 105
    stress and progression of, 109
Tumor necrosis factor (TNF), 64
Twins Heart Study, 68, 76
Twitter, 276
Type 2 diabetes, 74, 87, 146
Type A personality
    and cancer, 101
    and cardiac illness, 73
Type D personality, 73

UGT (uridine diphosphate
    glucuronosyltransferase), 209
Ultra-extensive metabolizers (UEMs), 181
Ultra-rapid cycling, and long-term
    prevention of depression, 41
United Kingdom, 101, 233
United States, 99
    antidepressants in, 196, 199
    depression in, 155, 269
    diagnosis of depression in, 233, 234–35
    long-term prevention of depression in, 45,
        46*t*, 47, 48, 49*f*, 50, 51
    mental health training for primary care
        in, 240–41, 249–50
    mood disorders in, 48*f*
    psychiatric disorders in, 62
University of Rochester, 247
University of Virginia, 247
University of West Virginia, 247
Uridine diphosphate
    glucuronosyltransferase (UGT), 209
U.S. Department of Health and Human
    Services, 256*f*
U.S. Food and Drug Administration (FDA),
    168, 190, 278
U.S./U.K. Diagnostic Project, 233

Vaccarino, V., 65
Vagal activity, in cardiac illness, 68

Validity
    in animal models, 2–3
    and diagnosis of depression, 229–30, 233
    in electronic health records, 261
Valproate, 44, 175
Valproic acid (VPA, Depakote, Depakene),
    133, 214*t*
Variability, drug, in drug-drug
    interactions, 176–81
Vascular depression, 130
Vascular endothelial growth factor
    (VEGF), 110
Vaughan, D., 182
Venlafaxine (Effexor), 183*t*, 186*t*, 191,
    194, 208
Ventral tegmental area, 5, 5*f*
Verapamil, 179*t*
Vietnam, 68
Vietnam Twins Registry, 76
Vigabatrin (Sabril), 215*t*
Vilazodone (Viibryd), 188*t*, 197
Vilazone, 197
Vinblastine, 104*t*
Vincristine, 104*t*
Vivactil. *See* Protriptyline
Voriconazole, 208
Vortioxetine (Brintellix), 188*t*, 197–98
VPA. *See* Valproic acid
Vraylar. *See* Cariprazine

WAIS Full-Scale and Verbal Scale IQ, 134
Wang, M. T., 88
Wang, Y., 66
Warfarin, 179*t*, 190
Weinberg, R. A., 110
Wellbutrin. *See* Bupropion
Whitehall II Cohort Study, 66, 70, 85
WHO (World Health Organization), 232
Wickramaratne, P., 50
Windle, M., 74
Windle, R. C., 74
WISE (Women's Ischemia Syndrome
    Evaluation), 63
Withdrawal symptoms
    paroxetine, 192
    SNRIs, 193
Wium-Anderson, M. K., 66